A Clinician's Guide to Reproductive Health

A Clinician's Guide to Reproductive Health

Editor: Sidney Alvarado

AMERICAN
MEDICAL PUBLISHERS
www.americanmedicalpublishers.com

AMERICAN
MEDICAL PUBLISHERS
www.americanmedicalpublishers.com

Cataloging-in-Publication Data

A clinician's guide to reproductive health / edited by Sidney Alvarado.
p. cm.
Includes bibliographical references and index.
ISBN 978-1-63927-468-0
1. Reproductive health. 2. Human reproduction. 3. Fertility, Human.
4. Reproductive health services--Guidebooks. I. Alvarado, Sidney.
RG133 .C55 2022
618.178--dc23

American Medical Publishers,
41 Flatbush Avenue,
1st Floor, New York,
NY 11217, USA

ISBN 978-1-63927-468-0 (Hardback)

Contents

Preface

This book has been a concerted effort by a group of academicians, researchers and scientists, who have contributed their research works for the realization of the book. This book has materialized in the wake of emerging advancements and innovations in this field. Therefore, the need of the hour was to compile all the required researches and disseminate the knowledge to a broad spectrum of people comprising of students, researchers and specialists of the field.

Reproductive health encompasses the major areas of adolescent health and maternal health that are subject to the social and cultural perspectives on contraception, abortion, child and forced marriage, etc. Current models of maternal health ideally encompass prenatal and postnatal care, family planning and preconception. During childbirth, severe bleeding, high blood pressure, delivery complications and infections place women at high risk. Such risks magnify with younger age. The field of reproductive medicine addresses the issues pertaining to reproductive health such as birth control, infertility, sexual dysfunction, puberty, sexual education, etc. The advancement in assisted reproductive technology, imaging, surgery and pharmacology has facilitated the necessary treatment and assessment for ensuring optimum reproductive health. This book studies, analyzes and upholds the pillars of reproductive health and its utmost significance in modern times. It includes some of the vital pieces of work being conducted across the world, on various topics related to reproductive health. For all those who are interested in this field, this book can prove to be an essential guide.

At the end of the preface, I would like to thank the authors for their brilliant chapters and the publisher for guiding us all-through the making of the book till its final stage. Also, I would like to thank my family for providing the support and encouragement throughout my academic career and research projects.

Editor

1

Characteristics of female sexual dysfunctions and obstetric complications related to female genital mutilation in Omdurman maternity hospital, Sudan

Khalid Yassin[1], Hadeel A. Idris[2] and AbdelAziem A. Ali[1,3*]

Abstract

Background: Female genital mutilation (FGM) is a major public health problem, especially in developing countries.

Method: This was a prospective observational cohort study conducted over six months duration (1st July-31st December 2015) at Omdurman Maternity Hospital, Khartoum, Sudan, primarily to determine whether exposure to FGM/C (exposed Vs. non-exposed) and degree of exposure (type III Vs. type I) are associated with impaired sexual function or not?. As secondary objective, the study also investigated the association between FGM/C and postpartum complications (eg: difficulties in cervical examination, episiotomy wound infection, postpartum bleeding) by following the participants from the time of admission at the hospital, through vaginal delivery and until the 6th post-partum week.

Results: A total of 230 (subjected to FGM/C) and 190 (not subjected to FGM/C) women were approached. The clinical examinations evidenced that the majority (67.8%) had FGM type *3*, while the remainder (32.2%) had type 1. The most common reported sexual complication was dyspareunia (76%). Bleeding following first attempt of sexual intercourse was reported in 35.2% followed by reduced sexual desire 62.6%, reduced sexual satisfaction 40.9% and need for surgery to release labial adhesions at first attempt of sexual intercourse 30.4%. With regard to FGM- related complications that occurred during labor 76.5% required an episiotomy, 61.7% experienced difficulties in cervical examination, 57.8% needed defibulations during second stage of labor, 26.5% complicated by episiotomy wound infection and 2.2% developed obstetric hemorrhage. In this study FGM/C was a significant factor increasing the risk of sexual complications. Interestingly when using logistic regression analysis the FGM-related complications were not significantly varied by FGM/C types.

Conclusion: Our observations indicate that FGM/C is a serious public health problem and there should be an urgent intervention such as planned health education campaigns to end FGM/C practice.

Keywords: Female genital mutilation, Circumcision, Women health, Sudan

* Correspondence: abuzianab73@yahoo.com
[1]Faculty of Medicine, Alnelain University, Khartoum, Sudan
[3]Department of Obstetrics and Gynecology, Faculty of Medicine, Kassala University, Kassala, Sudan
Full list of author information is available at the end of the article

Plain English summary

Female genital mutilation (FGM) is a major public health problem, especially in developing countries. It is a dangerous practice that leads to many serious complications including hemorrhage, sepsis, severe pain, sexual dysfunction, primary infertility and obstetric complications. This study investigated whether exposure to FGM/C and degree of exposure are associated with impaired sexual function or not?. It also investigated the association between FGM/C and postpartum complications by following the participants from the time of admission at the hospital, through vaginal delivery and until the 6th post-partum week. After taking informed written consent, structured questionnaires were administered in local language (Arabic) using closed-ended questions to gather the different variable from 420 primigravida in a labor ward of the largest maternity hospital in Sudan. The finding of this study showed that the FGM is strongly associated with sexual and obstetric complications. Another key finding of this study is that all the forms of FGM are responsible for a high percentage of sexual complications. This study indicates that FGM constitutes a major public health problem and subjecting the women and the girls to several serious health problems and there should be an urgent intervention such as planned health education campaigns to end FGM practice.

Background

Female genital mutilation (FGM) is a major public health problem, especially in developing countries [1]. Female genital mutilation is a cultural and traditional procedure and it is considered as a violation of the human rights of girls and women because of its negative impact on women health [2, 3]. Worldwide 200 million girls in 30 countries have undergone FGM and live with its health complications [4]. The procedure is outlawed in many countries [5, 6]. In Sudan girls typically undergo FGM between the age of 6 and 12 years and the cutting is always performed by the midwives without anesthesia, antibiotics or even sterilization, putting the girls in short and long term very serious consequences [7]. Female genital mutilation is highly prevalent in Sudan, it is reported in 83.3% among school girls and strongly associated with education [8], therefore the current study is directed to investigate the health complications associated with FGM and it is expected to provide the health planners and stakeholders with fundamental data for the development of strategic plan such as health education and good partnership towards the elimination of this practice.

Methods

Study design and study area

This was a prospective observational cohort study aimed, primarily, to determine whether exposure to FGM/C (exposed Vs. non-exposed) and degree of exposure (type III Vs. type I) are associated with impaired sexual function or not?. As secondary objective the study also investigated the association between FGM/C and postpartum complications (eg: difficulties in cervical examination, episiotomy wound infection, postpartum bleeding) by following the participants from the time of admission at the hospital, through vaginal delivery and until the 6th post-partum week. The study conducted over six months duration (1st July-31st December 2015) at Omdurman Maternity Hospital, Khartoum, Sudan which is the largest maternity hospital in Sudan established in 1957 and provide comprehensive obstetric and gynecological services to the public.

Participants

All primigravida (subjected and not subjected to FGM/C) who experienced vaginal delivery during the study period were invited to participate in this study. There was a 100% participation rate and participants were adequately informed about consent to participate and they were given the option of refusing to participate during the informed consent process. Structured self-administered questionnaires were administered in local language (Arabic) using closed-ended questions (yes and no) to gather socio-demographic data (age, residence, education and occupation) and sexual function history (dyspareunia, bleeding following first intercourse, need surgery to release labial adhesions at first sexual intercourse, reduced sexual desire and sexual satisfaction) (An additional movie file shows this in more detail see Additional file 1). Complications that occurred during labor (difficulties in cervical examination, need for performing episiotomy, defibulations during second stage of labor and obstetric hemorrhage) were obtained from the participant's clinical record. The types of FGM/C have been verified by physical examination. Ten female registrars in Obstetrics and Gynecology were selected to conduct the examination in the labor ward, they had been trained in relationship building, local cultures, believes, privacy, confidentiality, FGM/C typology and how to assist the respondents to fill the questionnaires. We used our own questionnaire which was constructed by the authors to consider different individual issues specific to our environment such as bleeding and need for surgery to release labial adhesion at time of first sexual intercourse, this is because the Female Sexual Function Index (FSFI) questionnaire was developed for the specific purpose of assessing domains of sexual functioning (e.g. sexual arousal, orgasm, satisfaction, pain). The questionnaire was revised by expert personnel in FGM/C, women health and right. We conducted one day session in which we discussed and approved the content of the questionnaire. This session was conducted by the authors and the expertise prior to the proposal approval. In this study the different sexual items were well explained for the respondents in local language. All women were followed for 6 weeks postpartum to report any complications happened (episiotomy wound infection). In this study we chose all the primigravida without exclusion criteria. Also we asked the women about whether the FGM/C is harmful or not and would they going to expose their daughter to the practice or not?. All women were examined to report the type of FGM. Female genital mutilation was defined according to the World Health Organization as all procedures involving partial or total removal of the external female genitalia or other injury to the female organs whether for cultural or other non-therapeutic reasons [9]. Again in this study we classified FGM according to WHO into four types: type1, also known as clitoridectomy: involves partial or total removal of the clitoris and/or prepuce; type2: involves partial or total removal of the clitoris and labia minora, with or without excision of the labia majora; type3: also known as infibulation, it entails removing part or all of the external genitalia and narrowing the vaginal orifice by re-approximating the labia minora and/or labia majora; type4: includes any form of other harm done to the female genitalia by pricking, piercing, cutting, scraping or burning [10].

Data analysis

Data were entered into a computer database and SPSS software (SPSS Inc., Chicago, IL, USA, version 21.0), double checked, cleaned and verified by statistician before analysis. Means and proportions for the socio-demographic characteristics were compared between the groups of the study using student t and ×2 test, respectively and $P < 0.05$ was considered significant. Logistic regression analysis was performed separately for dyspareunia, bleeding at first sexual attempt, reduced sexual desire, reduced sexual satisfaction and surgery to release labial adhesion to evaluate the effects of FGM\C on sexual function. Female genital mutilation was the independent variable and the sexual and obstetric complications were dependent variables. Confidence intervals of 95% were calculated and $P < 0.05$ was considered significant.

Results

Participant characteristics

A total of 420 primigravida delivered at Omdurman Maternity hospital were approached during this study, 230 were subjected to FGM/C and 190 were not subjected to FGM/C. There were no significant differences between the FGM/C group and non FGM/C group on socio-demographic characteristics. The mean age (SD) was not significantly different between the subjected to FGM/C group and those who were not, 27.2 (5.8) Vs. 26.0 (5.7), $P = 0.1$. The majority of the group who was subjected to FGM/C in comparison to the non-subjected to FGM/C group were of rural residence (61.7% Vs. 62.1%, $P = 0.371$), educated (57% Vs. 51.1%, $P = 0.550$) and housewives (84.7% Vs. 79.1%, $P = 0.371$), Table 1.

FGM types and attitude

The clinical examinations evidenced that the majority had FGM type 3 (156/230, 67.8%), while the remainder (74/230, 32.2%) had type 1. The vast majority of the women in the subjected to FGM/C group (76.5%, 176/230) mentioned that they are not going to expose their daughter for FGM in the future and 65% (150/230) of them affirmed that FGM is a harmful practice. There was no differences between women with FGM/C and without FGM/C in plans to subject their daughters to FGM/C (76.5%% Vs. 74.8%, $P = 0.411$).

Identified sexual complications

The majority (76.9%, $n = 177$) of women who have been subjected to FGM/C reported sexual complications. One hundred seventy seven women (76.9%) among them claimed that they had dyspareunia. Bleeding following first attempt of sexual intercourse was reported in 35.2% while reduced sexual desire, reduced sexual satisfaction and need for surgery to release labial adhesions at first attempt of sexual intercourse was reported in 62.6%, 40.9% and 30.4% respectively. Significantly more women in the group who have been subjected to FGM/C claimed that they have dyspareunia (76.9%% Vs. 46.2%, $P = 0.001$), reduced sexual desire (62.6%% Vs. 20%, $P = 0.004$) and reduced sexual satisfaction (40.9%% Vs. 6.3%, $P = 0.002$) compared with the other group, Table 2. Interestingly when using logistic regression analysis the FGM-related sexual complications were not significantly varied by FGM types, Tables 2 and 3.

Postpartum complications

With regard to FGM- related complications that occurred during labor 76.5% required an episiotomy, 61.7% experienced difficulties in cervical examination, 57.8% needed defibulations during second stage of labor, 26.5% complicated by episiotomy wound infection and 2.2%

Table 1 Basic characteristic of the women "subjected and not subjected" to FGM/C' and admitted to the labor ward at Omdurman Maternity Hospital, Sudan, 2015

Variable	Subjected to FGM/C ($n = 230$)	Not subjected to ($n = 190$)	P value
Age	27.2 (5.8)	26 (5.7)	0.100
Rural residence	142(61.7)	118 (62.1)	0.371
Illiteracy	99 (43)	93 (48.9)	0.550
Occupation, housewife	195 (84.7%)	151 (79.1)	0.371

Data was shown as number (%) as applicable

Table 2 Distribution of sexual and obstetric complications among primigravida 'subjected to FGM/C' and 'not subjected to FGM/C' and admitted to the labor ward at Omdurman Maternity Hospital, Sudan, 2015

Complication	Subjected to FGM/C (*n* = 230)	Not subjected to FGM/C (*n* = 190)	*P* value
Dyspareunia	177 (76.9%)	46 (24.2%)	0.001
Bleeding at first sexual attempt	81 (35.2%)	3 (1.5%)	<0.001
Reduced sexual desire	144 (62.6%)	38 (20%)	0.004
Reduced sexual satisfaction	94 (40.9%)	12 (6.3%%)	0.002
Surgery to release labial adhesion	70 (30.4%)	00 (00%)	<0.001
Difficulty in pelvic examination	142 (61.7%)	35 (18.4.%)	0.021
Episiotomy	176 (76.5%)	57 (30%)	0.011
Deinfibulation	133 (57.8%)	0 (00)	<0.001
Infection of episiotomy	61 (26.5%)	2 (1.1%)	<0.001
Hemorrhage	5 (2.2%)	3 (1.5%)	0.275

Data was shown as number (%) as applicable

developed obstetric hemorrhage. More proportion of the women among those who have been subjected to FGM/C had difficulties in cervical examination (61.7% Vs. 18.4%), required an episiotomy (76.5% Vs. 30%), needed defibulations during second stage of labor (57.8% Vs. 00) and developed episiotomy wound infection (26.5% Vs. 1.1%), Table 2.

Discussion

The finding of this study showed that the FGM is strongly associated with sexual and obstetric complications. Another key finding of this study is that all the forms of FGM are responsible for a high percentage of complications. This study indicates that FGM constitutes a major public health problem subjecting the women and girls to several serious health problems. In the present study dyspareunia (pain feel during sexual intercourse) was reported in 76.9% among the group subjected to FGM/C, while less than quarter (24.2%) of the other group reported dyspareunia. The FGM related health consequences have been investigated and reported. A more recent systematic review showing that women with FGM were more likely to experience dyspareunia, reduced sexual satisfaction and reduced sexual desire [11, 12]. Our result is in agreement with study which was conducted in Egypt, where the authors found that women with FGM have higher rates of dyspareunia and lack of sexual desire [13]. This could be explained by the fibrosis and rigid scar tissue following FGM which predispose to narrowing of the vaginal orifice and muscular spasm that make intercourse painful and difficult. These physical factors again contributed to psychological factor, where the painful sexual practice will drive women to lose both sexual desire and satisfaction. It might be difficult in the present time to reduce these risk and complications, this is because there is lack of knowledge regarding health consequences associated with FGM, even among local health professionals like nurses or midwifes in Sudan [14]. In this study difficulty in cervical examination during labor was reported in more than half (61.7%) of women who have been subjected to FGM/C, so pelvic examination on infibulated women can be challenging. The narrow introitus can made bimanual examination difficult, and if not impossible. Again this findings are supported by *De Silva* [15]. In the present study 76.5% of the women with FGM required an episiotomy and this is highly justifiable because performance of episiotomy may limit the degree of perineal laceration. About 57.8% of the women with FGM needed defibulations during second stage of labor to reduce the risks of delivery with infibulated scar which may lead to prolonged second stage of labor and increase risk of spontaneous laceration. Nearly one third (26.5%) of the women with FGM reported episiotomy wound infection. This possibly explained by the collection of blood and lochia behind the sutured skin and result in poor hygiene of the vagina and thus represent good media for the growth of the bacteria. Our study showed no association between obstetric hemorrhage and FGM and this is possibly explained by high incidence rate of performing episiotomy wound to prevent laceration and non linear tear during labor. This results

Table 3 Corrected odds ratio and 95% confidence interval for subjected women to FGM/C and those who were not subjected to FGM/C to evaluate the effects of FGM\C on sexual function (dyspareunia, bleeding at first sexual attempt, reduced sexual desire, reduced sexual satisfaction and surgery to release labial adhesion) in Omdurman Maternity Hospital, Sudan, 2015

Variables	Subjected to FGM/C		Not subjected to FGM/C	
	OR (95% CI)	*P*	OR (95% CI)	*P*
Dyspareunia	1.0 (0.9–1.0)	0.6	0.9 (0.9–1.0)	0.1
Bleeding at first sexual attempt	1.1 (1.0–1.1)	0.2	1.0 (1.0–1.2)	0.2
Reduced sexual desire	1.4 (1.0–1.2)	0.3	1.3 (0.7–2.4)	<0.2
Reduced sexual satisfaction	1.1 (0.9–1.0)	0.1	1.0 (1.0–1.1)	0.5
Surgery to release labial adhesion	1.5 (0.9–1.2)	0.6	1.2 (0.8–2.0)	0.2

is in contrast to the findings from six African countries including Sudan, where the authors reported that a loss of 130,000 life years is expected owing to FGM's association with obstetric hemorrhage [16]. One of the strength of this study is the use of close ended question regarding the sexual satisfaction and the answers rely on the participant's experience and feeling without scoring however we think one of the major limitation of this study is its inability to measure other sexual dysfunction items such as sexual arousal and orgasm. Again our results are limited by using a questionnaire instrument that has not been validated. Also we did not conduct separate analyses by type of FGM/C but rather just with FGM/C or without FGM/C.

Conclusion

Our observations indicate that FGM is a serious public health problem and there should be an urgent intervention such as planned health education campaigns to end FGM practice.

Abbreviations

CI: Confidence interval; FGM: Female genital mutilation; OR: Odds ratio; *P*: *P*- value; SD: Standard deviation; SPSS: Statistical Package for the Social Sciences; WHO: World Health Organization

Acknowledgements

We are grateful to the women who participated in this study, also we extend our thanks and appreciation to the staff of Omdurman Maternity Hospital for their great assistance and support.

Authors' contributions

Idris H A and Yassin K carried out the study and participated in the drafting of the manuscript. Ali AA supervised the work, participated in study design and drafting of the manuscript. All the author read and approved the final version of the manuscript.

Authors' information

Khalid Yassin K is a professor of Obstetric and Gynecology, Department of Obstetrics and Gynecology, Alneelain University, Sudan., Idris H. A is specialist of Obstetric and Gynecology, Fedral Ministry of Health, Sudan., Ali A. A is a professor of Obstetrics and Gynecology, Faculty of Medicine, Kassala University, Sudan.

Consent for publication

Not applicable

Competing interests

The authors declare that they have no competing interests.

Author details

[1]Faculty of Medicine, Alnelain University, Khartoum, Sudan. [2]Federal Ministry of Health, Khartoum, Sudan. [3]Department of Obstetrics and Gynecology, Faculty of Medicine, Kassala University, Kassala, Sudan.

References

1. WHO Press: World Health Organisation, Geneva, Switzerland Available from: http://www.who.int/reproductivehealth/publications/fgm/9789241596442/en/index.html. Accessed 13 June 2012.
2. Bjälkander O, Bangura L, Leigh B, Berggren V, Bergström S, Almroth L. Health complications of female genital mutilation in Sierra Leone. Int J Women's Health. 2012;4:321–31.
3. Yoder PS, Khan S. Numbers of women circumcised in Africa: the production of a Total. Calverton, Maryland: Macro International Inc; 2007.
4. UNICEF: Female genital mutilation/cutting: A global concern. 2016: New York. https://www.unicef.org/media/.../FGMC_2016_brochure_final_UNICEF_SPREAD.pdf.
5. Nour NM. Female genital cutting: a persisting practice. Revs Obstet Gynecol. 2008;1(3):135–9.
6. World Health Organization (WHO): Female genital mutilation (FGM). World Health Organization; 2008 [http://www.who.int\reproductive-health\fgm\index.html. Accessed September 2].
7. Nour N. Female genital cutting: clinical and cultural guidelines. Obstet Gynecol Surv. 2004;59:272–9.
8. Ali AA, Okud A, Mohammed AA. Prevalence and factors affecting female genital mutilation in eastern Sudan. Int Gynaecol obstet. 2013;120:288–9.
9. WHO: Female genital mutilation: a joint WHO\UNICEF\UNFPA statement. Geneva, Switzerland: World Health Organization; 1997.
10. WHO: Female genital mutilation (FGM). World Health Organization; 2008 [http://www.who.int\reproductive-health\fgm\index.html. Accessed September 2
11. Obermeyer CM. The consequences of female circumcision for health and sexuality: an update on the evidence. Cult Health Sex. 2005;7(5):443–61.
12. Berg RC, Denison E. Does female genitalmutilation/cutting (FGM/C) affect women's sexual functioning? A systematic review of the sexual consequences of FGM/C. Sex Res Soc Policy. 2012;9(1):41–56.
13. Ibrahim MA, Yasser AH, Mohamed MF, Shahin AY. prevalence and characteristics of female sexual dysfunction in sample of women from upper Egypt. Int j GynecolObstet. 2010;108:219–23.
14. Ali AA. Knowledge and attitudes of female genital mutilation among midwives in eastern Sudan. Reprod Health. 2012;9:23.
15. De Silva S. Obstetric sequelae of female circumcision. Eur J Obstet Gynecol Reprod Biol. 2000;32:233.
16. Adam T, Bathija H, Bishai D, Bonnenfant Y-T, Darwish M, Huntington D, Johansen E. Estimating the obstetric costs of female genital mutilation in six African countries. Bull World Health Organ. 2010;88:281–8.

2

Why ethnicity and gender matters for fertility intention among married young people: a baseline evaluation from a gender transformative intervention in rural India

Tina Khanna*, Murari Chandra, Ajay Singh and Sunil Mehra

Abstract

Background: Social inequities in early child bearing persist among young married people, especially among tribal populations in India. Rural women belonging to tribal groups and those coming from poor households are more likely to give birth before age 18. This paper explores the connection between ethnicity, gender and early fertility intention among young married people in rural India.

Methods: The data is drawn from a cross sectional baseline evaluation of an intervention programme in rural India. A sample of 273 married young people was taken. Respondents were selected using systematic random sampling. Logistic Regression was used to assess the effect of being a tribal on early fertility intention and also to determine if covariates associated with early fertility intention differed by tribal status. Qualitative data was analysed using deductive content analysis approach.

Results: Bivariate and logistic regression results indicated that young married people from tribal communities had higher odds of planning a child within one year of marriage than non-tribals (OR = 1.47, *p*-value-0.079). Findings further suggest that early fertility intention among tribals is driven by gender factors and higher education and among non-tribals, higher education and awareness on contraception are key predictors. Among tribals, the odds of planning a child within one year of marriage was strongly associated with inequitable gender norms (OR = 1.94, *p*-value-0.002). Higher education showed significant positive association with non-tribals (OR = 0.19, *p*-value-0.014) and positive association with tribals (OR = 0.56, *p*-value-0.416). Qualitative investigation confirms that fertility desires of young married people are strongly influenced by gender norms especially among tribal populations.

Conclusion: Early child bearing was underpinned by complex ethnic factors and gender norms. Preference for early child bearing was seen most among tribal communities. Gender attitudes were a cause of concern especially among tribal groups. These results suggest that efforts to improve early child birth will require changing gender norms related to fertility among tribals as well as social equity issues including higher education among non-tribals and tribals.

Keywords: Tribal, Fertility, Young men and women, Gender, Education, India

* Correspondence: tina@mamtahimc.org
MAMTA Health Institute for Mother and Child, B-5, Greater Kailash Enclave-II, New Delhi 110048, India

Plain English Summary

Despite increase in age of marriage and declining fertility, social inequities in early child bearing exist among young married women and men, especially among tribal populations in India. This study sought to understand ethnic variation in early fertility preference among young people in rural India. This study utilizes mixed method approach to assess the effect of being tribal on early fertility intention and also whether determinants associated with early fertility intention differed among tribals and non-tribals. The data was collected through a survey of young married women (ages 14–18) and men (ages 15–21) and also through qualitative interviews with young married women and men, community health workers and parents. Results showed that preference for early child bearing is significantly associated with tribal communities who had early marriages and low contraceptive use. This is attributable to inequitable gender norms associated with early child bearing among tribals. Also, the role of higher education in influencing fertility intention among non-tribal and tribal cannot be neglected. The analysis underscores the need to address gender inequitable attitude among tribals and to amplify efforts to promote higher education among tribals and non-tribals for delaying early child birth.

Background

In India, rates of early childbearing are persistently high, especially among ethnic and caste minorities and women from socio-economic disadvantaged backgrounds. Analysis of the National Family and Health Survey (NFHS-3) data indicates that rural women - those belonging to Scheduled Tribes (ST), and those coming from poor households were more likely to have had a birth before age 18 [1]. Fertility rates are higher for rural women in STs in comparison to Scheduled Caste (SCs), Other Backward Classes (OBCs), and general category [2]. Couples in tribal communities report some of the lowest rates of contraceptive use in India [2, 3].

Despite India's recent economic growth, health and human development indicators of STs or *Adivasi* lag behind the national averages [4, 5]. Among the social groups in India, tribes are the most socio-economically deprived groups with low literacy and poor economic conditions and low access to health services [4–6]. The latest NFHS-4 (2015–2016) data also highlighted that reproductive health services are least accessed by women from ST groups. Tribal women also had lower rates of antenatal care visits and institutional births among all social groups [7].

Although there is extensive literature on various aspects of population, fertility, and family planning, it is noteworthy that only a limited number of empirical studies have attempted to explain tribal reproductive health (especially among young people) systematically in India [8–10]. A recent study of adolescent fertility in Africa highlights that first birth among young people is most common among the poorest and least educated, and progress in reducing rates within this group has not been made over the last few decades [11]. It further highlighted that it is valuable to examine fertility behaviour of different cultural groups to target programmes at the people most at risk, in order to reduce young people's fertility [11].

A few micro-level studies in India demonstrate that being from a tribal community positively influenced the probability of early child bearing. Panel data from Andhra Pradesh [12] demonstrates that young married women from the tribal groups were 10.5% more likely to give birth by the time they were 19 years old than women from other castes [12]. Some studies in India highlighted that early age at marriage, son preference, lower education, and low access to services are some of the reasons for low contraceptive use among tribals [13]. Gender norms are an important aspect of early fertility desires, which are largely overlooked in interventions, especially for marginalised sections. Gender relations among Indian tribes have historically been more balanced and equitable; however there is an increasing trend of gender bias in tribal culture emerging due to the assimilation and modernising process [14]. In consonance with the recent declines of tribal female-male ratio (FMR) there is growing evidence to showcase the disadvantages that tribal females have been undergoing due to expansion of developmental activities and integration. A recent study suggests that the sharp drop in tribal FMR is due to assimilation into the patriarchal norms of higher castes through ongoing processes of sanskritisation and detribalisation -all contributing to an emerging culture of discrimination against women among tribal people [15, 16]. Therefore, the present paper tries to understand reproductive behaviour among young married people of tribal communities in India and explore the inter-connection between ethnicity and gender with early fertility intention, an important factor that has not been well established or investigated systematically.

The specific objectives of the paper are: (a) To explore fertility intention among tribal and non-tribal young married people (b) To assess the effect of being a member of tribal community on early fertility intention among young married people. (c) To assess gender and social determinants of early fertility intention among tribal and non-tribal young married people in rural India.

Method

Study design

This study involved analysis of cross-sectional baseline (using quantitative and qualitative methods) data from young married people[1] in a family planning evaluation study in rural India. This paper is based on the analyses of young married people living in marital home aged 14 to 21 (Total = 273, tribal = 108, non-tribal = 165). The survey was conducted in two states of India – Madhya Pradesh (MP) and Rajasthan (two districts each) where early marriage (55–60%) and total fertility rate in rural areas fertility was higher (3.3- MP and 3.6- Rajasthan) than national estimates (National Family Health Survey, 2007–08). A three-stage sampling design was implemented in selecting six blocks across study districts and further from each blocks, 10 villages were selected using Probability Proportion to Size. Systematic random sampling was used to randomly select the respondents from completed household list of selected villages.

Data

The quantitative data was collected through a structured questionnaire by trained male and female field investigators, taking an average time of 40 min. Male investigators interviewed young married men, and young married women were interviewed by female investigators. Survey data assessed determinants of fertility intention among these people by tribal and non-tribal groups. The survey tool contained questions on socio-demographic information (including age, sex, ethnic group, education, age at marriage) and also on fertility intention, decision making, gender attitudes, use of contraceptives etc. The instrument was verbally translated into Hindi and was field-tested to ensure language and cultural contexts.

Qualitative methods

A total of 40 in-depth interviews (IDIs) were conducted among young married men and women (10 each) and parents (10 each - father and mother). We also conducted key informant interviews (KIIs) (8) with health care providers. Under the National Rural Health Mission, the government of India has employed Accredited Social Health Activist (ASHA) and Anganwadi workers (AWW) who act as community health workers. They provide counselling to married couples for use of family planning methods and also support community to access public health services. ASHA and AWW were purposively selected for KIIs since they are first point of contact with young married people in village for health care counselling and services including family planning.

We included perspectives of both young men and women and parents of young men and women to better understand emergence of early fertility norms within their particular social environments. For IDIs it took approximately 60 min and around 40 min for KIIs. The qualitative instruments contained questions relating to cultural norms and practices around early marriage and fertility, knowledge, access and use of family planning methods, gender barriers, etc. Purposive sampling was followed to select participants for IDIs and KIIs. We selected married young girls (aged 14–18) and married young boys (15–21) who were married in last 1 year without any children/not currently pregnant (married young women and wife of married young men) from tribal and non-tribal communities. For the health care providers, we recruited community health workers who had more than two years of working experience in the community. The senior research team (qualitative) in collaboration with field team with extensive experience conducted interviews.

Ethics, consent and permissions

All study participants provided consent and/or assent to participate in the study. Verbal informed consent of parents, health care providers, young men and women was sought prior to the survey. Respondents aged below 18 provided assent, while verbal informed consent was sought from their parents. The questionnaires did not request the name or other identifying variables, to ensure anonymity of data for research purpose only. Participants did not receive any material compensation. Ethical permission was obtained from the Institutional Review Board (IRB) of MAMTA- Health Institute for Mother and Child (India) prior to data collection. Since young men and women aged 14–17 years are the most vulnerable populations in research, hence the study minimised all possible risks to the participants during the survey. Every effort was made to ensure protection and confidentiality and to reduce any potential adverse consequence to the participants.

Measurement

Outcome variable: The response (dependent) variable was chosen to investigate early child bearing plan among married young people. This was categorised into two levels: intention to have child within one year of marriage and after one year. Hence, the dependent variable was coded dichotomously within one year (coded as 1) and after one year (coded as 0).

Explanatory variables

Selected socio-demographic factors that may affect early child plan at young ages were controlled in an adjusted model. These variables were: gender of respondent, age at marriage, age at *gauna*, caste, education and economic status and gender attitudes. Since the data consists of young married men and women, hence fertility choices by genders was taken in an adjusted model. *Gauna* is a traditional custom in rural India (performed in marriage that occurs at very young age) where a married couple consummate their marriage and cohabit together. Education level was grouped as till primary level (0–5 years), secondary (6–10 years); and senior secondary and higher (11 years and above). Economic status was measured by household having Below Poverty Line (BPL) card or Antyodhaya card (extreme poor) provided by Government of India. Social-ethnic group was grouped/categorized as tribal (STs) and non-tribals (OBCs and SCs). Awareness of modern contraceptive method such as condoms, IUD, pills and injectable was computed. Anganwadi centers (AWC) is the nearest and the most feasible place that provides basic health care in Indian villages including contraceptive counseling and supply and reproductive health education hence awareness about AWC was coded as 1 and 0 otherwise. Exposure to mass media (measured as mobile/internet and books/magazine) was also computed.

Gender attitude of young married people was measured through Gender Equitable Men Scale (GEMS) on 10 statements related to early child bearing, contraceptive use, family planning, autonomy, reproductive rights, etc. The statements were a mix of attitudes that were gender equal and non-equal. For each statement, the response options were 'agree', 'partially agree' and 'do not agree'. All the statements were made unidirectional before assigning the scores to a gender discriminatory statement. A score of 0 was given to the most negative statement and a score of 2 was assigned to the most positive statement. Factor analysis was done using Principle Component Analysis (PCA) and factor loading was performed to identify the most important variables with highest variability explained (Eigenvalues) in particular factor (index) created with higher reliability value ($\alpha = 0.81$). Hence the predicted scores on the scale were distributed in three equal fragments assigning as low, moderate and high gender equitable attitudes. Of these, the two very relevant statements were chosen after bivariate tests were used in an adjusted model. This methodology of creating a GEM scale has been used and validated in previous research in India as well as other countries [17, 18].

Statistical analysis

Bivariate analysis and Chi square assessed associations between tribal status and selected socio-demographic variables, early fertility intention, contraceptive use and gender norms. Adjusted Logistic Regression was used to assess effect of tribal status on early fertility intention. Intention to conceive after one year was taken as a reference category. Further, separate models were developed to determine if covariates associated with early fertility intention differed by tribal status.

Qualitative analysis

For the qualitative data analysis, all the interviews were recorded, transcribed and subsequently translated into English. Professional translators well versed with English and Hindi translated the Hindi transcript into English. The first author (Indian speaking English and Hindi) cross checked all English translated transcripts with hindi transcripts (also checked with the audio files whenever necessary) to ensure quality of translation. Hindi transcripts were read several times to get acquainted with raw data and checked at random by the first author. The translated text was coded inductively, and ambiguities in meaning were resolved by consulting project staff. Data were organised using Atlas-ti software following a content analysis approach. Themes emerging during review of the transcripts were sorted and grouped according to key categories.

Results

Socio-economic characteristics, education and exposure

Participants ($n = 273$) were 39.5% tribal and 60.5% non-tribal. The mean age for tribal and non-tribal young people were 18.7 and 18.6 The socio-demographic characteristics varied among tribal and non-tribal groups. The majority of young married tribal people (77.8%) belonged to either poor or extremely poor families. Compared to non-tribal groups, young people from the tribal community received less education. More than 40% of the young tribal people had either no education or only primary education compared to nearly one-fourth of young non-tribal people. Only about 17% of the young tribal people reached education levels above class 10th as against one third of young non-tribal people (33.3%). The exposure to media through mobile/ internet and books/magazine was also very low among tribal as compared to non-tribal people. Young tribal people (55.6%) had less access to mobile and internet than their non-tribal counterparts (61.8%).

Early marriage, fertility preference and contraceptive use: Bivariate analysis

Tribal status of young people was significantly associated ($p < 0.001$) with younger age at marriage; and younger age at cohabitation with spouse *(Gauna)*. Around half of tribal young women (46.6%) were married before age 16 in comparison to non-tribal (27.1%). Also, the majority of young tribal men (63.5%) were married before age 18 as compared to nontribal (46.4%). Importantly, 23.3% of young tribal women and majority of young tribal men (42.8%) start cohabiting as married couples before age 16 and 18 years respectively in comparison to non-tribal young women (12.9%) and non-tribal young men (24.6%) as reflected in Table 1.

Data on fertility preference indicate a significant association between tribal status and intentions for early child bearing. Within the study sample, 27.4% of young married tribal people expressed the desire for having a child within one year of marriage compared to 18.7% of

Table 1 Socio demographic and family planning characteristics among tribals and non-tribals

	Tribal (n = 108)	Non-tribal (n = 165)	p-value
Mean age*	18.7 *.54	18.6 *.53	
Socio-Economic characteristics			
Below Poverty Line and extreme poor	77.8	52.1	0.001
Education			0.002
None	15.7	9.1	
Primary (1-5th standard)	25.9	13.3	
Up to Secondary (6-10th Standard)	41.7	44.2	
Higher secondary & above (10th Standard and above)	16.7	33.3	
Exposure to media			
Mobile/ Internet	55.6	61.8	0.303
Books/magazines	5.6	21.8	0.001
Marriage			
Young women married below 16 years	46.6	27.1	0.001
Young men married below 18 years	63.5	46.4	0.001
Age at *gauna* (young women) below 16 years	23.3	12.9	0.001
Age at *gauna* (young men) below 18 years	42.8	24.6	0.001
Family planning characteristics			
Plan to have child within one year of marriage	27.4	18.7	0.088
Awareness of modern contraception methods: condom	46.3	55.4	0.152
Awareness of modern contraception Methods: Pills	82.4	93.9	0.002
Awareness about place to get contraceptives near village (AWC)	27.8	45.4	0.003
Currently using any method	15.7	24.2	0.091
Methods of use (modern method)	14.8	23.0	0.096
Reasons for not using contraception			0.053
Lack of knowledge of modern contraceptive methods	24.7	14.1	
Planning to conceive	55.3	53.9	

*Standard deviation

their non-tribal counterparts. A difference was also observed on awareness of modern contraceptive methods (condoms and pills) between tribal and non-tribals. Also, less percentage of young married people who belonged to tribal families (27.8%) were aware of AWC as the place within or near the village where one could get modern contraceptives in comparison to non-tribals (45.4%). Likewise, the current contraceptive (modern method) use among tribals (15.7%) was less than among non-tribals (24.2%).

Gender Attitudes towards early child bearing among tribal and non-tribal young married people

Tribal and non-tribal young married people were asked whether they agree, partially agree or disagree with specific gender statements related to early child bearing which provides deeper insight into the effect of gender-related attitudinal differences among tribal and non-tribal young people, on fertility intention. Gender attitudes of young married people and especially in tribal groups were biased against women when it comes to planning for the first child. As reflected in Table 2, a vast majority of young married tribal people (68.5%) agreed to the statement that '*it is husbands who can decide when to have a first child*' in comparison to 50.3% of non-tribal young people. There was a difference in the attitudes of young people, especially among tribal groups towards the pressure of early child bearing for young women, with tribals displaying more rigid and biased attitudes. Half of young tribal people agreed that '*women should conceive within one year of marriage to avoid shame*' in comparison to only 31.5% non tribals. Also more than half of young tribal people were in agreement with the statement '*Early child bearing makes women valuable in family and society*,' than their non-tribal counterparts (37%).

Further, a Gender Equitable Men Scale (from the individual statements) was developed (as explained in methodology section) whereby individual scores of members were placed in one of three categories (low, moderate and high) reflecting their level of support for gender equity. The GEMS scale (Fig. 1) shows that a majority of young tribal people fall into low and moderate gender equity category, meaning that they hold attitudes that were less or moderately supportive of gender equity towards early child bearing ($p < 0.001$). As seen in Fig. 1, young non-tribal people were more gender equitable than their tribal counterparts.

Multivariate Analysis: Logistic regression (adjusted Model) for combined and separate ethnic groups

The logistic regression analyses showed that tribal status was a significant predictor for intention to have early child birth while adjusting with other confounders (Table 3). Young people from tribal communities had 47% higher odds to plan a child within one year of marriage than their non-tribal counterparts (OR-1.47, $p < 0.079$). In the combined model, gender measures (norms) and education were other significant predictors. Young married people with restrictive gender attitudes had higher odds to plan a child within

Table 2 Gender attitudes on early child bearing (percent who agreed to selected statements) among tribals and non-tribals young married people

Statements	Tribal %	Non-tribal %	*P*-value (Chi-square)
If a couple doesn't have a child then it's a woman's fault	27.8	18.2	0.061
It's a woman's responsibility to avoid getting pregnant	59.3	51.5	0.209
Women should conceive within one year of marriage to avoid shame	50.0	31.5	0.002
It is husbands who can decide when to have first child	68.5	50.3	0.003
The real man is the one who has child within one year of marriage	23.2	16.9	0.207
Early child bearing makes women valuable in family and society	51.9	37.0	0.015

one year of marriage. For example, young married people who agreed with the statement *'The real man is the one who has a child within one year of marriage'* had 78% higher odds of planning a child within one year of marriage than those who disagreed with the statement (OR = 1.78, $p < 0.004$), given that the other predictors in the model held constant. Also, overall, the young married women had higher odds to plan a child within one year of marriage as compared to men (OR-1.55, $p < 0.067$). Young married people with higher level of education (senior secondary and higher), had lower odds to go for early child bearing (both tribals and non-tribals in the combined model) than those who had low level of education (OR-0.39, $p < 0.025$).

Further, separate models were developed to determine if covariates associated with early fertility intention differed by tribal status. Among tribal groups, early fertility intention was significantly associated with gender factors unlike their non-tribal counterparts. Young people from tribal group who agreed with the statement *'The real man is the one who has a child within one year of marriage'* had 94% higher odds of early child bearing than those who disagreed with the statement (OR-1.94, $p < 0.002$). Within the tribal group, women had 82% higher odds of planning a child within one year of marriage as compared to their male counterparts (OR-1.82, $p < 0.020$).

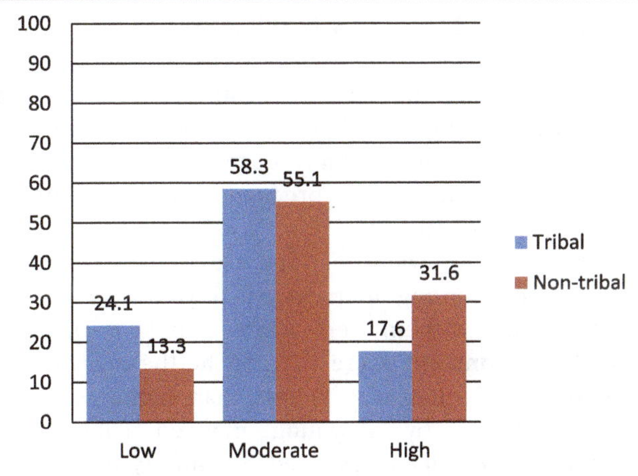

Fig. 1 Level of support for gender equity among tribal and non-tribals: Fertility Perception on Early Child Bearing (separate file attached)

Early fertility intention was positively associated with increase in education among both tribal and non-tribal groups. Table 3 reflects that with increase in level of education the odds of planning a child early after marriage decreased irrespective of ethnic groups. Among non-tribals higher education had positive and significant association (OR-0.19, $p < 0.014$) with early fertility intention, however among tribals it showed only positive association (OR-0.56, $p < 0.416$). Among non-tribals, young married people who were not aware of contraceptive methods had 71% higher odds of planning a child within one year of marriage (OR-1.71, $p < 0.026$). Thus among non-tribals, early fertility intention was significantly associated with education and awareness about contraception and not with gender factors.

Qualitative findings

The qualitative investigation found that the desire for young people to bear children early was influenced by social and gender norms, especially among tribal populations.

Social and family related factors

The pressure to fulfill the social demand to conceive early to prove their worth soon after marriage was found among young women, and this was particularly high for tribal women who were married early and had less education. Parents from both tribal and non-tribal communities shared that it is a common trend for a married couple to have a first child early, and therefore no birth control measures were taken. They were taken only after the second child for spacing. However, in the context of tribals, parents and families were more averse towards imparting family planning to newly married couples and feared using family planning methods. These respondents (parents) also had less education (primary education) and less exposure. They shared that talking about sexual relations, family planning issues is neither needed nor acceptable in the community. It is considered a cultural taboo and some parents even feared and

Table 3 Odds Ratio (OR) of Fertility Intention within one year by selected predictors for combined and separate ethnic groups

	Model 1: Combined ethnic groups	Model 2: Tribal	Model 3: Non-tribal
	OR	OR	OR
Gender			
Boy	1	1	
Girl	1.55*	1.82**	1.63
Caste			
Non-tribal	1	1	
Tribal	1.47*		
Education level			
Up to primary (0-5th standard)	1	1	1
Secondary (6-10th Standard)	0.88	0.80	0.93
Senior secondary & higher (10th standard and above)	0.39**	0.56	0.19**
Duration of cohabitation after marriage (years)	1.00	1.20	0.95
Awareness about contraception methods:			
Yes	1	1	1
No	1.52**	1.46	1.71**
Gender statements			
The real man is the one who has a child within one year of marriage			
Disagree	1	1	1
Agree	1.78***	1.94***	1.33
Early child bearing makes women valuable in family and society			
Disagree	1	1	1
Agree	1.08	0.37	1.42
Constant	0.015	0.0666	0.031
Adjusted R^2	0.115	0.2101	0.181

Note: Response outcome for early fertility preference 0(ref) = after 1 year, 1 = within 1 year, results are controlled for other predictors such as current age, BPL status, family support @reference category. *$p < 0.1$, ** $p < 0.05$, ***$p < 0.01$

questioned the relevance of providing this knowledge. As shared by an elder woman from the tribal community:

> *"No one talks about these things in a village. It is considered a wrong and sinful practice. You should not give this information otherwise newly married will know about ways to delay pregnancy and they will delay their first child. You should give this information to those who have at least one child."*

Young married tribal women shared that there is strong family pressure on them to conceive early especially for the first child. They explained that they have limited decision-making powers in family planning; these decisions are mostly taken by the husband. As shared emphatically by a married tribal girl (19):

> *I: What will you do if you don't want to have a child now?*
>
> *R: I/my husband will have to use birth control methods.*
>
> *I: Will you face any difficulty in using contraceptives?*
>
> *R: My in-laws can stop me; they will say we want to have a grandchild now.*
>
> *I: What will you do? What support would you need?*
>
> *R: I would definitely need my husband's support to refuse to have a child now. If my husband wants it, then I will have to conceive and deliver a child, and if he doesn't then I will not conceive.*

Young men were also influenced by social norms about early fertility and perceived attitudes of people in their social networks. Young married men also stated that there are negative repercussions that a woman has to bear if she doesn't conceive within two years of marriage, including facing negative remarks and abandonment. This was shared by both tribal and non-tribal men. The young tribal men who were married early (at 16–17 years) and had less education, were found more bound by traditional community norms for early child bearing.

> *"It is expected to have a child within one year of marriage. If she doesn't conceive within 1-2 years then such a woman is taunted, taken to doctors and may be abandoned."*

Married boy (19 years), Scheduled Tribe.

Among tribal populations, around two-thirds of interviewed young married tribal men and women ($n = 6$) lacked correct knowledge about pregnancy. Few of them thought that pregnancy can never occur in one sexual contact and it is possible after multiple contacts. The knowledge about use of contraception was also less among married tribal young people as less than half of them were aware of it ($n = 4$). Most of these respondents were married at the age of 15–16 years and had education less than higher secondary. As shared by a young married tribal man (18 years): *"No I have not used a condom, and I also don't know how to use it. In fact, I will never use; it looks horrible to me."*

Factors related to service provision/health care providers
The qualitative interviews with health care workers highlighted their apprehension to provide family planning knowledge and services to young married men and women and their limited outreach to tribal communities. Many village health care providers expressed disapproval at using contraceptive methods to delay the first pregnancy and spoke of community challenges and the non-acceptability of it.

> *"The first child should be born after two years - we can counsel the couple on this but we can't go against society. Even if the couple is educated and aware, they will be forced to have the first child soon. They can delay the second child not the first."*
>
> Community health worker (Female, 34 years).

Community health workers also expressed that young married men and women from tribal communities lacked awareness and access to health care services. They explained that they were not able to reach them as they lived on the periphery of the village, far from the health centre.

> *Tribal communities live far from the main village, and the health centre. We are less in contact with them and they also don't come to the centre.*
>
> Community health worker (Female, 28 years).

Discussion

The findings from bi-variate analysis and adjusted logistic regression also reinforced from qualitative analysis indicate that preference for early child bearing is significantly associated with tribals in comparison to non-tribal. The current findings indicate that young married people from tribal community have higher odds of planning a child early within one year of marriage. These findings have also been recognised in earlier studies that have found more cases of early marriage and child bearing among tribal populations than other socio-ethnic groups [1, 2, 12]. Studies on tribal population in south and west India have also found low contraceptive use, misconceptions and lack of access to various contraceptive methods to be the causes of early child bearing [2, 14, 19]. The tribal populations have less education, which further makes them vulnerable to low contraceptive use and high unmet need than other social groups [12, 19]. The bi-variate association between tribal status and gender inequitable attitudes was also significant. Overall, tribals had greater gender inequitable and patriarchal attitudes on early childbearing as compared with their non-tribal counterparts.

This study contributes to a growing body of studies on reproductive behaviour and is one of the few studies using the GEM scale to understand gender-equitable attitudes of tribals and non-tribals. Existing studies have reflected gender equitable attitude for equitable reproductive decision-making and increased contraceptive use [20, 21]. However, such linkages are explored less among tribal populations. While historically gender relations among tribals have been more egalitarian as compared to other social groups, anti-female patterns of discrimination are now increasing among some tribal communities as their lives become integrated into mainstream culture and social practices, generally through the conversion to Hinduism [11, 15]. These studies have pointed out the growing trend of gender deficit of females and gender bias among tribal communities [11, 15].

Further, findings also indicate that tribals who were more likely to plan child early was attributable to inequitable gender norms associated with early child bearing. This reflects that not only do gender attitudes influence the perception of young married people among tribals for early child bearing but they also impact the planning of a child within one year of marriage. The present findings have reaffrmed this connection on a firmer footing. This is particularly noteworthy in light of the current findings. Gender attitudes of young married people were a cause of concern especially among tribal groups and therefore support the need for involvement of both men and women for addressing traditional gender inequitable norms for reproductive behavior. This finding also corroborates with a recent study conducted among tribal populations in rural India on reproductive behavior, where tribals were less likely to practice spacing contraceptive use (SCU) than their non-tribal counterparts. The lower SCU among tribal was driven by gender inequalities and social vulnerabilities (higher son preference, higher fertility preference and low education) [19].

The finding also confirms that the pressures for early child bearing among tribals fall more on young married women than men. Young married women had higher odds of planning a child within one year in comparison to their male counterparts. Qualitative findings congruently found that young married women were more influenced by negative prejudices around delayed childbearing and obliged to have at least one child before seeking family planning services. This was also found in previous studies in India [22]. The role of higher education in influencing fertility intention among non-tribal and tribal cannot be neglected, although it was positively associated with tribal status however not significant. The results reflect that higher education (above class 10th) matters in determining fertility behavior among young married people in both non-tribal and tribal groups. Qualitative accounts further demonstrated that young married people from tribal communities had less access to health services and modern contraceptives. There was also poor outreach of reproductive services by community health workers to tribal communities. A review also highlights that tribal people face geographical isolation and limited interactions and exposure, along with poor access to healthcare in India [8].

Limitations of the study

The current findings should be viewed in context of certain limitations, which are important to state. The sample taken for the analysis was small ($n = 273$) and from the larger data on young men and women thus, the findings currently described may not hold true across other geographic and socioeconomic contexts and hence there can be limited generalisations. Further, the use of selective cross-sectional data limits our ability to make causal inferences at macro level. Therefore, further research will be required to extend and validate this analysis by including larger representative sample across different contexts.

Conclusion

This paper reaffirms that efforts need to be directed towards the tribal populations the most. These findings call for pursuing gender transformative strategies for promoting gender equitable attitudes for reproductive decision making especially among tribals. The focus of health and population interventions should not only be to target young married tribals, but also to improve their gender attitudes for the purpose of delaying early childbirth. Efforts should also be intensified for providing access to higher education among tribals and non-tribals as it can significantly influence fertility intention. There is also a need to reduce disparities in access to family planning health services that exist between tribals and other social groups, strengthening outreach for family planning programmes. The findings are relevant to design and tailor appropriate family planning interventions for young married people to meet their current and future fertility desire needs.

Endnotes

[1]Adolescence is defined by WHO as between 10 and 19 years, while youth refers to 15–24 years. Young people refer to the 10–24-year-old age group. For the purpose of this paper, we have used the term young people throughout to refer to 14–21 years of boys and girls in the study population.

Abbreviations

AWC: Anganwadi Center; BPL: Below Poverty Line; FMR: Female-male ratio; GEMS: Gender Equitable Men's Scale; IDIs: In-depth interviews; KIls: Key informant interviews; NHFS: National Family and Health Survey; OBC: Other Backward Classes; OR: Odds Ratio; SC: Scheduled Caste; SCU: Spacing Contraceptive Use; ST: Scheduled Tribes

Acknowledgements

First and foremost, the authors thank all the study participants and field staff. The authors would like to thank Dr. Rachana Patel for assisting with the analysis. The authors would also like to thank Mr. Praveer Goyal for coordinating the study in the field, Ms. Shilpa Jain, Mr. Mohammed Ahmed and Mr. Shubham Rai for ensuring quality checks during the data collection and assisting in field management.

Funding

The baseline study was conducted from the intervention project funded by American Jewish World Services (AJWS).

Authors' contributions

TK, MC, and SM conceived the study. TK and MC were involved in tool development and data acquisition. TK undertook the analysis and wrote the manuscript. AS and MC contributed to the interpretation of the findings providing inputs for the background, analysis and conclusion section. SM provided overall guidance and review of manuscript draft. All authors read and approved the final manuscript.

Ethics approval and consent to participate

All study participants provided informed consent and/or assent to participate in the study. Verbal informed consent was taken from parents, health care providers and young married men and women prior to the study. Respondents aged below 18 provided assent, while verbal informed consent was sought from their parents.

Ethical permission was obtained from the Institutional Review Board of MAMTA- Health Institute for Mother and Child for conducting research. The following members of the institutional ethics committee approved the study:

1. Dr. Ravi Verma, Chairperson, Ethics Committee, Regional Director (Expert in Gender and Research studies), International Centre for Research on Women (ICRW), Asia Regional Office, Delhi, India.
2. Dr. Sushanta Banerjee, (Expert in Social and behavioral sciences Senior) Advisor, IPAS, New Delhi, India.
3. Dr. U.V. Somayajulu: Expert in Biostatistics Statistics. CEO and Executive Director, SIGMA Research and Consulting Pvt. Ltd., New Delhi, India.
4. Dr. AK Sharma: (Expert in social and behavioral sciences) Professor of Sociology, Department of Humanities and Social Sciences, Indian Institute of Technology, Kanpur. India.
5. Dr. Anita Acharya, Associate Professor, Lady Harding Medical College, Delhi, India.
6. Ms. Sauda Begam, Community Member and Frontline Worker, India.
7. Dr. Sunil Mehra, (Medical Expert on RMNCH+A) Executive Director, MAMTA Health Institute for Mother and Child.

Consent for publication

Not applicable.

Competing interests

The authors declare that they have no competing interests.

References

1. Daniel EE, Masilamani R, Rahman M. The effect of community-based reproductive health communication interventions on contraceptive use among young married couples in Bihar, India. Int Fam Plan Perspect. 2008; 34(4):189–97.
2. National Family Health Survey (NFHS-3), 2005–06. India, vol. I. Mumbai: IIPS: International Institute for Population Sciences (IIPS) and Macro International; 2007.
3. Prusty RK. Use of contraceptives and unmet need for family planning among tribal women in India and selected hilly states. Journal of Health. Population and Nutrition (JHPN). 2014;32:342–55.
4. Sarkar S, Mishra S, Dayal H, Nathan D. Development and deprivation of Scheduled Tribes. Econ Polit Wkly. 2006;18:4824–7.
5. Subramanian SV, Davey Smith G, Subramanyam M. Indigenous health and socioeconomic status in India. PLoS Med. 2006;3:1794–804.
6. Agarwal S. Health and nutritional disadvantage among tribal women and children of Orissa, India: a situational analysis. Journal of Community Health

and medicine. 2013; 317-339. file:///C:/Users/newuser/AppData/Local/Packages/Microsoft.MicrosoftEdge_8wekyb3d8bbwe/TempState/Downloads/2.Heallthandnutritionaldisadvantage%20(2).pdf.
7. National Fact Sheet BF. NFHS-4 (National Family Health Survey-4). International Institute for Population Studies. 2016.
8. Mohindra KS, Labonté R. A systematic review of population health interventions and Scheduled Tribes in India. BMC Public Health. 2010;10:438.
9. Maharatna A. Fertility, mortality and gender bias among tribal population: an Indian perspective. Soc Sci Med. 2000;50:1333–51.
10. Maharatna A. Tribal fertility in India: Socio-cultural influences on demographic behaviour. Econ Polit Wkly. 2000;19:3037–47.
11. Neal SE, Chandra-Mouli V, Chou D. Young people first births in East Africa: disaggregating characteristics, trends and determinants. Reprod Health. 2015;12(1):13.
12. Singh A, Revollo PE. Teenage Marriage, Fertility, and Well-being: Panel Evidence from India. 2016.
13. Susuman SA. Son preference and contraceptive practice among tribal groups in rural south India. Studies of Tribes and Tribals. 2006;4:31–40.
14. Maharatna A. How Can 'Beautiful 'Be' Backward'? Tribes of India in a Long-term Demographic Perspective. Econ Polit Wkly. 2011;22:42–52.
15. Xaxa V. Women and Gender in the Study of Tribes in India. Indian Journal of Gender Studies. 2004;11:345–67.
16. Bramley D, Hebert P, Tuzzio L, Chassin M. Disparities in indigenous health: a cross-country comparison between New Zealand and the United States. Am J Public Health. 2005;95(5):844–50.
17. Barker G, Contreras M, Heilman B, Singh A, Verma R, Nascimento M. Evolving Men: Initial Results from the International Men and Gender Equality Survey (IMAGES). In. Washington, DC and Rio de Janeiro: International Center for Research on Women (ICRW) and Instituto Promundo; 2011. p. 47.
18. Verma RK, Pulerwitz J, Mahendra VS, Khandekar S, Singh AK, Das SS, Nura A, Barkar G. "Promoting Gender Equity as a Strategy to Reduce HIV Risk and Gender-Based Violence among Young Men in India". In Horizons Final Report. Washington, DC: Population Council; 2008.
19. Battala M, et al. Association between tribal status and spacing contraceptive use in rural Maharashtra, India. Sexual & Reproductive Healthcare. 2016:78–80.
20. Mishra A, Nanda P, Speizer IS, Calhoun LM, Zimmerman A, Bhardwaj R. Men's attitudes on gender equality and their contraceptive use in Uttar Pradesh India. Reprod Health. 2014;4; 11(1):41.
21. Khan ME, Patel BC. Male Involvement in Family Planning: A Knowledge Attitude Behaviour and Practice Survey of Agra District. New Delhi: Population Council, June 1997. https://pdfs.semanticscholar.org/95b5/c9516040efc472f6dde5f777abccc5a40fe6.pdf. Accessed 2 Feb 2017.
22. Mathur S, Greene M, Malhotra A. Too Young to Wed: The Lives, Rights, and Health of Young Married Girls. International Centre for Research on Women. 2003; Accessed 10 Feb 2017.

3

Sexual and reproductive health services utilization and associated factors among secondary school students in Nekemte town, Ethiopia

Wakgari Binu[1], Taklu Marama[2*], Mulusew Gerbaba[3] and Melese Sinaga[3]

Abstract

Background: Despite policy actions and strategic efforts made to promote sexual and reproductive health service uptake of youths in Ethiopia, its utilization remains very low and little information was found on the extent to which school youths utilize available reproductive health services in Nekempt town. This study was aimed to assess utilization of Sexual and Reproduactive Health (SRH) services and its associated factors among secondary school students in Nekemte town, Ethiopia.

Method: A school based cross-sectional study design was conducted from April 18 to 22, 2016. Multistage cluster sampling technique was used to select a total of 768 students who attended secondary schools. Sexual and reproductive health services utilization was measured using one item asking whether they had used either of sexual and reproductive health services components during the last one year or not. The data was entered using EpiData Manager with Entry Client and further analysis was done using SPSS version 21 software. Descriptive statistics, cross tabulations, biviarate and multivariate logistic regression analyses were used. All variables were set by *p*-values less than 0.05 and reported by Adjusted Odds Ratio with its 95%CI.

Result: Out of the 768 study subjects, 739 participants underwent all the study components giving response rate of 96%. About 157 (21.2%) school youths reported that they utilized SRH services. On multivariable logistic regression analysis after adjusting for other variable, discussion with health workers (AOR 3.0, 95%CI [1.7–5.2]), previous history of perceived Sexually transmitted infections (STIs) symptoms (AOR 2.6, 95%CI [1.2–5.5]), being ever sexually experienced (AOR 5.9, 95%CI [3.4–10.2]) and exposure to information from school teachers (AOR 0.36, 95%CI [0.2–0.6]) were found to be independent determinants of sexual and reproductive services utilization among secondary school youths. Inconvenient times, lack of privacy, religion, culture, and parent prohibition were barriers to SRH service uptake cited by the school youths.

Conclusions: The overall utilization of sexual and reproductive services was low among school youths in the town. Discussion with health workers, history of perceived STIs symptoms, sexual experience and information were the association factors of sexual and reproductive service utilization among secondary school youths.

* Correspondence: mtaklu2002@gmail.com
[2]Department of Midwifery, College of Health Sciences and Medicine, Wolaita Sodo University, Wolaita Sodo, Ethiopia
Full list of author information is available at the end of the article

Plain English summary

Even if policy actions and strategic efforts made to promote sexual and reproductive health service uptake of youths in Ethiopia, few literatures showed its utilization remains very low. So, this study was aimed to assess utilization of Sexual and reproductive Health (SRH) services and its associated factors among secondary school students in Nekemte town, Ethiopia.

Students' utilized as well as utilizing Sexual and reproductive Health services before and during April 18th to 22nd, 2016 are included in the study. Among 12 above grade 9 schools, two government and 2 non-government schools were selected using lottery methods. For this study, a total of 768 students were needed. To have these, students from each grade and sections were randomly selected from their attendance lists. On the day of data collection the randomly selected students were told to remain in their classes. Sexual and Reproductive Health services utilization was measured if the students utilized one of the six given components. To keep data quality first data was entered to EpiData Manager and exported to SPSS version 21 software to have the required output. The result was described in table and figures, and cross tabulated. Bivariate logistic regression model was used to see association between utilization and other factors.

In this study, only 157 (21.2%) of students reported their utilization of Sexual and Reproduction Health services. Students who discussed with health workers, perceived history of Sexually transmitted infections (STIs) symptoms previously, experienced sex ever and exposed to information from school teachers were found to be better utilized Sexual and Reproductive Health services.

When summarized, the overall utilization of SRH services was low among school youths in the town.

Background

There were 1.8 billion young people aged 10–24 years among which 1.2 billion youth aged 15–24 years globally in 2015, accounting for one out of every six people worldwide in which Africa comprises 19% (above 226 million) of the global youth population [1]. Young people make up the greatest proportion of the population in sub-Saharan Africa, with more than one-third of the population 10–24 ages [2], and 33.8% of the total population in Ethiopia is between the age of 10–24 [3].

Since the International Conference on Population and Development Key Informant Interview held in Cairo in 1994, governments have pledged to improve the SRH of adolescents by providing access to comprehensive, appropriate information and education and youth friendly health services. Most regions of the world however, still fall short of these commitments, especially for unmarried young people [4].

Even though the comprehensive knowledge of HIV and other Reproductive Health (RH) problems is increasing around the world, many young people do not have the information or means to protect themselves from these problems [5]. Many health problems are contributed by adolescents and young people worldwide: 8.7 million abortions undergone, 41% of new HIV infection, high rate of early marriage and STIs, and high proportion of stillbirth and newborn deaths [6].

In Africa, 430,000 young people are infected with HIV per year; 2.6 million young people are living with HIV; teenage pregnancy rates still remain high and maternal mortality is among the leading causes of death for adolescent girls in this region [7]. Studies done in Ethiopia also show that there was 42.1% sexual risk behavior [8], 19% of youths reported having had premarital sexual intercourse with the mean age of 16.48 years at the first sexual intercourse [9], self-reported STIs prevalence was 19.5% [10] and abortion rate was also 65 per 1000 women [11].

Concerning the utilization of SRH services, it is not enough as expected from the efforts tried in Ethiopia. The SRH services utilization has great variation, 21.5% in Hadya [12] to 96.1%in Harar [13], that refers different factors are affecting the utilization differently in different part of the country. The SRH services utilization is high in areas where youth friendly services are available and accessible at community level [13]. It is evidenced that high school students were visiting SRH services to receive SRH information, for counseling service, to obtain a condom, for treatment of STI, for postabortion care [14] while others were not using SRH services because of inconvenience service hour, feel fear to be seen by others, too long waiting hours, providers are judgmental and unfriendly, feel embracement at seeking RH services [15]. Even, the utilizationof SRH services among secondary school students is not well explored in the country and the existing studies do not show enough information about the SRH situation of secondary school students, resulting in the absence of sustainable school based intervention for secondary chool students. So, additional study that assesses the magnitude and factors affecting SRH service utilization is very crucial to improve SRH service utilization of secondary school young people in the study area in the way that reduce morbidities and disabilities related to sexual and reproductive health.

Methods

Institution based cross-sectional study design was conducted in Nekemte town, East Wallaga zone, Western Ethiopia from April 18th to 22nd, 2016. Nekemte Town is situated 331 km from Addis Ababa city. The town covers an area of 5480 ha. According to data from

Central Statistics Agency Branch in the town, the total population of the town is projected to be 97,289 and young people in the town is estimated to be 37,796 (male = 19,626, female = 18,170) in 2016 [16].

According to the information from Nekemte Town Education Office, the total number of young people enrolled to secondary school (grade 9–12) in 2015/16 was 11,428 (male = 5539, female = 5867) students in seven government secondary schools 9771(85.5%) and five none-government (two Non-Governmental Organizations (NGO) and three Private) secondary schools 1657(14.5%). The government schools are free of charge for educational purposes. From the estimated total population of young people, only 30.24% (28.22% of male and 32.29% of female) of young people were attending schools. The data from Nekemte Town Health Office showed that the town has one general hospital, two government health centers, one higher and twelve medium private clinics, twelve NGO health facilities that are serving the society. From these health facilities, one government health centre and two NGO clinics were delivering SRH services and youth friendly services separately which is free of charge.

All secondary school students enrolled in the year 2015/2016 in the town were the source population and all the students in randomly selected secondary schools were the study population. Sample size was calculated using single population proportion formula by taking the proportion (p) of SRH services utilization by school youths to be 32% taken from the study conducted in Bahir Dar Town (19) [17] with the conservative assumptions in order to get enough sample size that would allow the study to look into various aspects of school youths. The assumptions of 95% confidence level (level of significance, $z_\alpha = 1.96$), 5% margin of error, design effect of 2.0 and 15% non-response were used to determine the sample size. Accordingly, the total sample size was 768.

Concerning Sampling Techniques, Multistage cluster sampling technique was used in order to select a representative sample of students. Four schools (two from government ant two from non-government) were selected randomily. Samples were selected from government and non-government schools proportional to their size of the student population. The total sample was allocated to each grade from grade 9 to 12 proportionate to their student population size; Then four (2 government and 2 non-government) schools were selected using simple random sampling to recruit the allocated subjects for each grade. From each grade, sections were selected randomly and finally the study subjects were selected by using lottery method in SPSS using their attendance lists in the respective schools. On the day of data collection the randomly selected students were told to remain in their classes.

The dependent variable in this study was whether a participant had utilized SRH services within the last 12 months anywhere whether in government or private health institutions. This was measured through the dichotomous response (yes or no). The positive response was further validated with questions on the type of SRH services utilized. This included information and counseling on SRH issues, family planning, voluntary testing and counseling on HIV, abortion care, maternal and child care, testing and treatment of STIs. A positive ("yes") response to any one of these services was regarded as service utilization. The questionnaire was developed by collecting and adopting after customizing into the study context from various literatures [18–20].

The quality of data were assured by translating questionnaires from English to Afan Oromo then back to English by another expert using properly designed and pretested questionnaire. The data was collected by two Diploma Nurses and supervised by 1 BSc Nurse who were trained for two days. The pretest was done on 5 % of the sample size in Gimbi secondary school, a 100 km Town from Nekemte and some modifications such as skipping pattern and sequence sections in the questionnaire were made. To maintain confidentiality, each participant took a single sparsely arranged seat and the participant put the questionnaire on separate table arranged at corner of the room.

The questionnaires were designed by using Epidata manger and entry-client. Regarding data analysis and management, all returned questionnaires were checked for completeness and consistency manually. Thereafter, data was coded, entered into EPI-data entry client 2.0.8.56 and exported to Statistical Package for the Social Sciences (SPSS) version 21. Frequencies and percentages were used to summarize descriptive statistics. Bivariate logistic regression analysis was done by entering variables that were found to affect SRH utilization. Variables with the *p*-value of less than or equal to 0.25 were entered into multivariate logistic regression. Those variables statistically significant at p-value less than 0.05 in multivariate logistic regression analysis were found to be taken as statistically significant. Adjusted odds ratio with the confidence level of 95% was considered to assess the strength of the association between dependent and independent variables.

Some phrases are Operationed as follows:

Attitude

Respondents has favorable attitude if they score equal or above mean score (66.48) of the total 24 attitude questions with 1–5 likert scale points.

Knowledge of SRH services

First knowledge about the SRH services was assessed by asking participants whether they were aware of SRH service components or not. Then SRH knowledge was assessed through 8-item scale on knowledge of SRH service components and the sum of scores ranging from one (minimum) to eight (maximum) for subjects were used in the analysis.

SRH services utilization

This was measured through the dichotomous response (yes or no) by asking whether a participant had utilized one or more of SRH service components within the last 12 months. The positive response was further validated with questions on the type of SRH services utilized. A positive ("yes") response to any one of these services was regarded as service utilization.

Results

Out of the total of 768 study participants, 739 of students took part in the survey giving a response rate of 96.0%. Out of these, 349(47.2%) were males, 665 (90.0%) and 74(10.0%) falls under the age group of 15–19 and 20–24 years respectively with the mean age of 17.3(SD = ±1.7); 25(3.4%) and 136(18.4%) were single and in relationship respectively. Majority of them 925(97.4%) were Oromo by ethnic group, and protestant 525(55.5%) followers. Regarding their current educational status, h 82.9% and 17.1% of them were attending government and private schools respectively. The result also shows that the fathers 666(91.1%) and mothers 573(77.5%) of respondents were formally educated and 291(39.4%) of fathers and 220(29.8%) of mothers were employed. Majority of the students 486(65.8%) were living with their family (Table 1).

Knowledge, attitudes towards SRH services and sexual practices

Three hundred fifteen (42.6%) and 30 (4.1%) of the respondents know at least one and eight SRH service components respectively. Six hundred eighty six of participants have an information on SRH services and 564 (76.3%) of participants were aware of at least one health facility where SRH services could be delivered. Government health facilities, private health facilities, NGO health facilities and traditional facilities were SRH services delivery points as cited by 509(68.9%), 286(38.7%), 187(25.3%) and 50(6.8%) of the respondents respectively. Majority of the respondents (72.7%) have involved in the available school clubs and 400 (54.3%) had discussed on SRH issues with friends followed by health workers 163 (22.1%). 387(52.4%) of respondents had favorable attitude towards the SRH services. A total of 140 (18.9%) of respondents had ever experienced sexual intercourse and 101 (13.7%) of respondents had sexual contact within the last 12 months. The mean age at first sexual contact of respondents was 15.14 (SD = ±2.98) years. This study also showed that 70 (69.3%) of the sexually active respondents were male and 16 (15.8%) of them had more than one sexual partners (Table 2).

Table 1 Socio-demographic, community and family characteristics of secondary school students in Nekemte Town, Ethiopia, April 18–22, 2016

Socio-demographic characteristics		Frequencies	Percentage
Age	15–19	665	90.0
	20–24	74	10.0
Sex	Male	349	47.2
	Female	390	52.8
Marital status	Married	25	3.4
	In a love relationship	136	18.4
	Single	578	76.0
Ethnicity	Oromo	719	97.3
	Others	20	2.7
Religion	Protestant	405	54.8
	Orthodox	155	21.0
	Wakefata	140	18.9
	Muslim	28	3.8
	Others***	11	1.4
Educational status	Grade 9	297	40.2
	Grade 10	173	23.4
	Grade 11	134	18.1
	Grade 12	135	18.3
School type	Government	613	82.9
	Private	126	17.1
Pocket money in ETB	No money	224	30.3
	1–500	450	60.9
	> 500	65	8.8
Mother's education	No formal education	166	22.5
	Formal education	573	77.5
Father's education	No formal education	73	9.9
	Formal education	666	91.1
Mother's occupation	Unemployed	519	70.2
	Employed	220	29.8
Father's occupation	Unemployed	448	60.6
	Employed	291	39.4
Living arrangement	Living with family	486	65.8
	Not living with family	253	34.1
Family residence	Urban	534	72.3
	Rural	205	27.7

Others = Amhara, Guraghe, Tigrie Others*** = Adventist, Catholic, Jhoba

Respondents answered media 333(45.1%), teachers 305(41.3%), health workers 271(36.7%), friends 198(26.8%) as their potential sources of information for SRH services (Fig. 1).

Utilization of SRH services

This study result showed that 157(21.2%) of overall study subjects had received at least one component of

Table 2 Knowledge, Attitudes towards SRH services and Sexual practices among secondary school youths in Nekemte Town, 2016

SRH services and sexual related		Frequencies	Percentage
Awareness of SRH services(*n* = 739)	Yes	686	92.8
	No	53	7.2
Awareness of Health facilities(*n* = 687)	Yes	564	76.3
	No	123	16.6
Source of information on SRH services (Multiple Response)	Parent talk	116	12.2
	Friends	198	26.8
	Relatives	60	8.1
	Health workers	271	36.7
	School teachers	305	41.3
	School clubs	149	20.2
	Medias	333	45.1
	Printed materials	154	20.8
Participated in school clubs	Yes	537	72.7
	No	202	27.3
Discussion on SRH topics with (Multiple Response)	Mother	88	11.3
	Father	32	4.3
	Brother/sister	66	9
	Friends	400	54.3
	Health workers	163	22.1
	Relatives	34	4.6
Awareness of health facilities where to get SRH services (Multiple Response)	Government	509	68.9
	Private	286	37.8
	Non-government	187	25.3
	Traditional	50	6.8
Sexually ever experienced	Yes	140	18.9
	No	599	81.1
Currently sexually active	Yes	101	13.7
	No	638	86.3
Currently sexually active	Male	70	69.3
	Female	31	29.7
Partners for sexually actives	Only one	85	84.2
	More than one	16	15.8
Attitude towards SRH services use(*n* = 737)	Unfavorable	350	47.5
	Favorable	387	52.5

the SRH services in the last twelve months. Majority of the participants 116(54.8%) reported government health facilities from where they received SRH services followed by NGO health facilities 46(29.3%) (Table 3).

The most frequently utilized SRH services was Volunteer Test and Counseling 93(59.2%) followed by information and counseling on SRH issues 80(51%) and condom service 46(29.3%). The result also showed 27(26.7) of the sexually active respondents had utilized family planning methods in the last twelve month (Fig. 2).

In this study, 582(78.8%) of the study participants did not use SRH services in the last twelve months. The most frequently reported reasons for not utilizing SRH services, are not encountering any problem 249(42.8%) ,and believing that the services were not necessary 135 (23.2%) majorly (Fig. 3).

Factors associated with utilization of SRH services

During bivariate analysis, being in 20–24 age (COR 2.36, 95%CI [1.34 to 4.16]), being married (COR 2.69, 95%CI [1.14 to 6.34]), history STIs (COR 4.41, 95%CI [2.46 to 7.91]),

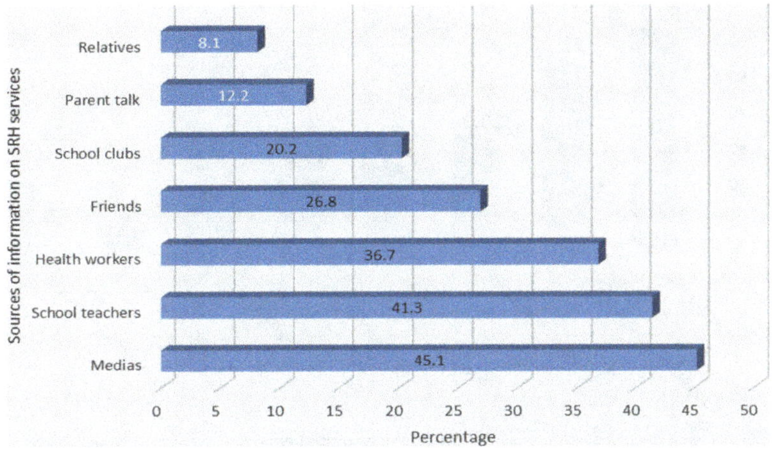

Fig. 1 Sources of information on SRH services for secondary school youths in Nekemte Town, April 18-22, 2016

having ever sexual contact (COR 7.51, 95%CI [4.87 to 11.6]), and having favorable attitude towards SRH services (COR 1. 46, 95%CI [1.01 to 2.13]), heard SRH information from school teachers (COR 0.4, 95%CI [0.27, 0.59]) discussing on SRH issues with friends (COR 0.46, 95%CI [0.3, 0.72]), discussing on SRH issues with health care workers (COR 2.78, 95%CI [1.8, 4.3]) and attending non-government schools (COR 0.46, 95%CI [0.27–0.79]) were found to be associated with SRH services utilization (Table 4).

After controlling the effects of confounding, multivariate logistic regression analysis showed that the likelihood of SRH service utilization among secondary school was about 3 times (AOR = 3, 95%CI [1.72 to 5.24]) higher among respondents who discussed SRH issues with health workers than their counterparts. Students who had heard SRH issues from their school teachers were 64% (AOR = 0.36, 95%CI [0.21 to 0.61]) less likely to utilize SRHS than those who had not heard SRH related

Table 3 SRH service utilization and reasons don't use the services by secondary school youths in Nekemte Town, April 18–22, 2016

Characteristics		Frequency	Percentage
Utilized at least one SRH service (n = 739)	No	582	78.8
	Yes	157	21.2
SRH services utilized in the last 12 months ($n = 157$)			
Information and counseling on SRH issues		80	51
Family planning services		34	21.7
Pregnancy test		15	9.6
Pregnancy care		7	4.5
Abortion care services		5	3.2
Condom services		46	29.3
STIs treatment services		28	17.8
Voluntary testing and counseling for HIV		93	59.2
Sexually actives utilized FP methods ($n = 101$)	Yes	27	26.7
	No	74	74.3
Facilities where SRH services received (n = 157)			
Government		86	54.8
Private		35	22.3
Non-government		46	29.3
Traditional		6	3.8

N.B. System missed values were excluded from analysis, some observations may exceed 100% due to multiple options and others may be less than 100% due to missed values

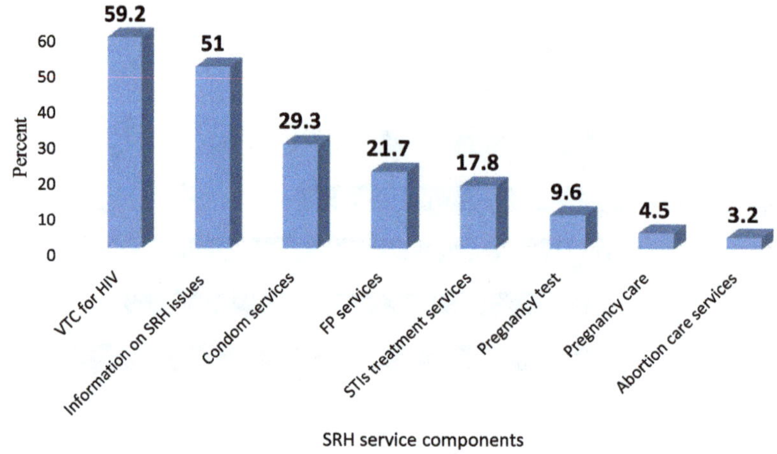

Fig. 2 Components of SRH services utilized by secondary school youths in Nekemte Town, 2016

issues from their school teacher. The odds of SRH service utilization was about 6 times [AOR = 5.87, 95%CI [3.38 to 10.19)] higher among respondents who ever had sexual contact than their counterparts. Respondents who had history of perceived STIs symptoms were 2.6 times (AOR 2.61, 95%CI [1.24 to 5.49]) more likely to utilize the SRH services.

Discussion

The overall utilization of SRH among school youths was 21.2% (95% CI[18.3–24.0]). It is similar with the cross-sectional study conducted in Mekele Town and East Gojjam zone [21, 22]. However, this finding was less than findings from Harar Town, Bahir Dar Town and Hadiya zone [12, 15, 23]. The possible reason for the discrepancy might be due to respondent characteristics, socio-demographic backgrounds and time reference used in the definition of SRH service utilization [24].

Around 13.7% of the students (9.5% male) were found to be sexually active within the last 12 month. Even though it seems low percentage of respondents, sexual behavior may have been masked because of the socio-cultural context, where sexual intercourse out of marriage is taboo.This result was consistent with another study from Mekele and Nepali [22, 25]. But this percentage is lower than studies in Bahir Dar and Hadiya [17, 26]. The difference might be due to socio-cultural background in which early marriage is encouraged in the two areas. In addition, the number of sexually active male students is greater than of female student. This might indicate that male are having sex with out of school females. The mean age at first sexual contact of respondents was 15.14 indicating early initiation of sexual

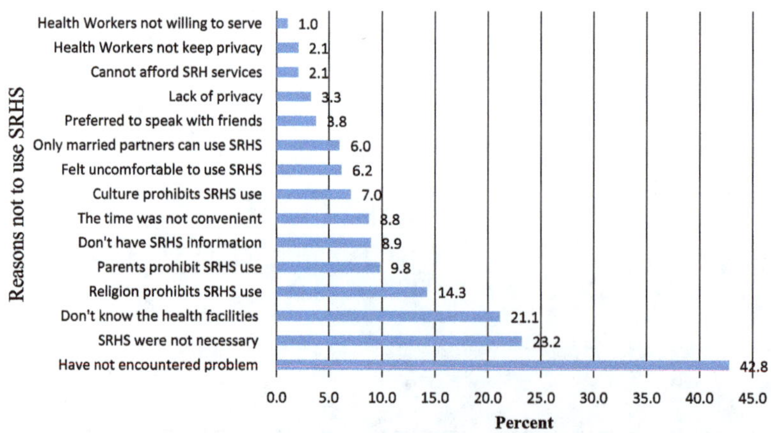

Fig. 3 Reasons not to utilize SRHS by secondary cchool youths in Nekemte Town, 2016

Table 4 Bivaraite and Multivariate logistic regression analysis of factors associated with SRH services utilization among secondary school students, Nekemte, April 18–22, 2016

Variables		SRH service utilization		COR (95%CI)	COR (95%CI)
		Yes (%)	No (%)		
Age					
15–19		132(84.1)	374(92.6)	1	1
20–24		25(15.9)	30(7.4)	2.36 (1.34–4.16)*	1.15(0.51-2.57)
Marital status					
Married		11(7.0)	11(2.7)	2.69(1.14–6.34)*	1.9(0.58-6.48)
Single		146(93.0)	393(97.3)	1	1
School type					
Government		139(88.5)	315(78.0)	1	1
Non-government		18(11.5)	89(220)	0.46(0.27–0.79)*	0.56(0.26-1.20)
Discussion on SRH					
With friends	Yes	76(60.3)	239(76.6)	0.46(0.3–0.72)*	0.73(0.39-1.37)
	No	50(39.7)	73(23.4)	1	1
With health workers	Yes	59(46.8)	75(24.0)	2.78(1.8–4.3)*	3(1.72-5.24)***
	No	67(53.2)	237(76.0)	1	1
Sources of SRH services					
School teachers	Yes	47(29.9)	209(51.7)	0.4(0.27–0.59)*	0.36(0.21-0.61)***
	No	110(70.1)	195(48.3)	1	1
History of STIs	Yes	33(24.3)	22(6.8)	4.41(2.46–7.91)*	2.61(1.24-5.49)**
	No	103(75.7)	303(93.2)	1	1
Sexually ever experienced	Yes	79(50.3)	48(11.9)	7.51(4.87–11.6)*	5.87(3.38-10.19)***
	No	78(49.7)	356(88.1)	1	1
Attitude for SRH services					
Unfavorable attitude		62(39.7)	198(49.1)	1	1
Favorable attitude		94(60.3)	205(50.9)	1.46(1.01–2.13)*	1.21(0.69-2.10)

*significant at bivatiat e ** significant at multivariate, $p < 0.05$ *** significant at multivariate, $p < 0.001$

intercourse. Sixteen (15.8%) of sexually active respondents had multiple sexual partiner that may pose them for risky sexual behavior and these are important indicators of exposure to risk of pregnancy and STI during adolescence. This finding was in line with the study conducted in Mekele Town [22].

Majority of sexually active respondents 62(61.4%) had received at least one component of the SRH services in the last twelve months. This finding goes in line with the finding from Hadiya zone [14]. The possible justification of this may be sexually active respondents were more exposed for SRH problems so that they were concerned about their sexual and reproductive healths than sexually inactive respondents.

The commonly utilized SRH service component was voluntary testing and counseling service (59.2%) which is almost similar with the findings of studies done in Goba Town and Gondar Town [27, 28]. Information and counseling on SRH issues, condom services and STIs services were also commonly recieved by 51.0%, 29.3% and 17.8% of the SRH services seekers respectively. This finding somewhat goes in line with the finding in Mekele Town [22]. Family planning service was utilized by 26. 7% of the sexually active respondents which was similar to the findig from Nepali [25, 29] but less than findings in Gondar Town and Goba Town [27, 28]. The possible explanation for this difference might be due to more implimentation opportunities at the community than at school level and information gap among school youths of the study area as more government and non-government facilities are designed and implementing at community level.

The findings of this study indicated that school youths used various health facilities in which government health facilities most frequently cited (50.9%) followed by NGO health facilities similar to those previous studies conducted in Bahir Dar [17]. The possible explanation for this could be the services in governmental and NGO health institutions were given either free of charge or with a minimal payment.

This study also showed that a small proportion (3.8%) of the participants used traditional health service that goes in line with Bahir Dar and East Gojjam study [17, 21]. Even if this proportion seems insignificant, it needs a special concern because unless it is confirmed by health experts traditional treatments may pose health risks to individuals.

For the successfulness of the YSRH program appropriate and relevant information about SRH should be delivered to youths. In this study, Medias (45.1%), teachers (41.3%) and health workers (36.7%) were found to be the main source of information about SRH services which was in line with the finding from Mekele [22].

The result of this study showed that majority of the respondents had not utilized SRH services diferrent reasons. Absence of SRH problems for a moment and the service was not necessary for the moment were most commonly cited reasons not to use SRH services. Religion, cultural and parent prohibition, inconvenience service hour and lack of privacy at delivery point were also barriers to SRH services utilization. This finding was consistent with the findings of East Gojjam, Bahir Dar and Mtwara Tanzania [17, 21, 30]. This implies that there is a need of tackling the barriers by dealing with the community leaders, religious leaders, families and health service systems.

In this study, discussion with health workers, previous history of perceived STIs symptoms, being ever sexually experienced and exposure to information from school teachers were found to be independent determinants of SRH services utilization among school youths.

This study revealed that discussion of the service with health care workers had a significant association with SRH service utilization. This can be justified by the fact that discussion of services with people allows youths to create more opportunities to exchange information, experiences, and build comprehensive knowledge about SRH. It can also create opportunities to deal with adolescent problems associated with SRH service utilization so that health professionals might be the source of accurate information for youths which help them for appropriate decision making in health services seeking behavior.

School youths who had encountered at least one of STIs symptom were more likely to utilize SRH services than who did not encounter the problem. And also individuals who had ever sexual contact were more likely to utilize SRH services than abstainers. This finding goes in line with study conducted in Hadiya, Nepali and Bahir Dar [12, 15, 29] This might be explained as youths were more concerned about their health when they encounter SRH problems that triggered them to use SRH services and youths who engaged in sexual intercourse were more vulnerable to SRH problems that might increase the need for SRH services utilization. This implies that youths need an access to a wide range of health information and services as well as health professional support to engage in healthy and safe behavior.

The students who had heard SRH related issues from their school teachers seemed to be 64% less likely to utilize SRH service than students who had not heard from school teachers in contrary to the fact that school teachers were the main sources of information for SRH. The justification of this finding is not simple and difficult to hypothesize that information leads to less SRH service utilization. In fact school teachers may strictly disseminate information that early sexual initiation can lead to risk of unwanted pregnancy and STIs. Therefore, before formulating hypotheses about information from school teachers, additional studies using qualitative designs are needed to dig out the deeper meaning and to identify type of information delivered by school teachers.

Limitation

Since this study examines personal and sensitive issues, obtaining honest responses among adolescent students might have been difficult. Therefore this data might have prone to respondent bias. The quantitative study design did not allow for probing into certain areas which needed further qualitative description. Finally, the study was conducted in schools of only one town, which means the findings may not be generalizable to the overall Ethiopian adolescent and youth population, who are socio-economically, linguistically, and ethnically diverse. In addition factors at community (e.g. parental attitude and control over the children) and health system are needed to be included in the future researches.

Conclusion

This study had showed that low proportion of the school youths visited different health facilities to utilize SRH services in the last 12 months. The most frequently utilized SRH service component was voluntary testing and counseling service followed by information and counseling on SRH issues. Media was the potential source of information on SRH services for school youths followed by teachers and health workers. Discussion with health workers, previous history of perceived STIs symptoms, being ever sexually experienced and exposure to information from school teachers were found to be independent determinants of SRH services utilization among school youths.

Abbreviations

NGOs: Non-Governmental Organizations; RH: Reproductive Health; SPSS: Statistical Package for the Social Sciences; SRH: Sexual and Reproductive Health; SRHS: Sexual and Reproductive Health Services

Acknowledgements
We would like to pass our thanks to Jimma University with its respective College of Health sciences, Department of Population and Family Health. Our thanks also go to the school teachers who devoted their time from the busy schedule during data collection, all the study participants for giving us their busy time of study and who had took part in the survey, data collection facilitation and supervisions.

Funding
Sponsored by Jimma University.

Authors' contributions
*These authors contributed equally to this work. All authors of this paper have read and approved the final version before submission.

Ethics approval and consent to participate
Ethical clearance was obtained from Jimma University, Collage of Health Sciences ethical review committee. Then letter of permission was written from the Oromia Regional Health Bureau to Nekemte Town Health and Education Offices. Cooperation letter was taken to each selected School Directors of the randomily selected schools from which the data is to be collected. Verbal informed consent was obtained from the selected individuals after objective of the study was communicated in detail. The respondents were assured that they have the right to be involved or not in the study, and that their non-involvement will not affect them in any way. Participants were not requested for name or any identifier on the questionnaire.

Competing interests
The authors declare that they have no competing interests.

Author details
[1]Department of Midwifery, Arba Minch College of Health Sciences, Arba Minch, Ethiopia. [2]Department of Midwifery, College of Health Sciences and Medicine, Wolaita Sodo University, Wolaita Sodo, Ethiopia. [3]Department of Population and Family Health, College of public Health and Medical Sciences, Jimma University, Jimma, Ethiopia.

References

1. United Nations Development of Economic and Social Association, *Youth population trends and sustainable development*. 2015.
2. United Nations Population Fund, *Status Report on Adolescents and Young People In Sub-Saharan Africa; Opportunities and Challenges*. 2012: 7 Naivasha Road, Sunninghill, Johannesburg, 2157 South Africa.
3. Central Statistical Agency of Ethiopia, *Ethiopia Mini Demographic and Health Survey*. 2014: Addis Ababa.
4. Siegrid Tautz *The Youth to Youth Initiative: an assessment of results in Ethiopia and Kenya*. 2011.
5. Population Reference Bureau, *The World's Youth*. 2013.
6. United Nations, Framework of actions for the follow-up to the Programme of action of the international conference on population and development beyond. 2014.
7. United Nations Education Social and Culture Organization, *One Year in Review | 2013–2014 Eastern And Southern; The Eastern and Southern Africa (ESA)* Commitment,. 2014.
8. Abebe M, Tsion A, Netsanet F. Living with parents and risky sexual behaviors among preparatory school students in Jimma zone, south West Ethiopia. African Halth Sci. 2013;13(2):498–506.
9. Bogale A, Seme A. Premarital sexual practices and its predictors among in-school youths of shendi town, west Gojjam zone, north western Ethiopia. BIOMED Cent Reprod Heal. 2014;11(1):1–9.
10. Yohannes B, Gelibo T, and T. M, Prevalence and Associated Factors of Sexually Transmitted Infections among Students of Wolaita Sodo University, Southern Ethiopia.. Int J Sci Technol Res, 2013. 2(2): p. 86–94.
11. Gelaye, A.A., KNT, and TM, Magnitude and risk factors of abortion among regular female students in Wolaita Sodo University, Ethiopia BMC Womens Health, 2014. 14(50): p. 1–9.
12. Cherie, N., G. Tura, and N. Teklehaymanot, Reproductive health needs and service utilization among youths in West Badewacho Woreda, Hadiya. **7**(April): p. 145–153.
13. Harar Bulletin of Health Sciences Extracts Number 4. Youth-friendly health services utilization and factors in Harar, Ethiopia Aboma Motuma. In: 4; January 2012.
14. Bilal, S.M., et al., *Sexual & Reproductive Healthcare Utilization of Sexual and Reproductive Health Services in Ethiopia-Does it affect sexual activity among high school students ?* Sexual & Reproductive Healthcare. 6(1): p. 14–18.
15. Abebe, M. and W. Awoke, *Utilization of Youth Reproductive Health Services and Associated Factors among High School Students in Bahir Dar, Amhara Regional State*. (May): p. 69–75.
16. International, C.S.A.E.a.I., Ethiopia Demographic and Health Survey 2011. 2012, Central statistical agency and ICF international: Addis Ababa, Ethiopia and Calverton, Maryland, USA. p. 450.
17. Abebe M, Awoke W. Utilization of youth reproductive health services and associated factors among high school students in Bahir Dar, Amhara regional state. Open J Epidemiol. 2014;4:69–75.
18. Hynes, M., Et al., Reproductive Health Assessment Toolkit for Conflict-Affected Women. 2007: Atlanta, GA.
19. J., C., Illustrative Questionnaire for Interview Surveys with Young People.
20. Control, C.O.D., Reproductive health assessment questionnaire for conflict-affected WomenCDC. 2011.
21. Abajobir AA, Seme A. Reproductive health knowledge and services utilization among rural adolescents in east Gojjam zone, Ethiopia : a community-based cross-sectional study. BMC Health Serv Res. 2014;14(1):1–11.
22. Bilal SM, et al. Sexual & Reproductive Healthcare Utilization of sexual and reproductive health Services in Ethiopia – does it affect sexual activity among high school students ? Sex Reprod Healthc Elsevier BV. 2015;6(1):14–8.
23. Malarcher S, Social determinants of sexual and reproductive health. 2010: Geneva Swizerland;.
24. Motuma A, Youth-friendly Health Services Utilization and Factors in Harar, Ethiopia. Harar Bull Heal Sci., 2012. **4**(5.).
25. Bam K, et al. Perceived sexual and reproductive health needs and service utilization among higher secondary school students in urban Nepal. Am J Public Heal Res. 2015;3(2):36–45.
26. Cherie N, Tura G, Teklehaymanot N. Reproductive health needs and service utilization among youths in west Badewacho Woreda, Hadiya zone, Ethiopia. J Public Heal Epidemiol. 2015;7(4):145–53.
27. Feleke SA, et al. Reproductive health service utilization and associated factors among adolescents (15 – 19 years old) in Gondar town, northwest. BMC Health Serv Res. 2013;13(1):1.
28. Gebreselassie B, et al., Assessment of Reproductive Health Service Utilization and Associated Factors Among Adolescents (15–19 Years Old) in Goba Town, Southeast Ethiopia. 2015. 3(4): p. 203–212.
29. Bam, K., et al., Perceived Sexual and Reproductive Health Needs and Service Utilization among Higher Secondary School Students in Urban Nepal. 3(2): p. 36–45.
30. Mbeba RM, et al. Barriers to sexual reproductive health services and rights among young people in Mtwara district, Tanzania : a qualitative study. Pan Afr Med J. 2012;13(1):1–6.

4

Determinants of antenatal care attendance among women residing in highly disadvantaged communities in northern Jordan

Heba H. Hijazi[1*], Mohammad S. Alyahya[1], Amer M. Sindiani[2], Rola S. Saqan[3] and Abdulhakeem M. Okour[4]

Abstract

Background: One of the major reproductive health challenges among disadvantaged populations is to provide pregnant women with the necessary antenatal care (ANC). In this study, we suggest applying an integrated conceptual framework aimed at ascertaining the extent to which attendance at ANC clinics may be attributed to individual determinants or to the quality of the care received.

Methods: Using a cross-sectional design, data were collected from a sample of 831 women residing in nine sub-districts in three northern governorates of Jordan and designated according to national categorization as persistent poverty pockets. All of the sampled women were recruited from public maternal and child health centers and interviewed using a structured pre-tested survey. This tool covered certain predictors, ranging from the user's attributes, including predisposing, enabling, and need factors, to the essential components of the experience of care. These components assessed the quality of ANC in terms of five elements: woman–provider relations, technical management, information exchange, continuity of care, and appropriate constellation of services. Adequate ANC content was assessed in relation to the frequency of antenatal visits and the time of each visit.

Results: The results of multivariate logistic regression analyses show that the use of ANC facilities is affected by various factors related to the quality of service delivery. These include receiving information and education on ANC during clinic visits (OR = 9.1; 95% CI = 4.9–16.9), providing pregnant women with opportunities for dialogue and health talks (OR = 7.2; 95% CI = 4.1–12.8), having scheduled follow-up appointments (OR = 6.5; 95% CI = 3.5–12.0), and offering dignified and respectful care (OR = 5.7; 95% CI = 2.5–13.1). At the individual level, our findings have identified a woman's education level (OR = 1.2; 95% CI = 1.1–1.3), desire for the pregnancy (OR = 1.7; 95% CI = 1.1–2.7), and living in a district served by an ANC clinic (OR = 4.3; 95% CI = 2.3–8.1) as determinants affecting ANC utilization.

Conclusion: Taking women's experiences of ANC as a key metric for reporting the quality of the care is more likely to lead to increased utilization of ANC services by women in highly disadvantaged communities. Our findings suggest that the degree to which women feel that they are respected, informed, and engaged in their care has potential favorable implications for ANC.

Keywords: Utilization, Antenatal care, Disadvantaged communities, Poverty, Experience of care, Quality, Jordan

* Correspondence: hhhijazi0@just.edu.jo
[1]Department of Health Management and Policy, Faculty of Medicine, Jordan University of Science and Technology, P.O. Box 3030, Irbid 22110, Jordan
Full list of author information is available at the end of the article

Plain English summary

Millions of women in developing countries are more likely to experience life-threatening and pregnancy-related complications because of a lack of access to adequate and good-quality antenatal care (ANC). Indicators of adequate care, as recommended by the World Health Organization (WHO), include providing pregnant women with four antenatal visits, of which the initial contact should be scheduled during the first trimester of pregnancy. In Jordan, remarkable progress has been made to expand the coverage of ANC; however, disparities and inequity in access to quality ANC services among different socioeconomic groups are still evident and subject to debate. Thus, our study aims to explore barriers that prevent women who live in low-income settings from utilizing antenatal services adequately.

This study collected quantitative data from women aged 15–49 years residing in highly disadvantaged sub-districts in three northern governorates of Jordan. Data were gathered by means of a face-to-face interview using a health facility-based survey.

Among the 831 enrolled women, 36.6% had inadequate attendance at ANC services. Our findings indicate that utilization of ANC is embedded in the context of the healthcare delivery system, in which women's access to the necessary health education and engagement in one-to-one consultations were found to be significant predictors. Treating women with respect and dignity and providing them with scheduled follow-up appointments were also associated with ANC attendance.

As a result, to achieve significant changes in the delivery of ANC, it is extremely important for health authorities to pay more attention to the woman–provider interaction in increasing utilization of ANC and enhancing women's experience of pregnancy.

Background

ANC is a key strategy for reducing maternal morbidity and mortality directly by affording increased chances of the timely identification of high-risk pregnancies [1–3]. It also represents an entry point for the integrated use of skilled health personnel [4]. Empirical studies of preventive services have often found that regular monitoring of women during pregnancy is vital to reduce birth-related complications, provide supportive care, and promote safer motherhood [5, 6]. In contrast, low health service utilization throughout the prenatal period breaks the critical link in the continuum of care and contributes to poor birth outcomes [7].

In low- and middle-income countries (LMICs), ANC utilization has increased since the introduction of the 2002 WHO ANC model, known as 'focused' ANC (FANC) [8]. This model aims at delivering 'reduced but goal-orientated' clinic visits, at which essential interventions should be provided to pregnant women at specified intervals. With the FANC model, healthy women with no underlying pregnancy complications should be scheduled a minimum of four ANC visits, and more than four in the case of danger signs or pregnancy-related illnesses. For many of the essential interventions in FANC, it is crucial to initiate the care during the first trimester of pregnancy (up to 12 weeks of gestation), and schedule the second visit at 24 to 28 weeks of gestation and the third and fourth visits at 32 weeks and between 36 and 38 weeks of gestation, respectively [8, 9].

During the last decade, considerable research attention has been paid to determining the routine number of visits that are necessary to optimize the health of mothers and babies and enhance safety during pregnancy. Recently, however, a 2015 systematic review of randomized controlled trails has raised concerns that the reduced number of antenatal contacts is associated with an increased risk of perinatal mortality, particularly stillbirth [10]. Accordingly, in November 2016, the WHO began promoting a new model of ANC aimed at reducing perinatal deaths and improving women's experience of care by recommending a minimum of eight contacts [8].

While many may argue that increasing the frequency of antenatal visits would positively influence the health of mothers and newborns [8, 10], related literature has indicated that a reduced number of visits, but with targeted interventions at each visit, proved to be equally effective as monthly ANC visits [11]. In many resource-limited settings, increasing the number of ANC visits for women with uncomplicated pregnancies to more than four has not been found to be associated with improved birth outcomes [12, 13]. Considering that the optimum number of ANC visits in low-income settings depends not only on effectiveness but also on feasibility and other barriers to ANC access and supply [7], our study placed particular emphasis on investigating the delivery of 'reduced and goal-orientated' ANC.

In Jordan, only a few studies have examined factors that predict the utilization of ANC services. Importantly, previous research has generally focused on studying the association between the use of ANC facilities with a range of individual characteristics, such as a woman's age, occupation, parity, and level of education [14–17]. However, this may be imprecise and offers little insight into the context in which utilization occurs. Other attributes, including the accessibility, availability, and quality of ANC services, are also significant factors to consider. Hence, the main objectives of our study are to explore barriers that prevent women who live in highly disadvantaged communities from utilizing ANC services adequately, and to ascertain the extent to which their attendance may be attributed to the quality of the ANC service delivery or to the individual determinants of these women. Addressing such barriers is considered a matter of equality, social justice, and ethics, requiring policymakers to think differently about the poor and those at risk of social exclusion.

Jordan overview

The current national coverage rate for ANC is high in Jordan; almost all women (99%) receive ANC from medically trained personnel (doctors, nurses, or midwives) at least once during pregnancy [18]. While it is obvious that Jordan is on track to achieving its goal of expanding coverage of ANC services, most efforts to enhance the use of these services have focused on quantifiable issues, such as increasing the number of prenatal visits. Data on ANC are obtained mostly from household surveys, in which women who have had a live birth during the last five years preceding the survey are asked whether and from whom they received care. However, no information on the quality of ANC services is provided by the national surveys. Further, no specific data on ANC utilization are available for those who live in highly disadvantaged communities (i.e., poverty pockets).

To facilitate the geographic targeting of the poor, Jordan has developed a system for mapping poverty, using the Small Area Estimation Method to identify 'poverty pockets' across the country [19]. A poverty pocket represents a district or sub-district, which may be a village, a desert oasis, or a large, low-income locality within a metropolitan city or in the suburbs, where more than 25% of the population is below the poverty line [19]. Based on the Household Expenditure and Income Surveys (HEIS) data, most recently updated in 2010/2011, the absolute poverty line amounted to 814 Jordanian Dinars (JDs) annually or 67.8 JD per capita per month [19]. This measure continues to be used as the principal measure of poverty in Jordan, and the majority of the poor are still clustered around this line [19].

During the last decade, Jordan has made strenuous efforts in fighting poverty, within its limited resources and in the context of the global political and economic upheavals. However, figures released by the Ministry of Planning and International Cooperation (MoPIC), with the technical support of the United Nations Development Program (UNDP), show an increase in poverty rates from 13.3% in 2008 to 14.4% in 2010 [20]. The number of poverty pockets also increased from 22 pockets in 2006 to 32 and 36 poverty pockets in 2008, 2010, respectively [20].

Another worrisome finding reported by the United Nations Children's Fund (UNICEF) in 2016 is that a notable variation in the source of services across all social classes is apparent in Jordan. Women from lower wealth quintiles represent a larger share of women who access ANC services and deliver their babies at public facilities [21]. According to the National Strategy for the Health Sector in Jordan for the years 2015–2019, there are significant disparities with respect to the quality of health services between the health sector institutions and between different geographic regions [22]. This raises concerns about equitable access to quality ANC services among different socioeconomic groups within the country.

Conceptual framework

A woman's decision to seek ANC is not simply a matter of personal preference; the accessibility of services that either facilitate or impede utilization also has an important influence [23]. As outlined by the WHO, access to ANC services consists of several elements, including distance and/or time to a facility, the physical availability of services, cultural and social factors that may impede access, economic and other costs associated with use of services, and the quality of the services offered [24].

In a healthcare context, the use of services is a complex human behavioral phenomenon [25]. It reflects a point at which patients' needs meet the professional system [26]. During the last few decades, a number of models have been developed to identify factors affecting the utilization of healthcare services, the most widely used being the 1995 version of the Andersen's behavioral model [26]. According to this model, an individual's use of a service is considered to be a function of three components. These include predisposing factors, which represent the sociocultural characteristics of individuals that exist prior to their illness or condition; enabling factors in terms of the logistical aspects of obtaining care; and need factors that generate the necessity for healthcare services, such as the presence of diagnosed medical conditions and self-perception of health status.

Despite the importance of individual determinants affecting the utilization of care, it is well known that service attendance is strongly dependent on the quality of care experienced at healthcare facilities [26]. The philosophy behind providing pregnant women with FANC is to ensure access to goal-oriented and high-quality care for all women, not only those at risk, with targeted interventions at each visit [11]. Achieving improvements in the quality of ANC is multidimensional and requires increased attention to the process of care delivery, in which the experience of care should be evaluated based on globally determined and locally feasible criteria. In 2016, the WHO released a global framework for improving the quality of care throughout pregnancy, childbirth, and the postnatal period, quality being understood as the provision and experience of care from a health systems perspective [27].

Recent evidence has acknowledged that, if the quality of ANC is poor and women's experience is negative, women will not attend ANC services, regardless of the recommended number of contacts in the model [8, 28]. Accordingly, our study provides an additional consideration for identifying gaps in the experience of care that may lead to poor delivery of adequate care. Within the WHO framework, the experience of care consists of effective communication between healthcare providers with pregnant women; care that involves respect and the preservation of dignity; and access to social and emotional support that is sensitive to women's needs [27].

Inspired by the 2016 WHO framework and taking into account the study's main objectives, we suggest applying an integrated conceptual framework that incorporates both individual determinants for seeking care and the contextual characteristics of ANC service delivery. Specifically, our study aims to explore the effects of quality of care on the utilization of ANC and how the experience of care can lead to different access outcomes for women from lower-income backgrounds. As per Fig. 1, individual determinants are categorized as predisposing, enabling, and need factors; while variables related to the quality of ANC capture the essential components of the experience of care.

To assess the quality of ANC experienced, our study is directed by Bruce's framework for conceptualizing the quality of care in the provision of reproductive health services [29]. Within this framework, evaluating the quality of ANC requires the examination of five main elements, namely interpersonal relations between healthcare providers and clients; technical management; information exchange; continuity and follow-up; and an appropriate constellation of services [29].

Methods

Study design and sample

This study collected quantitative data from 14 sub-districts, identified by the MoPIC as poverty pockets, in northern Jordan. These sub-districts are spread over three northern governorates (the administrative division in the country), Irbid, Mafraq, and Jerash, and classified as rural and desert towns/villages. The modeling of the 14 sub-districts is compatible with the sampling frame of the HEIS 2011 and the social data pilot module survey launched by MoPIC and UNDP to measure vulnerability risk and social exclusion in the country. Over the last decade, nine of these sub-districts are classified as persistent poverty pockets, and five are classified as fluctuating ones [20]. To ensure that all poverty pockets shared the same characteristics, only persistent ones were included in our study. Furthermore, all of the sampled sub-districts are broadly similar in their level of socioeconomic wealth (i.e. sanitation, electricity, and water service) and age/gender structure.

Out of the nine selected sub-districts, five were served by public Maternal and Child Health (MCH) centers; however, the remaining four had no such service. Given that the target population of this study was users of reproductive health services at public MCH centers, and that these centers provide services to well-defined geographic

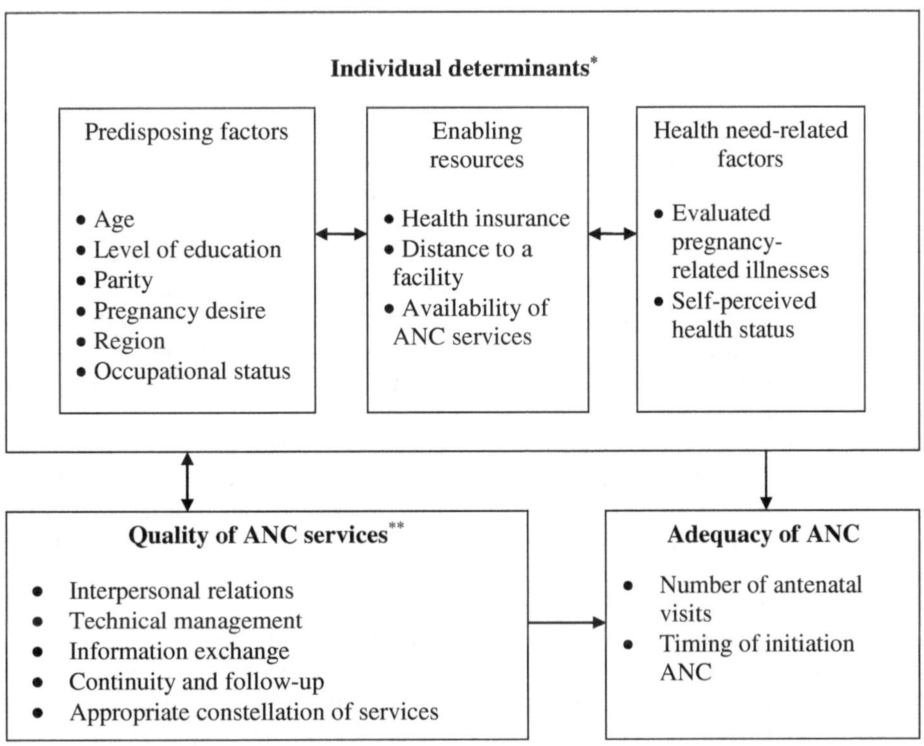

Fig. 1 Conceptual framework for analyzing determinants of ANC utilization among women residing in highly disadvantaged communities in northern Jordan
*Adapted from Andersen's behavioral model for health service use (Andersen, 1995)
**Adapted from Bruce's framework for assessing the quality of care (Bruce, 1990)

areas, the nearest center in each of the underserved sub-districts was targeted. Before starting the fieldwork, the names of MCH centers were obtained using a list provided by the Jordanian Ministry of Health (MoH). During this phase, new maps of all sub-districts were prepared, and the numbers of MCH centers were updated, listed, and documented.

The field work stage of data collection started in June 2015 and ended in July 2016. Using purposive sampling, efforts were made to ensure that all participating women met a number of inclusion criteria. In particular, a woman was eligible to participate only if she was a currently married woman, aged 15–49 years, had been living in one of the chosen highly disadvantaged sub-districts for at least the preceding four years, and had a household monthly income of 68 JDs or less per person and was receiving no other type of assistance. The primary users of services provided at the public MCH centers are married women of childbearing age from the middle and low socioeconomic classes, and thus most of the facilities' attendees were eligible for participation. Since the main focus of this study was to assess the quality of care as perceived by the women receiving the care, a number of exclusion criteria were applied. These included any currently married woman within the specified age group who had not had a live birth in the last two years preceding the survey ($n = 136$), was pregnant at the time of the survey ($n = 118$), did not have at least one ANC visit during the last pregnancy ($n = 21$), initiated ANC visits after the first trimester ($n = 190$), and obtained ANC from multiple/other facilities, or was a new registry ($n = 215$). Of the total 1511 women interviewed in the survey, with a 96% response rate, data from 831 participants were eligible for analysis.

The study instrument and variables

Data collection instrument

This study is based on original cross-section data collected by means of a face-to-face interview using a structured, pre-tested survey. The survey was adopted after reviewing the literature in the relevant research area. Prior to data collection, several steps were taken to assess the validity and reliability of the instrument. To examine content validity, a panel of eight experienced perinatal personnel was asked to review and refine each item in the instrument. This panel was composed of three obstetricians, three senior community midwives, and two researchers in the field of reproductive health. Further, the Pearson correlation coefficient was calculated to examine the test–retest reliability of the survey for a sub-sample of participants ($n = 28$). The questionnaire was administered again to the same sample three weeks later. The test–retest correlation coefficient for the instrument was 0.78 ($p < 0.001$), which is indicative of acceptable stability over time.

Outcome variable

In our analysis, the utilization of ANC services is classified into adequate versus inadequate as the outcome variable. To assess the overall adequacy of ANC, reviews of the medical records of respondents were conducted to obtain more accurate information about the basic ANC components received (i.e., frequency of antenatal visits and timing of each visit). Keeping in mind that this study was limited to the sample of women who initiated antenatal visits during the first trimester, ANC was defined as adequate if the woman with a normal pregnancy had at least four antenatal visits and more than four in case of complications; otherwise, it was defined as inadequate.

Explanatory variables

The study's explanatory variables consist of a number of covariates and predictors. Based on the previous conceptual framework and a review of the literature, several covariates were taken into consideration. These covariates embodied the background determinants of respondents: predisposing characteristics (i.e., age, education, parity, occupation, desire for the pregnancy, and region); enabling resources (i.e., health insurance, living in an area served by a MCH center, and the time taken to get to the nearest center); and need factors (i.e., evaluated pregnancy-related illnesses and self-perceived health status). Using a list of pregnancy-related complications, the participating women were asked to self-report the main illnesses that they had had during their last pregnancy. This list was identified by obstetricians and involved a number of medical conditions, including hypertension, diabetes, anemia, respiratory distress, abnormal vaginal discharge, pre-eclampsia, joint problems, and urinary tract infection.

Factors related to the perceived quality of ANC were included in the analysis as the main predictors of interest. These involved interpersonal relations (i.e., communication, understanding, and the presence of privacy); technical management (physical examination, availability of vaccines/supplements, and clinical tests); information exchange (clarity of providers' explanations, consultation time, and obtaining information and counseling on ANC); follow-up and continuity (i.e., scheduling of appointments and the sincerity of the provider); and an appropriate constellation of services (i.e., waiting time and opening hours).

Statistical analyses

Summary statistics were carried out to describe the study participants according to different characteristics. Differences in ANC attendance (i.e., adequate vs. inadequate use) were reported using chi-squared tests and two sample t-tests for categorical and continuous variables, respectively. Standardized residuals were examined for categorical variables to determine which cell contributed to the statistically significant difference between the observed frequency and the expected one. Binary logistic regression models were performed to obtain adjusted odds ratios (ORs) for the outcome variable, using the SPSS 20.0 statistical package. Statistical significance was set at $p < 0.05$.

Results

Descriptive analysis

Analyses for characteristics of mothers using ANC services are presented in Table 1. The ages of the women at the birth of their last child ranged from 16 to 45 years, with a median age of 31 years. Forty-eight percent had received 10 or fewer years of schooling. The average total number of living children was 3.6, giving a range between 1 and 12 children. The majority of the respondents was housewives (85.4%) and had public sector insurance coverage (69.8%). The health status of 48.5% of participants was average during the last pregnancy, and 33.6% of the sample had had a high-risk pregnancy. Urinary tract infection, joint problems, and anemia were the three most common pregnancy-related illnesses among respondents, respectively. Concerning ANC attendance, 63.4% of women received the recommended care components, while 36.6% received inadequate ANC.

Table 1 Baseline characteristics of the sample population ($N = 831$)

Variable	n (%)	Mean; SD
Age (years)		30.99; 7.47
≤ 23	185 (22.3)	
24–31	293 (35.3)	
32–39	229 (27.6)	
≥ 40	124 (14.9)	
Education (years)		10.41; 2.71
≤ 6	69 (8.3)	
7–9	240 (28.9)	
10–12	430 (51.7)	
> 12	92 (11.1)	
Parity		3.56; 2.06
1	154 (18.5)	
2–3	284 (34.2)	
4–5	254 (30.6)	
≥ 6	139 (16.7)	
Region		-
Irbid	213 (25.6)	
Jerash	170 (20.5)	
Mafraq	448 (53.9)	
Employment status		-
Unemployed	710 (85.4)	
Employed	121 (14.6)	
Health insurance		-
Uninsured	251 (30.2)	
Insured	580 (69.8)	
Total number of pregnancy-related illnesses		-
No health problems	380 (45.7)	
1–2 health problems	172 (20.7)	
≥ 3 health problems	279 (33.6)	
Self-perceived health status		-
Poor	208 (25.0)	
Average	403 (48.5)	
Excellent	220 (26.5)	

Differences in the usage of antenatal care services

Table 2 presents a comparative analysis of the differences between women who received the recommended basic ANC service components and those who did not, by individual determinants. Overall, there were statistically significant associations between all of the individual determinants and ANC attendance, except for employment and health status variables ($p = 0.644$ and $p = 0.837$, respectively). On bivariate analysis, the means of age and the number of living children variables were significantly lower among women who attended ANC adequately. Being more educated was also found to be positively associated with receiving adequate ANC services. Likewise, the proportions of women who had adequate use of ANC services were significantly higher among those who had wanted the pregnancy (67.6%), resided in Irbid governorate (72.8%), were insured (68.1%), lived in a neighborhood served by MCH services (71%), required less than 15 min to get to the nearest center (68.9%), and had a high-risk pregnancy (70.3%).

Differences in the overall ANC service adequacy were also observed by a number of factors related to the quality of care. As per Table 3, the highest percentages of adequate ANC attendance were among women who were often treated in a humane, respectful, supportive environment (82.7%) and those who were able to discuss their health problems/concerns with healthcare providers (81.0%). However, maintaining privacy during consultations was not significantly associated with the outcome variable ($p = 0.880$).

In relation to the technical management features, no significant differences were noticed between the two groups of interest, with the exception of the physical examination variable. Women who reported that a comprehensive physical exam was often performed at the center represented the highest rate of adequate ANC attendees (78.1%). Availability of vaccines/supplements at the facility and conducting clinical tests during the antenatal period were not found to be significantly associated with the utilization of ANC ($p = 0.404$ and $p = 0.879$, respectively).

Table 2 Comparison between adequate and inadequate utilization of ANC by individual determinants

Variables	Utilization of ANC		t-test/chi2	*p*-value
	Inadequate *n* = 304 n (%)	Adequate *n* = 527 n (%)		
Predisposing Characteristics				
Age in years[a] (Mean; SD)	(32.49; 7.04)	(30.12; 7.58)	4.45	<0.001
Years of education[a] (Mean; SD)	(9.69; 2.51)	(10.82; 2.73)	-5.91	<0.001
Parity[a] (Mean; SD)	(3.97;2.05)	(3.33; 2.04)	4.33	<0.001
Desire for the pregnancy				
Unwanted	128 (44.4)	160 (55.6)	11.74	0.001
Wanted	176 (32.4)	367 (67.6)		
Region				
Irbid	58 (27.2)	155 (72.8)	17.33	<0.001
Jerash	54 (31.8)	116 (68.2)		
Mafraq	192 (42.9)	256 (57.1)		
Employment status				
Unemployed	262 (36.9)	448 (63.1)	0.21	0.644
Employed	42 (34.7)	79 (65.3)		
Enabling Resources				
Health insurance				
Uninsured	119 (47.4)	132 (52.6)	18.17	<0.001
Insured	185 (31.9)	395 (68.1)		
Time taken to get to the nearest MCH center in minutes				
< 15 min	122 (31.1)	270 (68.9)	24.06	<0.001
15 -30	123 (36.6)	213 (63.4)		
>30	59 (57.3)	44 (42.7)		
Availability of ANC services				
Underserved	155 (48.7)	163 (51.3)	32.83	<0.001
Served	149 (29.0)	364 (71.0)		
Health Needs				
Total number of pregnancy-related illnesses				
No health problems	153 (40.3)	227 (59.7)	8.48	0.014
1-2 health problems	68 (39.5)	104 (60.5)		
≥ 3 health problems	83 (29.7)	196 (70.3)		
Self-perceived health status				
Poor	74 (35.6)	134 (64.4)	0.36	0.837
Average	146 (36.2)	257 (63.8)		
Excellent	84 (38.2)	136 (61.8)		

[a]t-test was run on the following variables: age, education, and parity
Bold text represents categories that are over-represented, indicating that they were more likely to utilize ANC services adequately

It is also interesting to note that there were statistically significant differences in the adequacy of ANC in terms of information exchange. In particular, the proportion of women who utilized ANC adequately was significantly higher among those who reported that the procedures and the diagnosis were often explained clearly by providers (73.2%), received enough information about ANC (86.9%), and had enough consultation time (78.7%).

By continuity and follow-up variables, the highest percentages of adequate ANC users were among women who often had follow-up appointments scheduled by health

Table 3 Comparison between adequate and inadequate utilization of ANC by factors related to the quality of service delivery

Variables	Utilization of ANC		chi2	*p*-value
	Inadequate *n* = 304 n (%)	Adequate *n* = 527 n (%)		
Interpersonal relations				
Dignified and respectful care was offered by healthcare providers				
Rarely	157 (62.5)	94 (37.5)	141.42	<0.001
Sometimes	77 (43.8)	99 (56.3)		
Often	70 (17.3)	334 (82.7)		
Providers were ready to discuss health problems/concerns with women				
Rarely	171 (58.6)	121 (41.4)	105.85	<0.001
Sometimes	70 (33.8)	137 (66.2)		
Often	63 (19.0)	269 (81.0)		
Privacy was maintained during consultations				
Rarely	94 (37.5)	157 (62.5)	0.26	0.880
Sometimes	36 (34.6)	68 (65.4)		
Often	174 (36.6)	302 (63.4)		
Technical management				
Comprehensive physical exams were performed				
Rarely	117 (50.4)	115 (49.6)	63.68	<0.001
Sometimes	105 (46.7)	120 (53.3)		
Often	82 (21.9)	292 (78.1)		
Vaccines/supplements were available at the facility				
Rarely	108 (39.6)	165 (60.4)	1.81	0.404
Sometimes	36 (33.0)	73 (67.0)		
Often	160 (35.6)	289 (64.4)		
Clinical tests were routinely conducted				
No	196 (36.8)	337 (63.2)	0.02	0.879
Yes	108 (36.2)	190 (63.8)		
Information exchange				
Information received on ANC was				
Little	175 (61.2)	111 (38.8)	171.19	<0.001
Fair	80 (46.8)	91(53.2)		
Enough	49 (13.1)	325 (86.9)		
Provider explanations were easily to understand				
Rarely	86 (65.6)	45 (34.4)	78.85	<0.001
Sometimes	68 (48.2)	73 (51.8)		
Often	150 (26.8)	409 (73.2)		
Consultation time was				
Short	136 (60.7)	88 (39.3)	101.62	<0.001
Average	78 (42.4)	106 (57.6)		
Enough	90 (21.3)	333 (78.7)		

Table 3 Comparison between adequate and inadequate utilization of ANC by factors related to the quality of service delivery *(Continued)*

Variables	Utilization of ANC		chi2	*p*-value
	Inadequate *n* = 304 n (%)	Adequate *n* = 527 n (%)		
Continuity and follow-up				
Follow-up appointments were regularly scheduled by providers				
Rarely	180 (61.2)	114 (38.8)	157.43	<0.001
Sometimes	78 (40.2)	116 (59.8)		
Often	46 (13.4)	297 (86.6)		
A return visit was encouraged by healthcare providers				
Rarely	123 (55.4)	99 (44.6)	46.95	<0.001
Sometimes	23 (34.3)	44 (65.7)		
Often	158 (29.2)	384 (70.8)		
Appropriate constellation of services				
Time had to wait was				
Short	21 (33.9)	41 (66.1)	0.22	0.894
Average	124 (37.0)	211 (63.0)		
Long	159 (36.6)	275 (63.4)		
Hours of service were				
Inconvenient	76 (38.0)	124 (62.0)	0.23	0.633
Convenient	228 (36.1)	403 (63.9)		

Bold text represents categories that are over-represented, indicating that they were more likely to utilize ANC services adequately

workers (86.6%), and those who reported that they were encouraged by providers to make a return visit (70.8%). In contrast, no significant differences in the utilization of care were observed according to the appropriateness of the constellation of services, such as waiting time and service hours ($p = 0.894$ and $p = 0.633$, respectively).

Predictors of antenatal care attendance

Following the study's objectives, three models were employed to estimate the association between the explanatory variables (i.e., covariates and predictors) and the response variable (i.e., adequacy of ANC attendance). Table 4 summarizes the logistic regression estimation results for the three models. Each factor showing a statistically significant association with the response variable was interpreted controlling for the effects of other explanatory variables included in the model.

Initially, the first model was developed to investigate which of the individual's determinants are associated with receiving sufficient contents of ANC, and therefore only covariates were included in this model. As the figures in Table 4 indicate, the years of education showed a significant association with the use of ANC (95% CI = 1.09–1.23). For a one-year increase in women's education, the odds of utilizing ANC services increased by a factor of 1.15. Women's desire to become pregnant was also found to have a positive association with the use of care, in which women who had a desire to get pregnant were 1.82 times more likely to attend ANC adequately compared to those who had an unwanted pregnancy (95% CI = 1.31–2.52). According to this model, mothers residing in the governorate of Mafraq were 52% less likely to have an adequate usage of ANC services than those living in Irbid (95% CI = 0.29–0.77). Our results also illustrated that, as the travel time to the nearest center increased, the odds of reporting an adequate use of ANC declined by a factor of 0.42 (95% CI = 0.26–0.69). Women who lived in a neighborhood served by MCH services were 2.73 times more likely to report adequate use of ANC (95% CI = 1.85–4.03). In respect of health needs variables, women who had experienced three or more previous pregnancy-related illnesses were 2.14 times more likely to attend ANC adequately compared to those had had a normal pregnancy (95% CI = 1.47–3.13).

To ascertain the extent to which the utilization of ANC services may be attributed to the quality of the ANC service delivery, only the predictors of interest were included in the second model. The results of this model demonstrated that women who often received dignified and respectful treatment from healthcare providers were 5.54 times more likely to utilize ANC adequately compared to

Table 4 Multivariate regression analysis predicting the utilization of ANC among women in highly disadvantaged communities in northern

Variables	Individual determinants (Model 1)	Quality of service delivery (Model 2)	Both (Model 3)
	Adjusted OR (95% CI)	Adjusted OR (95% CI)	Adjusted OR (95% CI)
Predisposing factors			
Age in years	0.98 (0.95-1.01)		0.98 (0.93-1.03)
Years of education	**1.15** (1.09-1.23)**		**1.16* (1.06-1.27)**
Parity	0.94 (0.84-1.05)		0.92 (0.77-1.09)
Desire for the pregnancy: (unwanted)			
Wanted	**1.82** (1.31-2.52)**		**1.70* (1.06-2.72)**
Region: (Irbid)			
Jerash	0.92 (0.57-1.51)		1.73 (0.86-3.51)
Mafraq	**0.48* (0.29-0.77)**		0.61 (0.30-1.23)
Employment status: (unemployed)			
Employed	0.80 (0.51-1.26)		1.45 (0.75-2.81)
Enabling recourses			
Health insurance: (uninsured)			
Insured	0.81(0.50-1.32)		0.72 (0.35-1.48)
Time taken to get to the nearest MCH center in minutes: (< 15 min)			
15-30	0.92 (0.66-1.29)		0.97 (0.60-1.56)
≥30	**0.42* (0.26-0.69)**		**0.35* (0.17-0.70)**
Availability of ANC services: (underserved)			
Served	**2.73** (1.85-4.03)**		**4.34** (2.34-8.07)**
Health needs			
Total number of pregnancy-related illnesses: (no health problems)			
1-2 health problems	1.01 (0.67-1.50)		0.80 (0.45-1.44)
≥ 3 health problems	**2.14** (1.47-3.13)**		1.66 (0.97-2.84)
Self-perceived health status: (poor)			
Average	1.03(0.70-1.51)		1.48 (0.85-2.59)
Excellent	0.94(0.61-1.44)		1.41 (0.76-2.60)
Patient-provider relations			
Dignified and respectful care was offered by healthcare providers: (rarely)			
Sometimes		2.09 (0.61-7.08)	1.80 (0.43-7.52)
Often		**5.54** (2.60-11.81)**	**5.68** (2.45-13.13)**

Table 4 Multivariate regression analysis predicting the utilization of ANC among women in highly disadvantaged communities in northern *(Continued)*

Variables	Individual determinants (Model 1)	Quality of service delivery (Model 2)	Both (Model 3)
	Adjusted OR (95% CI)	Adjusted OR (95% CI)	Adjusted OR (95% CI)
Providers were ready to discuss health problems/concerns with women: (rarely)			
Sometimes		**2.37* (1.41-3.97)**	**2.28* (1.27-4.07)**
Often		**5.38** (3.28-8.82)**	**7.22** (4.06-12.82)**
Privacy was maintained during consultation: (rarely)			
Sometimes		0.56 (0.12-2.63)	0.46 (0.09-2.52)
Often		0.70 (0.21-2.25)	0.38 (0.09-1.58)
Technical management			
Comprehensive physical exams were performed: (rarely)			
Sometimes		1.08 (0.61-1.93)	1.19 (0.61-2.33)
Often		1.45 (0.82-2.54)	1.58 (0.84-2.97)
Vaccines/supplements were available at the facility: (rarely)			
Sometimes		1.86 (0.41-8.43)	2.24 (0.43-11.82)
Often		1.87 (0.58-5.99)	3.63 (0.89-14.83)
Clinical tests were regularly conducted: (no)			
Yes		1.29 (0.84-1.97)	1.27 (0.77-2.08)
Information exchange			
Information received on ANC was: (little)			
Fair		1.11 (0.56-2.22)	1.16 (0.54-2.51)
Enough		**7.34** (4.26-12.66)**	**9.12** (4.91-16.92)**
Consultation time was:(short)			
Average		1.04 (0.29-3.69)	1.11 (0.26-4.81)
Enough		0.65 (0.29-1.46)	0.51 (0.21-1.27)
Provider explanations were easily to understand: (rarely)			
Sometimes		1.02 (0.53-1.96)	0.77 (0.37-1.62)
Often		**1.97* (1.12-3.46)**	**2.38* (1.22-4.66)**
Continuity and follow-up			
Follow-up appointments were regularly scheduled by providers: (rarely)			
Sometimes		**3.03* (1.46-6.29)**	**3.65* (1.61-8.28)**
Often		**6.05** (3.51-10.43)**	**6.51** (3.52-12.01)**

Table 4 Multivariate regression analysis predicting the utilization of ANC among women in highly disadvantaged communities in northern *(Continued)*

Variables	Individual determinants (Model 1)	Quality of service delivery (Model 2)	Both (Model 3)
	Adjusted OR (95% CI)	Adjusted OR (95% CI)	Adjusted OR (95% CI)
A return visit was encouraged by healthcare providers: (rarely)			
Sometimes		1.90 (0.89-4.07)	1.66 (0.72-3.83)
Often		**2.42** (1.53-3.83)**	**1.82* (1.08-3.06)**
Appropriate constellation of services			
Time had to wait was: (short)			
Average		0.86 (0.39-1.94)	0.63 (0.25-1.57)
Long		0.68 (0.31-1.50)	0.65 (0.27-1.57)
Hours of service were: (inconvenient)			
Convenient		0.94 (0.59-1.51)	0.96 (0.56-1.63)
Nagelkerke R^2	0.205	0.574	0.660

*$p < 0.05$; **$p < 0.001$
The reference category is in parentheses

those who rarely had positive communication with providers (95% CI = 2.60–11.81). Additionally, the odds of reporting an adequate use of ANC services increased by factors of 2.37 (95% CI = 1.41–3.97) and 5.38 (95% CI = 3.28–8.82) for women who were sometimes and often able to discuss their health problem/concerns with healthcare providers, respectively.

According to the second model, women who received enough information and counselling on ANC were 7.34 times more likely to attend the targeted care as recommended compared to those who obtained little information (95% CI = 4.26–12.66). The odds of reporting adequate use of ANC also increased by a factor of 1.97 for women who perceived that the provider's explanations on pregnancy-related issues were clear compared to those who had poorer explanations (95% CI = 1.12–3.46).

Analysis of factors associated with the continuity of services revealed some significant results. The odds of reporting the adequate use of ANC were increased by factors of 3.03 (95% CI = 1.46–6.29) and 6.05 (95% CI = 3.51–10.43) for women who sometimes and often had regular follow-up appointments scheduled by healthcare providers, respectively. Women who were often encouraged to make a return visit were 2.42 times more likely to utilize ANC adequately compared to those who were rarely encouraged to come back (95% CI = 1.53–3.83). In contrast, variables related to technical management and the appropriateness of the constellation of services included in the second model did not show statistically significant associations with the outcome variable (Table 4).

All of the study's covariates and predictors were included in the third and final model, to identify if the quality of care was associated with the adequacy of ANC attendance, controlling for the influences of individual determinants. Based on this model, certain variables related to predisposing factors and enabling resources remained significant; however, health needs no longer had statistically significant associations with the response variable. As per Table 4, for a one-year increase in the woman's education, the odds of utilizing ANC services adequately increased by a factor of 1.16 (95% CI = 1.06–1.27). Likewise, women who had wanted the pregnancy were 1.7 times more likely to attend ANC adequately than those who had an unplanned pregnancy (95% CI = 1.06–2.72). Women who lived in a neighborhood served by MCH services were 4.34 times more likely to report adequate use of ANC (95% CI = 2.34–8.07). Our analysis also revealed that, as the travel time to the nearest center increased, the odds of reporting adequate utilization of ANC declined by a factor of 0.35 (95% CI = 0.17–0.70).

The results of the final model also illustrated that dimensions related to women–provider relations, information exchange, and follow-up and continuity were all significant predictors for the utilization of ANC services. Specifically, women who often received respectful and friendly treatment from healthcare providers were 5.68 times more likely to utilize ANC adequately compared to those who rarely had positive communication with providers (95% CI = 2.45–13.13). The odds of reporting adequate use of ANC services were also increased by factors of 2.28 (95% CI = 1.27–4.07) and 7.22 (95% CI = 4.06–12.82) for women who sometimes and often had opportunities for dialogue and health talks with staff, respectively.

Women's exposure to enough information, education, and advice on ANC during clinic visits had a significant positive association with ANC attendance (OR = 9.12; 95% CI = 4.91–16.92). Compared to mothers who reported limited understanding of providers' explanations on issues related to diagnosis and procedures, the odds of reporting adequate utilization of care increased by a factor of 2.38 for those who often received clear explanations (95% CI = 1.22–4.66).

Women who were often encouraged by health workers to continue antenatal visits at the same facility were 1.82 times more likely to utilize ANC adequately compared to those who were rarely encouraged to come back (95% CI = 1.08–3.06). Our analysis also indicates that the odds of reporting the adequate use of ANC were increased by factors of 3.65 (95% CI = 1.61–8.28) and 6.51 (95% CI = 3.52–12.01) for women who sometimes and often had regular follow-up appointments scheduled by healthcare providers, respectively. Similarly to the second model, technical management and the appropriateness of the constellation of services were not found to be significant predictors of ANC utilization (Table 4).

Discussion

This paper suggests applying an integrated conceptual framework to ascertain the extent to which the attendance at ANC clinics may be attributed to individual determinants among women from disadvantaged backgrounds or to the quality of service delivery. Empirical research on healthcare utilization has shown that users' characteristics account for an estimated 20 to 25% of the variance explained [30]. This is consistent with our findings, in which individual determinants (model 1) accounted for 21% of the systematic explained variance compared to 57.4% of the variance explained by the quality of ANC (model 2). Once the two models have been merged, the variance explained by the final model increased to 66.0%. This implies that the variations in the use of ANC facilities were mainly attributable to the quality of service as experienced by women at healthcare facilities.

One of the major concerns of current research is to explore the barriers that prevent women in highly disadvantaged communities from attending ANC adequately. According to the final model, adequacy of ANC coverage is affected by a number of health service and individual factors. In particular, our findings illustrate that the increase in the woman's level of education is a significant motivator for increasing the likelihood of her ANC attendance. This concurs with other studies demonstrating that the low level of a woman's education is associated with infrequent and no ANC, as well as delay in accessing medical help [1, 2, 9, 12, 31]. It makes sense that educated women are more likely to appreciate the benefits of ANC for their health and their children's well-being and to exercise autonomy and decision-making power. More years of schooling may also promote women's ability to approach health staff to ask questions and to discuss any possible health concerns.

The actual desire of women to become pregnant was also found to be an important factor in determining the adequacy of ANC. A study by Muhwava et al. [12] also supports this finding, revealing that wanted pregnancy was associated with increased odds of early initiation and adequate ANC attendance compared to unwanted pregnancy. Another study, done in Holeta in central Ethiopia [32], showed that women who reported an unplanned pregnancy were 67% less likely to attend ANC than those who reported they had planned the pregnancy. Researchers argue that unplanned pregnancy is highly likely to reflect a lack of access to education on family planning during antenatal visits [32, 33].

Not surprisingly, women's decision to use ANC services is affected by having the means available to utilize these services. Research findings from resource-poor sites (i.e., Malawi and Kenya) have indicated that a large distance to reach a health facility was associated with delayed initiation of ANC use and low frequency of care attendance [9]. One explanation for such behavior is women's desire to minimize the number of journeys to the facility and thereby their total expenditure on ANC. In the case of Jordan, in spite of policies promising free ANC, many women in disadvantaged communities tend to avoid clinic visits because they are unable to afford the associated travel costs. Considering that the actual ANC is being provided free of charge, this might explain the non-significant finding of the association between health insurance and ANC attendance in the study's models.

In the same context, our study revealed that living in a district served by an MCH clinic was a potential contributing factor to increasing the use of ANC among poor women in northern Jordan. These findings are in agreement with previous research conducted in underserved populations, where living closer to a health facility was found to be a motivator for ANC use, as absence from work and transportation costs might be minimized [34, 35].

At the health service level, our study highlights the importance of several factors in enhancing the frequency of ANC attendance, the most prominent of which is the information and education women received on ANC during one-to-one consultations. This assertion is supported by the literature, in which the provision of maternal health information by healthcare professionals has been reported to be an effective means of encouraging the use of ANC during pregnancy [9, 31]. Research has shown that improving women's access to the necessary health education is fundamental for increasing their knowledge of ANC benefits and helping them make informed decisions about their care [1, 36]. In a study by Asfawosen et al. [37], the mother's knowledge about pregnancy danger signs had the potential to impact positively on ANC utilization. A study by Erlindawati et al. [38] also illustrated that pregnant women who obtained enough information about ANC services had a lower percentage of inadequate utilization compared to those who received fair but limited information. In the literature, it has been reported that pregnant women with low quality of ANC and no counseling services were at risk of pregnancy complications owing to the lack of relevant information [39, 40]. According to a study by Ejigu et al. [40], receiving incomplete information about ANC was also among the reasons for mothers' dissatisfaction with the overall perceived quality of care offered in ANC clinics in northwest Ethiopia.

Women's attendance at ANC facilities was also found to be related to ease of understanding the provider's explanations on pregnancy-related issues. Researchers have asserted that the limited understanding women received during their visit to a health facility represents a 'missed opportunity' to inform women about the possible complications of pregnancy [41–43]. The delivery of clear advice and messages that explain how to prevent and manage problems (i.e., miscarriage, multiple births, and abnormal position of the baby) can result in better recognition of the importance of attending ANC in improving health outcomes for mothers and children.

It was not a surprise to find an association between the woman–provider relationship and the use of ANC services. This link is most apparent in studies showing that building a positive rapport with pregnant women can contribute to their achieving the recommended number of antenatal visits. In contrast, researchers have pointed out that having low-quality care because of providers' poor communication skills (which may include an abusive attitude on the part of staff) may negatively influence ANC attendance [32, 40, 44]. In the study by Birmeta et al. [32], one of the participating women stated that the reason for underutilization of ANC was that, "If you go to a health institution you will find a low quality of services and a lack of respect and mistreatment from some of the healthcare providers". Obviously, the lack of women's desire to return to the clinic could be largely based on their expectations about the care provided, which may depend on previous experience.

Similarly, this study demonstrated that providing pregnant women with opportunities for dialogue and health talks during visits had a central role in increasing their motivation to attend ANC adequately. Many have argued that allowing women to communicate their concerns to health staff may encourage them to start ANC earlier and to have at least four ANC visits [9]. It is also important to mention that women who have good relations with health staff may feel more supported to ask questions and talk about their reproductive concerns and problems [45].

Interestingly, our study illustrated that scheduling follow-up appointments is likely to have an impact on women's decision about future visits. It is widely known that healthcare providers exercise significant authority and their advice is generally trusted by women. In view of that, instructions about when to attend ANC communicated by health staff apparently influence ANC utilization. Similarly, a lack of encouragement to attend upcoming appointments can result in delays to accessing ANC [9]. In Jordan, a study conducted by Al-Qutob et al. [35] found that almost 80% of the women were satisfied with ANC when the return visit was scheduled by the midwife; moreover, their satisfaction level had improved when providers explained to them the advantages of the timed follow-up visit.

Policy considerations

Health education and information exchange

Our study provides additional evidence that it is critical for health authorities to put considerable efforts into enhancing the quality of ANC by providing pregnant women with proper counseling that includes supportive listening, advice giving, and relevant information. Engaging mothers as active participants in consultations would also help make changes in healthcare delivery from one based on provider-dominated dialogues to one that involves users in the decision-making process. This requires a transition in the role of health workers from one characterized by authority to one that depends on collaboration and partnership between patients and providers.

Antenatal information should also be given in a form that is easy to understand and accessible to the users of ANC services. Medical providers' explanations of reproductive health matters should be tailored to the different social contexts, including those with low levels of education and income. Healthcare workers at MCH centers need to ascertain that the pregnant women understand the information received during consultation well enough to make an informed decision.

Since the desire to have a pregnancy was found to be a significant factor in determining adequacy of ANC attendance, it may therefore be useful to focus on informing women about effective contraceptive methods that help prevent unintended pregnancy in these populations. Promoting family planning education and more widely disseminating knowledge on contraception need to be an integrated component of ANC coverage. This research also proposes that the MoH appoint a person in each of the MCH centers to work as a reproductive health counselor. This person would be able to present clear information about birth preparedness, complications readiness, danger signs, nutrition, breastfeeding, and maternal stress.

Our study suggests using radio reports and television spots as a means of raising public awareness regarding the benefits of antenatal visits for improving babies' and mothers' health. Such information could provide just enough knowledge to initiate action before the women's exposure to health education at clinics. Displaying educational posters in a prominent place at MCH centers is highly recommended.

Follow-up appointments and continuity of care

Given that women generally place trust in health staff's recommendations, repeated, structured follow-up appointments and encouragement for return visits are suggested as an effective approach to improve the continuation of ANC attendance. Issuing appointment cards showing the times of upcoming ANC visits would be one possible way to remind women about the date of attendance. The relevance of this schedule also needs to be explained by health workers.

Women's interpersonal relations with health staff

Recognition must be also given to the impact on women's willingness to attend ANC of respectful and friendly treatment offered by providers. This would call for special training courses targeted at improving the communication skills of health staff on how to deal with the centers' referents and how be more mindful, informative, and empathic. Treating women kindly and having sound interpersonal relations with them would be a key means of increasing the numbers of those turning to antenatal clinics to receive care.

It is also hugely important for healthcare providers to ensure an effective approach by giving women a chance to be heard and to encourage free discussion on their physical and psychological well-being. This study highly recommends health workers to spend more time with clients to obtain their medical histories, and to ask if they have previously experienced pregnancy-related complications. For this purpose, it is essential to increase the number of health staff working at ANC clinics.

Accessibility to antenatal care facilities

To achieve significant changes at the health service level, this research strongly suggests that the public sector develop health policies aimed at expanding the availability of MCH centers to cover underserved areas. Increasing the number of ANC clinics that are physically close to those who live in disadvantaged conditions would help enhance their use. Likewise, the MoH can introduce mobile ANC in order to increase utilization of perinatal services and eliminate associated travel costs.

Conclusion

Whereas some researchers may consider the utilization of ANC services as a reflection of individual determinants, our study provides proof that this behavior is also embedded in the context of the healthcare delivery system. Specifically, our research has identified that attendance at ANC services was influenced by a number of factors, the most prominent of which are information exchange, follow-up and continuity of care, interpersonal relations with healthcare providers, and the availability of health facilities.

The results of this study have clarified that the interaction between women and providers is a key metric for the reported quality of ANC. The degree to which women feel that they are respected, informed, and engaged is considered an essential component of a successful strategy for improving mothers' experience with ANC and a way to motivate them to attend MCH clinics. In conclusion, our study reveals the strong association between how women perceive quality of care and their decision to attend reproductive health services. Strengthening the role of healthcare providers in counseling and health education would result in greater acceptance and sustained use of ANC.

Strengths and limitations

The potential limitations of this research were that the study may have been subject to recall bias, limited to women who were visiting the participating MCH centers at the time of the survey, and the tool did not include variables related to women's psychosocial and cultural factors. Future studies may also try to contact women who are not attending ANC at all and those who initiate ANC late (i.e., in the second or third trimester). Considering the importance of adaptation and implementation of the new ANC model within different health systems, clinical research investigating the contribution of the updated model to increasing the likelihood of positive pregnancy outcomes should be given priority. A need for research addressing the acceptability, feasibility, and cost-effectiveness of implementing the eight-contact model in low-resource settings is also obvious.

The strengths of this study include the use of a conceptual framework that takes contextual characteristics of ANC service delivery into account, the potential impact of such factors having been little explored in literature to date. Importantly, targeting contextual factors represents an opportunity to find areas that can be improved by policy formulation and implementation, unlike individual determinants, which are difficult to change. Analyzing women's perceptions of the care they have experienced by engaging stakeholders from disadvantaged communities would make the quality of care assessment more applicable to the expectations of users than that of health providers. By reviewing the medical records of respondents, the risk of recall bias is reduced, especially for measurement of the outcome variable.

Abbreviations

ANC: Antenatal Care; CI: Confidence Interval; DoS: Department of Statistics; FANC: Focused Antenatal care; HEIS: Household's Expenditure and Income Survey; JD: Jordanian Dinar; LMICs: Low and Middle Income Countries; MCH: Maternal and Child Health; MoPIC: Ministry of Planning and International Cooperation; OR: Odds Ratio; UNDP: United Nations Development Program; UNICEF: United Nations Children's Fund; WHO: World Health Organization

Acknowledgements

The authors would like to sincerely thank all women for their willingness to participate in this study. Special thanks are directed to Amneh Mohammad and Heba Abu-Awad for their efforts in data collection stage.

Funding

This research received no specific grant from any funding agency in the public, commercial or not-for-profit sectors. All the authors dedicated their additional working hours to develop this paper.

Authors' contributions

All authors contributed to study design, overall analysis and writing-up. All authors read and approved the final manuscript.

Competing interests

The authors declare they have no potential conflicts of interest with respect to the research, authorship, and/or publication of this article.

Author details

[1]Department of Health Management and Policy, Faculty of Medicine, Jordan University of Science and Technology, P.O. Box 3030, Irbid 22110, Jordan. [2]Department of Obstetrics and Gynecology, Faculty of Medicine, Jordan University of Science and Technology, P.O. Box: 3030, Irbid 22110, Jordan. [3]Department of Pediatrics and Neonatology, Faculty of Medicine, Jordan University of Science and Technology, P.O. Box: 3030, Irbid 22110, Jordan. [4]Department of Public Health and Community Medicine, Faculty of Medicine, Jordan University of Science and Technology, P.O. Box: 3030, Irbid 22110, Jordan.

References

1. Asamoah BO, Agardh A. Inequality trends in maternal health services for young Ghanaian women with childbirth history between 2003 and 2014. BMJ Open. 2017;7:e011663. https://doi.org/10.1136/bmjopen-2016-011663.

2. Aminur R, Monjura KN, Tahmina B, Sayem A, Nurul A, Iqbal A. Trends, determinants and inequities of 4+ ANC utilisation in Bangladesh. J Health Popul Nutr. 2017;36:2. https://doi.org/10.1186/s41043-016-0078-5.
3. Bitew T, Hanlon C, Kebede E, Medhin G, Fekadu A. Antenatal depressive symptoms and maternal health care utilisation: a population-based study of pregnant women in Ethiopia. BMC Pregnancy and Childbirth. 2016;16:301. https://doi.org/10.1186/s12884-016-1099-1.
4. Liu X, Behrman JR, Stein AD, Adair LS, Bhargava SK, Borja JB, et al. Prenatal care and child growth and schooling in four low- and medium-income countries. PLoS One. 2017;12(2):e0171299. https://doi.org/10.1371/journal.pone.0171299.
5. Kifle D, Azale T, Gelaw YA, Melsew YA. Maternal health care service seeking behaviors and associated factors among women in rural Haramaya District, eastern Ethiopia: a triangulated community-based cross-sectional study. Reprod Health. 2017;14:6. https://doi.org/10.1186/s12978-016-0270-5.
6. United Nations Development Program. A social determinants approach to maternal health:discussion paper. 2011. http://www.undp.org/content/dam/undp/library/Democratic%20Governance/Discussion%20Paper%20MaternalHealth.pdf. Accessed 18 July 2017.
7. Lincetto O, Mothebesoane-Anoh, Gomez P, Munjanja S. Chapter 2: Antenatal care. In: Lawn J, Kerber K, editors. Opportunities for Africa's newborns: practical data, policy and programmatic support for newborn care in Africa. Geneva: World Health Organization. 2006, 51–62. http://www.who.int/pmnch/media/publications/aonsectionIII_2.pdf. Accessed 22 June 2017.
8. World Health Organization. WHO recommendations on antenatal care for a positive pregnancy experience. 2016.http://apps.who.int/iris/bitstream/10665/250796/1/9789241549912-eng.pdf. Accessed 20 February 2017.
9. Pell C, Meñaca A, Were F, Afrah NA, Chatio S, et al. Factors affecting antenatal care attendance: results from qualitative studies in Ghana, Kenya and Malawi. PLoS One. 2013;8(1):e53747. https://doi.org/10.1371/journal.pone.0053747.
10. Dowswell T, Carroli G, Duley L, Gates S, Gülmezoglu AM, Khan-Neelofur D, Piaggio G. Alternative versus standard packages of antenatal care for low-risk pregnancy. Cochrane Database Syst Rev. 2015;7:CD000934. https://doi.org/10.1002/14651858.CD000934.pub3.
11. Miltenburg AS, van der Eem L, Nyanza EC, van Pelt S, Ndaki P, Basinda N, et al. Antenatal care and opportunities for quality improvement of service provision in resource limited settings: a mixed methods study. PLoS One 2017; 12(12): e0188279. https://doi.org/10.1371/ journal.pone.0188279.
12. Muhwava LS, Morojele N, London L. Psychosocial factors associated with early initiation and frequency of antenatal care (ANC) visits in a rural and urban setting in South Africa: a cross-sectional survey. BMC Pregnancy and Childbirth. 2016;16:18. https://doi.org/10.1186/s12884-016-0807-1.
13. Low P, Paterson J, Wouldes T, Carter S, Williams M, Percival T. Factors affecting antenatal care attendance by mothers of pacific infants living in New Zealand. N Z Med J. 2005;1216:1–10.
14. Abbas AA, Walker GJ. Determinants of the utilization of maternal and child health services in Jordan. Int J Epidemiol. 1986;15(3):404–7.
15. Obermeyer CM, Potter JE. Maternal health care utilization in Jordan: a study of patterns and determinants. Stud Fam Plan. 1991;22(3):177–87.
16. Shakhatreh FM, Abbas AA, Issa AA. Determinants of infant mortality and the use of maternity services in Jordan. Dirasat medical and biological sciences. 1996;23(2):59–69.
17. Alkhaldi SM. Predictors of antenatal care utilization in Jordan: findings from a national survey. Jordanian medical. Journal. 2016;50(2):69–79.
18. Department of Statistics [Jordan] and ICF International. Jordan population and family health survey 2012. 2013. https://dhsprogram.com/pubs/pdf/FR282/FR282.pdf. Accessed 15 July 2017.
19. United Nations Development Program. Jordan poverty reduction strategy: final report. 2013.http://www.jo.undp.org/content/dam/jordan/docs/Poverty/Jordanpovertyreductionstrategy.pdf. Accessed 15 July 2017.
20. United Nations Development Program, Department of Statistics, and Ministry of Planning and International Cooperation. Thinking differently about the poor "Findings from Poverty Pockets Survey in Jordan". 2012. http://www.undp.org/content/dam/jordan/docs/Poverty/Jordan_Poverty%20Pocket%20Report.pdf. Accessed 16 July 2017.
21. United Nations Children's Fund. Analyzing equity in health utilization and expenditure in Jordan with focus on maternal and child health services. 2016. https://www.unicef.org/jordan/ExecSummary_Analysing_equity_in_MCH_health_JordanMay2016.pdf. Accessed 16 July 2017.
22. The Higher Health Council. The national strategy for health sector in Jordan 2015–2019. 2016.http://www.hhc.gov.jo/uploadedimages/The%20National%20Strategy%20for%20Health%20Sector%20in%20Jordan%202015-2019.pdf. Accessed 19 July 2017.
23. Byrd TL, Law JG. Cross-border utilization of health care services by United States residents living near the Mexican border. Rev Panam Salud Publica. Pan Am J Public Health. 2009;26(2):95–100.
24. World Health Organization. Antenatal care in developing countries: promises, achievements and missed opportunities. 2003. http://apps.who.int/iris/bitstream/handle/10665/42784/9241590947.pdf?sequence=1. Accessed 19 July 2017.
25. Andersen RM. Revisiting the behavioral model and access to medical care: does it matter? J Health Soc Behav. 1995;36(1):1–10. https://doi.org/10.2307/2137284.
26. Babitsch B, Gohl D, Re-revisiting Andersen v LT. S behavioral model of health services use: a systematic review of studies from 1998–2011. GMS. Psychosoc Med. 2012; https://doi.org/10.3205/psm000089, URN: urn:nbn:de:0183-psm0000891.
27. World Health Organization. Standards for Improving Quality of Maternal and Newborn Care in Health Facilities. 2016. http://www.who.int/maternal_child_adolescent/documents/improving-maternal-newborn-care-quality/en/. Accessed 20 February 2018.
28. De Masi S, Bucagu M, Tunçalp Ö, Pablo Peña-Rosas J, Lawrie T, Oladapo OT, et al. Integrated person-centered health care for all women during pregnancy: implementing World Health Organization recommendations on antenatal care for a positive pregnancy experience. Global Health Sci Pract. 2017;5(2):197–201.
29. Bruce J. Fundamental elements of the quality of care: a simple framework. Stud Fam Plan. 1990;21(2):61–91.
30. Davidson PL, Andersen RM, Wyn R, Brown ERA. Framework for evaluating safety-net and other community-level factors on access for low-income populations. Inquiry. 2004;41:21–38.
31. Moore N, Blouin B, Razuri H, Casapia M, Gyorkos TW. Determinants of first trimester attendance at antenatal care clinics in the Amazon region of Peru: a case-control study. PLoS One. 2017;12(2):e0171136. https://doi.org/10.1371/journal.pone.0171136.
32. Birmeta K, Dibaba Y, Woldeyohannes D. Determinants of maternal health care utilization in Holeta town, Central Ethiopia. BMC Health Serv Res. 2013; 13:256.
33. Peer N, Morojele N, London L. Factors associated with contraceptive use in a rural area in western Cape Province. S Afr Med J. 2013;103:406–12.
34. Simkhada B, Teijlingen ER, Porter M, Simkhada P. Factors affecting the utilization of antenatal care in developing countries: systematic review of the literature. J Adv Nurs 2008; 61(3):244–260. doi: https://doi.org/10.1111/j.1365-2648.2007.04532.x PMID: 18197860.
35. Al-Qutob R, Mawajdeh S, Bin Raad F. The assessment of reproductive health services: a conceptual framework for prenatal care. Health Care Women Int. 1996;17(5):423–34.
36. Association of Reproductive Health Professionals. Breaking the contraceptive barrier: techniques for effective contraceptive consultations. Washington, DC: Association of Reproductive Health Professionals; 2008. http://www.arhp.org/Publications-and-Resources/Clinical-Proceedings/Breaking-the-Contraceptive-Barrier/System-Barriers. Accessed 2 August 2017.
37. Asfawosen A, Mussie A, Huruy A, Wondeweson T. Factors associated with maternal health care services in Enderta District, Tigray, northern Ethiopia: a cross sectional study. Am J Nurs Sc. 2014;3(6):117–25.
38. Erlindawati CJ, Isaranurug S. Factors related to the utilization of antenatal care services among pregnant women at health centers in Aceh Besar district, Nanggroe Aceh Darussalam province, Indonesia. J public health Dev. 2008;6(2):99–108.
39. Nwaeze IL, Enabor OO, Oluwasola TA, Aimakhu CO. Perception and satisfaction with quality of antenatal care services among pregnant women at the university college hospital, Ibadan. Nigeria Ann Ibd Pg Med. 2013; 11(1):22–8.
40. Ejigu T, Woldie M, Kifle Y. Quality of antenatal care services at public health facilities of Bahir-Dar special zone, Northwest Ethiopia. BMC Health Serv Res. 2013;13:443.
41. Nikie'ma B, Beninguisse G, Haggerty JL. Providing information on pregnancy complications during antenatal visits: unmet educational needs in sub-Saharan Africa. Health Policy Plan. 2009;24:367–76.
42. Anya S, Hydara A, Jaiteh L. Antenatal care in the Gambia: missed opportunity for information, education and communication. BMC Pregnancy and Childbirth. 2008;8:9.

43. Magoma M, Requejo J, Merialdi M, Campbell O, Cousens S, et al. How much time is available for antenatal care consultations? Assessment of the quality of care in rural Tanzania. BMC Pregnancy and Childbirth. 2011;11:64.
44. Ndwiga C, Warren CE, Ritter J, Sripad P, Abuya T. Exploring provider perspectives on respectful maternity care in Kenya: "work with what you have". Reprod Health. 2017;14:99. https://doi.org/10.1186/s12978-017-0364-8.
45. Sharan M, Valente TW. Spousal communication and family planning adoption: effects of a radio drama serial in Nepal. Int Fam Plan Perspect. 2002;28(1):16–25.

Client satisfaction with family planning services in the area of high unmet need: evidence from Tanzania Service Provision Assessment Survey, 2014-2015

Deogratius Bintabara[1,2*], Julius Ntwenya[1], Isaac I. Maro[2], Stephen Kibusi[1], Daniel W. Gunda[3] and Bonaventura C. T. Mpondo[4]

Abstract

Background: Client satisfaction has been found to be an important factor for the uptake and continuation of family planning services. This study aimed to examine the current status of and factors associated with client's satisfaction with family planning services in Tanzania, which has a high unmet need for family planning.

Methods: The study used data from the Tanzania Service Provision Assessment survey of 2014–2015. A facility was classified as having high service readiness for FP if it scored at least 67.7% on a composite score based on three domains (staff training and guidelines, basic diagnostic equipment, and basic medicines), following criteria developed by the World Health Organization. The exit interview questionnaire was used to collect information from women about their level of satisfaction, whether "very satisfied," "more or less satisfied," or not satisfied with the services received. The response was dichotomized into "Yes" if the woman reported being very satisfied with services received otherwise coded as "No". Unadjusted and adjusted logistic regression models were used to assess the association between the client satisfaction and covariate variables; service readiness, facility type, managing authority, location, management meetings, supervision, provider's sex, and working experience, clients' age and education. All analyses were weighted to correct for non-response, disproportionate and complex sampling by using the "SVY" command in Stata 14.

Results: Out of the 1188 facilities included in the survey, 427 (35.9%) provided family planning services. A total of 1746 women participated in observations and exit interviews. Few (22%) facilities had a high readiness to provide family planning services. While most facilities had the recommended equipment available, only 42% stocked contraceptives (e.g. oral pills, injectable contraceptives and/or condoms). Further, trained staff and clinical guidelines were present in only 30% of services. Nevertheless, the majority (91%) of clients reported that they were satisfied with services. In the multivariate analysis, a high service readiness score [AOR = 2.5, 95% CI; 1.1–6.0], receiving services from private facilities [AOR = 2.3, 95% CI; 1.1–5.0], and being in the age group 20 to 29 years [AOR = 0.3, 95% CI; 0.1–0.7] were all significantly associated with clients' satisfaction with family planning services.

(Continued on next page)

* Correspondence: bintabaradeo@gmail.com
[1]Department of Public Health, College of Health Sciences, The University of Dodoma, P.O Box 395, Dodoma, Tanzania
[2]Department of Global Health Entrepreneurship, Division of Public Health, Graduate School of Tokyo Medical and Dental University, 1-5-45 Yushima, Bunkyo-ku, Tokyo 113-8519, Japan
Full list of author information is available at the end of the article

(Continued from previous page)

Conclusion: There is a high level of client satisfaction with family planning services in Tanzania. Maintaining and exceeding this level will require improvements in the provision of staff training and the availability of contraceptives in existing services.

Keywords: Client satisfaction, Family planning, Service readiness, Tanzania

Plain English summary

Client satisfaction is a crucial indicator that measures the extent to which a client is gratified with the services received from healthcare providers. Several studies pointed out that client satisfaction is among the factors which influence the use of family planning services. In this study, we examine the current status of and factors associated with client satisfaction with family planning services in Tanzania, which has a high unmet need for family planning. The exit interviews were performed to family planning clients for providing their opinions on the services they had received. A total of 1746 study participants were involved in this study. Since this survey employed several stages to obtain study participants, the estimates were adjusted during analysis to minimize errors due to complex sampling.

The results presented here indicated the high proportion of clients who had satisfied with the services received. The possible factors identified for client satisfaction with family planning services were; readiness of the facility to provide the service, service provided by privately-owned facilities and client's age. In conclusion, there is high client satisfaction with family planning services in Tanzania. However, there is a need for improving services provided by publicly-owned facilities in order to increase and sustain client satisfaction.

Background

Rapid population growth resulting from high fertility rate and reduced mortality has become a new challenge of concern in sub-Saharan Africa (SSA) [1]. Projections show that the population in SSA will have increased by 128 and 290% by the year 2050 and 2100 respectively [1, 2]. Family planning (FP) is among the effective strategies that not only slow the population growth but also reduce maternal and child mortality due to outcomes of unintended pregnancies [2–4]. This led many developing countries in the 1960s to establish several programmes that promotes FP use [2, 5]. Between 1960 to the year 1996, the number of developing countries providing FP services had increased from 2 to 115 [6].

Despite the global emphasize on FP use so as to reduce the burden of overpopulation, Tanzania is still placed among the SSA countries with high fertility rate (5.2 births per women) [7], that is above the African average of 4.7 births per woman reported in 2015 [8]. In response, the Ministry of Health, Community Development, Gender, Elderly and Children (MoHCDGEC) of Tanzania developed the National Family Planning Costed Implementation Program (NFPCIP) which was officially launched in March 2010 [9]. The main goal of the program was to increase the contraceptive prevalence rate among women of reproductive age from 28% in 2010 to 60% by the year 2015. Despite this effort, the target has not been met in Tanzania; as the current uptake of any modern contraceptive (that includes; female sterilization, intra-uterine device, pills, injectable, implants and male condoms) is still low (32%) [7]. Among the reasons for this low uptake of contraceptive is client satisfaction with FP services provided within the health facilities [10–12]. Therefore assessing client satisfaction will help to understand the quality of FP services offered as the crucial aspect for improving utilization of FP services.

Generally, quality of healthcare can be assessed by using several measures but all of them falls under four broad attributes: structure, process, outcome and client experience [13, 14]. Structure; that assesses characteristics of care setting, process; that assesses the service provided to patients, outcome; that evaluate patient health as the results of care received, and client experience; that provides feedback on patient experiences of care. Since the satisfaction explains client experience and opinion regarding services received, this measure help to inform how facility and provider meeting clients' expectations. Therefore, it is considered as an important measure for assessing the level of services provided by facility or provider [15–17].

Despite the fact that several studies examining client satisfaction with FP services in SSA [10, 18–20] yet, only limited studies explored the relationships between structural (facility organizational characteristics and setting) factors and clients satisfaction. But some factors have been explained to influence the client satisfaction which such as waiting time, kind of provider, privacy, staff motivation, poor quality of care, availability of medicines and equipment, and some demographic characteristics like age and education of client [10, 19, 21]. However, some factors such as the type of managing authority and readiness of facility to provide services were left unstudied, that we think they might have some contribution to client's satisfaction. Therefore, this study aimed to examine the current status of and factors associated with client satisfaction with FP services in Tanzania, which has a high unmet need for FP services. The obtained findings may provide a broad spectrum of policymakers, and public health specialists to design appropriate interventions for strengthening the quality of FP services.

Methods

Data source

This study analyzed data from the 2014–15 Tanzania Service Provision Assessment (TSPA) Survey dataset. This survey was undertaken by Tanzania's National Bureau of Statistics (NBS) in collaboration with the Office of the Chief Government Statistician (OCGS), Zanzibar, the Ministry of Health, Community Development, Gender, Elderly, and Children (MoHCDGEC), Tanzania Mainland, and the Ministry of Health (MOH), Zanzibar. The technical assistance for the survey was provided by ICF International through the United States Agency for International Development (USAID)-funded Demographic and health survey (DHS) program.

Sample size and sampling procedure

The 2014–15 TSPA was a sample survey of all the formal sector health facilities in Tanzania. The MoHCDGEC in Tanzania mainland and the Ministry of Health (MOH) in Zanzibar provided the list that included all the hospitals, health centers, dispensaries, and clinics. The list consisted of 7102 verified (active) health facilities and used as a sampling frame. From the list, a total of 1200 facilities were randomly selected for inclusion in the survey. The sample was designed to provide nationally representative results according to the facility type, managing authority, and regions for both Tanzania Mainland and Zanzibar. Though of 1200 health facilities sampled, seven refused to participate, four had closed down, and one could not be reached. Finally, a total of 1188 facilities were successfully surveyed. But, the analysis for this study was based on 427 health facilities that reported to provide FP services. These included 106 hospitals, 34 health centers, and 287 dispensaries/clinics. Thereafter, a total of 1746 women clients who received FP services were systematically selected in FP exit interviews based on the number of clients present at service site on the day of the visit. In case many clients were present and eligible for the interviews, a maximum of five clients for each provider and 15 clients for each selected facility were observed. Then all observed clients were included in an exit interview soon after receiving FP services from providers.

Data collection

The 2014–2015 TSPA survey data were collected between October 20, 2014, and February 21, 2015, and revisit of some facilities that were not covered previous were conducted between March 2 to 13, 2015. The exit interviews were performed by health workers (nurses) selected from different institutions trained and qualified to be interviewers. The 2014–2015 TSPA used four main types of data collection tools: facility inventory questionnaire, health provider interview questionnaire, and observation protocols for antenatal care (ANC), FP, and services for sick children, exit interview questionnaires for ANC and FP clients and for caretakers of sick children whose consultations were observed. The information collected for each questionnaire is stored in a different file.

Data processing and management

The current study used data from Facility inventory, Health Provider, and Observation/client files. The data in these files were edited and cleaned and later were merged together into the new file (dataset) by using the facility and provider identification as a unique identifier of these three files. During merging process, the Observersion/client file was used as the master file, while the others as using files. The merge command in Stata was performed at M:1 (many-to-one); therefore, the unit of analysis of the merged file remained at the client level.

Definition of variables

Outcome variable: client satisfaction with FP services

Client satisfaction This was the primary outcome variable in which during the exit interviews client was asked to provide their opinion about the FP services they either received or provided at that facility on the day of the interview. The responses were "very satisfied," "more or less satisfied," and "not satisfied" with the services received. Later, the responses were dichotomized into "Yes," if the client reported "very satisfied" with the FP services received or provided and "No," if client reported either "less or more satisfied" or "not satisfied" with FP services received or provided.

Key independent variable (proximate factor)

FP service readiness

FP services readiness This variable was measured based on the score of FP service readiness index. The score was constructed by using the World Health Organization (WHO) approach and FP readiness indicators were identified according to the WHO Service Availability and Readiness Assessment (SARA) Manual. Through this approach, the FP service readiness indicators were categorized into three domains. The first domain included staff and guideline, which had two indicators, i.e., the guideline on FP and staff trained to provide FP services. The facilities with guidelines and at least one provider that had received in-service training in FP within 2 years were coded as "Yes," while those without such guidelines or at least one provider had received in-service training in FP within 2 years were coded as "No." The second domain was equipment, which had one indicator, i.e., the presence of blood pressure (BP) apparatus. Facilities with BP apparatus were coded as "Yes," while those without such item were coded as "No." The third domain was medicine and commodities, which had four indicators, i.e., the availabilities of progestin-only pills, combined oral pills, injectable contraceptives (combined or progestin-only), and condoms. Facilities with the availability of these methods of contraception were coded as "Yes," while those without were coded as "No." The FP readiness index was then summed by adding the presence of each indicator, with equal weight given to each of the domains and each of the indicators within the domains. As the target was 100%, each domain accounted for 33.3% (100%/3) of the index. The percentage for each indicator within the domain was equal to 33.3% divided by the number of indicators in that domain. The FP service readiness index for each facility was then calculated by adding the percentages. The similar approach has been used elsewhere [22]. The facilities with the score "less than 33.3%," "between 33.3% and 66.7%," and "more than 66.7%" were considered to have low, medium and high readiness for offering FP services respectively.

Other independent variables (background factors)

These were categorized into provider characteristics (sex, qualification, and years of experience), facility characteristics (location, facility type, managing authority, routine management meetings and external supervision) and client characteristics (age and level of education).

Statistical analysis

Data were analyzed using Stata 14 (StataCorp, College Texas). Since the facilities sampled were not evenly distributed and the response rate might be very different by regions or facility type, then over and under-sampled in the regions with fewer and more facilities respectively were performed before data collection. Therefore, before analysis, client weight was used to restore the actual representativeness and to correct for sampled data (weighting). Furthermore, the "SVY" set command was used to adjust for the complex sampling design employed in the TSPA survey so that to obtain the accurate estimates.

Descriptive statistics were presented as frequency listings and percentages because our variables are categorical. We fitted an unadjusted logistic regression model to assess whether there were any associations between the outcome and key independent variable, also, with other variables from the health facility, provider, and client separately. All variables with a P-value less than 0.2 were considered for inclusion into the multiple logistic regression (Adjusted) model using the stepwise (backward elimination) method to test for the association of each variable with the outcome variable. The obtained final model included all the variables that determined client satisfaction with FP services. The P-value < 0.05 and 95% confidence interval (CI) for the odds ratio (OR) were used to confirm the significance of the associations.

Ethical considerations

The original 2014–2015 TSPA survey was approved by Tanzania's National Institute for Medical Research (NIMR), the Zanzibar Medical Ethics and Research Committee (ZAMREC), and the Institutional Review Board of ICF International in the USA. The informed consent was obtained from the manager, the person-in-charge of the facility, or the most senior health worker responsible for client services present at the facility, and women received FP services within the facilities surveyed. The respondents were adequately informed regarding all relevant aspects of the study, including its aim and interview procedures.

Results

Background characteristics of observed consultations according to facilities, health providers, and clients

Out of the 1188 facilities included in the survey, 427 offered FP services with a total of 1746 observations and exit interviews. Majority of the FP consultations (1497, 85.7%) were performed in public facilities, more than half (954, 54.6%) were performed either in clinics or dispensaries, while 974 (55.8%) were performed in rural settings. About nine-tenths (1541, 88.3%) of the consultations were performed by female health providers. Furthermore, 1049 (63.5%) consolations were performed by providers with experience of 5 years or less, while only 55 (3.2%) consultations were performed by clinicians. The majority (931, 53.3%) of the consultations involved women between the age of 20 to 29 years (Table 1).

Client satisfaction with FP services

Out of 1746 observed FP consultations, the majority (1592, 91%) of consultations clients reported that had satisfied with the services received or provided to them; only 153 (9%) of the consultations the clients reported not being satisfied with the services.

Indicators of service readiness by managing authority

About third-quarters of public (75.1%) and private (73.3%) facilities reported having equipment for providing FP services while only 42% stocked contraceptives (e.g. oral pills, injectable contraceptives and/or condoms). Further, trained staff and clinical guidelines were present in only 30% of services. When the indicators for service readiness were compared by managing authority,

Table 1 Characteristics of health facilities, health providers and clients in the FP exit interviews ($n = 1746$)

Variable	Number (n)	Percentage (%)
Health facility characteristics		
Managing authority		
Public	1497	85.7
Private	249	14 3
Facility type		
Hospital	298	22.8
Health center	394	22.6
Clinic & dispensary	954	54.6
Facility location		
Urban	772	44.2
Rural	974	55.8
Routine management meetings		
No	214	12.2
Yes	1532	87.8
External supervision		
Not done	359	20.6
Yes, < 3 months	1052	60.2
Yes, > 3 months	335	19.2
Health provider characteristics		
Sex of provider		
Male	205	11.7
Female	1541	88.3
Working experience (years)[a]		
0–5	1048	63.5
> 5	696	36.5
Qualification		
Clinicians	55	3.2
Nurses	1691	96.8
Client characteristics		
Age		
< 20	158	9.1
20–29	931	53.3
30–39	535	30.7
> =40	121	6.9
Formal education		
No	280	16.1
Yes	1466	83.9
Level of formal education[b]		
Primary	1221	83.4
Secondary	223	15.2
Tertiary	22	1.4

[a]Do not add up to 1746 because some providers did not remember the year they started working in the facility
[b]Do not add up to 1746 because some clients did not have any formal education

it was found that availability of the indicators was comparable between public and privately owned facilities. A major difference was in the presence of trained staff and clinical guideline that was high in private (36%) than public (28%) facilities ($P < 0.05$). However, when the overall FP service readiness was compared according to managing authority, the scores were comparable between public and privately owned facilities, especially in the medium and high scores categories. In the low category of service readiness, public facilities were found to perform poor (7.1%) than private facilities (11.2%) (Fig. 1).

Factors associated with client satisfaction

Table 2 presents the results of unadjusted and adjusted analyses. In adjusted analysis, high FP service readiness and receiving services from private owned facilities were significantly associated with client satisfaction with FP services [AOR = 2.5; 95% CI, 1.1–6.0] and [AOR = 2.3; 95% CI, 1.1–5.0] respectively. Additionally, compared with clients who were < 20 years, clients with the age between 20 to 29 years were significantly less likely to be satisfied with FP services [AOR = 0.3; 95% CI, 0.1–0.7].

Discussion

This study aimed to examine the current status of and factors associated with client satisfaction with FP services in Tanzania, which has a high unmet need for FP. It found the high proportion of women had satisfied with the FP services. In addition, FP service readiness and its individual indicators except for trained staff and clinical guideline were comparable between the publicly and privately-owned facilities. Furthermore, high FP service readiness and privately-owned facilities were significantly associated with client's satisfaction with FP services.

The high proportion of client's satisfaction with FP services observed in this study was higher than earlier studies performed in Tanzania [23], South Ethiopia [3], Nigeria [19], and Kenya but comparable to the study performed in Mozambique [20]. The high proportion of clients' satisfaction with FP services in the current study can be explained by the increased number of health facilities that provide FP services compared to before, provision of in-service training to health care providers and important supplies (contraceptives and commodities) from governmental and some non-governmental organizations that operate in Tanzania. Also, the study found no significant difference in FP service readiness between private and public facilities. This finding was in agreement to that of the previous study performed in Tanzania using the 2006 Service Provision Assessment survey [23].

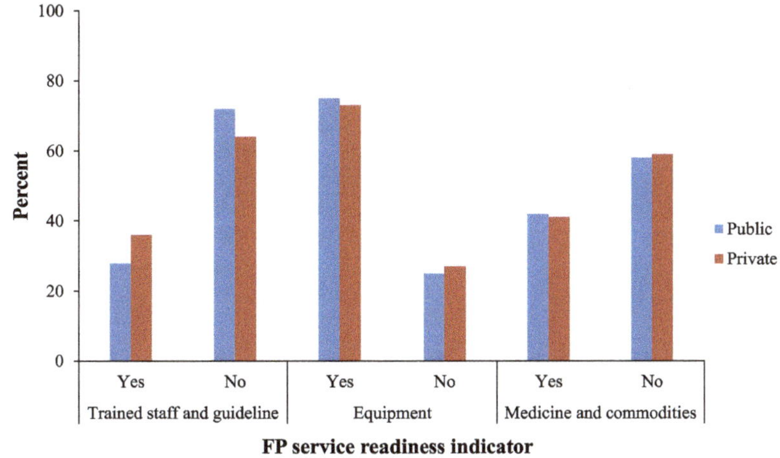

Fig. 1 Individual indicators of service readiness by managing authority

Understanding the factors associated with client's satisfaction with services received or provided could help the health providers and policy-decision makers to design programmes that will meet the client needs [24]. This study revealed that client's satisfaction with services was associated with a high FP service readiness scores. Due to lack of studies that assessed the association between FP service readiness and clients' satisfaction with FP services it becomes difficult to compare this finding. However, previous studies performed in Kenya and Mozambique found that availability of essential equipment as the important domain of FP service readiness was associated with client's satisfaction [18, 20]. These findings are not in agreement with the findings from the previous study that did not find any association between FP service readiness and client's satisfaction [10]. The difference in findings might be due to that the previous survey analyzed data that were collected more than 10 years ago, while the current study analyzed data that collected 2014–2015. Therefore ten-year deference in this era of globalization could explain the change of some of the socio-economic and demographic factors.

Evidence from the previous study suggests that client's satisfaction differs by type of managing authority [25]. In agreement with this, the current study found that the odds of clients being satisfied with FP services were two times higher for privately-owned facilities than publicly-owned one. These findings are in agreement with those of previous studies performed in Kenya [10, 18, 25, 26] and in West African countries [27]. The similarity of these findings might be explained by the fact that privately-owned facilities are more responsible and committed to the patients since are operated for profit basis compared to publicly-owned facilities, therefore, tend to provide better and complete services in order to gain more clients and profit [28]. Additionally, privately-owned facilities are not crowded and clients could quickly receive service and spent plenty of time with health providers during consultations hence more likely to be satisfied. On the other hand, publicly-owned facilities are characterized with the long queue, staffs that have low morale or relatively poor performance and attendance [29]. These facilities usually have the shortage of staff, medicines and functioning equipment required to provide standard services [30, 31].

The current study found that clients in the age between 20 to 29 years were less likely to report being satisfied with FP services compared to those less than 20 years. This observation was in agreement with those of the previous studies performed in Kenya and Egypt [18, 32]. This finding might be explained by the fact that younger clients are more likely to have more expectations compared to older ones; also, younger clients are more likely to be new FP clients with first-time visits that do not know components of FP services that should be provided to them. One previous study found that repeat FP clients were more likely to be satisfied than first-time clients [3]. Other studies, however, have found no association between clients' age and satisfaction with FP services [3, 27, 33, 34].

Unlike in other previous studies performed elsewhere, that found an association between clients' level of education and satisfaction with FP services, the current study found no association between those variables. Some of those previous studies found that clients with the higher level of education were more likely to be satisfied with the services they receive [10, 33], while others found that less educated ones were more likely to be satisfied [18]. Furthermore, the current study found that providers' years of experience were not significantly associated with client satisfaction. This finding was in contrast to those of previous studies performed in Kenya and Senegal [18, 34]. However, the current study found that facility type and location were not

Table 2 Bivariate and Multivariate analysis of factors associated with client satisfaction to family planning services

Variable	Client satisfied Number (%)	Unadjusted OR [95% CI]	Adjusted OR [95% CI]
Service readiness			
Low	163 (10.2)	Ref.	Ref.
Medium	1079 (67.8)	1.3 [0.6–2.7]	1.3 [0.6–2.7]
High	351 (22.0)	2.7 [1.1–6.3]	2.5 [1.1–6.0]
Managing authority			
Public	1355 (85.1)	Ref.	Ref.
Private	238 (14.9)	2.1 [0.9–4.9]	2.3 [1.1–5.0]
Facility type			
Hospital	362 (22.7)	Ref.	Ref.
Health center	348 (21.9)	0.8 [0.5–1.2]	0.8 [0.4–1.5]
Clinic & dispensary	883 (55.4)	1.2 [0.7–2.3]	1.2 [0.5–2.3]
Facility location			
Rural	887 (55.7)	Ref.	Ref.
Urban	706 (44.3)	1.1 [0.6–1.7]	1.1 [0.6–2.0]
Routine management meetings			
No	194 (12.2)	Ref.	Ref.
Yes	1399 (87.8)	1.1 [0.4–3.1]	1.1 [0.4–3.4]
External supervision			
No	323 (20.3)	Ref.	Ref.
Yes, < 3 months	955 (59.9)	1.1 [0.6–2.0]	1.2 [0.7–2.2]
Yes, > 3 months	315 (19.8)	1.8 [0.9–3.8].	2.0 [0.9–4.2]
Sex of the Provider			
Male	1403 (88.1)	Ref.	Ref.
Female	190 (11.9)	1.3 [0.6–2.6]	1.2 [0.5–2.8]
Working experience			
5 years and less	961 (60.4)	Ref.	Ref.
More than 5 years	630 (39.6)	0.9 [0.5–1.4]	0.9 [0.5–1.3]
Qualification			
Clinician	51 (3.2)	Ref.	Ref.
Nurses	1542 (96.8)	0.8 [0.3–2.6]	0.8 [0.3–2.8]
Age of client			
< 20	153 (9.6)	Ref.	Ref.
20–29	834 (52.4)	0.3 [0.1–0.7]	0.3 [0.1–0.7]
30–39	495 (31.0)	0.4 [0.2–0.9]	0.4 [0.2–1.1]
> =40	111 (7.0)	0.4 [0.1–1.4]	0.4 [0.1–1.5]
Education			
No	258 (16.2)	Ref.	Ref.
Yes	1335 (83.2)	0.9 [0.5–1.6]	0.9 [0.5–1.7]

associated with client's satisfaction. Similar findings have been reported in previous studies conducted in Ethiopia, Nigeria, and Mozambique [3, 19, 20].

The strength of the current study is that it analyzed the data with a nationwide representative sample of health facilities, with a response rate of 99%. The use of such data suggests that the findings accurately reflect the current situation regarding FP services in the study area. By considering the complex sampling techniques involved in the TSPA survey, the findings were adjusted for clustering effect and weighted to correct for non- response and disproportionate sampling. However, the study has some limitations, due to its cross-sectional nature, it fails to explain the causality assumptions hence results should be interpreted with caution. Additionally, the outcome variable "client satisfaction" in the current study was assessed by using a single question with response of "very satisfied," "more or less satisfied," and "not satisfied", this might be not very sensitive enough that is why we found high proportion of client who was satisfied with FP services. Furthermore, since exit interviews were based on prior direct observations between client and provider, our findings might be subjected to social desirability bias, observation bias, and Hawthorne effect; that is the change of behavior by the subjects of a study due to their awareness of being observed [35]. However, we minimized these biases by restricted to a maximum of five observations per each provider.

Conclusion

There is a high level of client satisfaction with FP services in Tanzania. High FP service readiness score, privately-owned facilities, and client's age matter on client's satisfaction with FP services. Maintaining and exceeding this level will require improvements in the provision of staff training and the availability of contraceptives in existing services.

Abbreviations

AOR: Adjusted odds ratio; BP: Blood pressure; COR: Crude odds ratio; DHS': Demographic health survey; FP: Family planning; MOHCDGEC: Ministry of Health, Community Development, Gender, Elderly and Children; NFPCIP: National family planning costed implementation program; SARA: Service availability and readiness assessment; SSA: Sub-Saharan Africa; TSPA: Tanzania service provision assessment; WHO: World Health Organization

Acknowledgments

We acknowledge DHS program for data accessibility, Dr. Wenjuan Wang, Dr. Michelle Winner, Dr. Rebecca Winter and ICF international for TSPA data analysis training.

Authors' contributions

DB originated the design of the study; DB&BCT performed statistical analysis and interpretation of data; DB, JN, IM, SK, DWM, and BCT drafted the manuscript and critically revised the drafted manuscript. All authors read and approved the final draft of the manuscript.

Consent for publication

N/A

Competing interests

The authors declare that they have no competing interests.

Author details

[1]Department of Public Health, College of Health Sciences, The University of Dodoma, P.O Box 395, Dodoma, Tanzania. [2]Department of Global Health Entrepreneurship, Division of Public Health, Graduate School of Tokyo Medical and Dental University, 1-5-45 Yushima, Bunkyo-ku, Tokyo 113-8519, Japan. [3]Department of Internal Medicine, Catholic University of Health and Allied Sciences, P.O. Box 1464, Mwanza, Tanzania. [4]Department of Internal Medicine, College of Health Sciences, The University of Dodoma, P.O Box 395, Dodoma, Tanzania.

References

1. Bongaarts J, Casterline J. Fertility transition: is sub-Saharan Africa different? Popul Dev Rev. 2013;38:153–68.
2. Cleland J, Bernstein S, Ezeh A, Faundes A, Glasier A, Innis J, et al. Family planning: the unfinished agenda. Lancet (London, England). 2006;368:1810–27. Elsevier
3. Argago TG, Hajito KW, Kitila SB. Client's satisfaction with family planning services and associated factors among family planning users in Hossana Town Public Health Facilities South Ethiopia: Facility-based cross-sectional study. Int J Nurs Midwifery. 2015;7:74–83.
4. Loha E, Asefa M, Jira C, Tessema F, Loha E, Asefa M, Chali Jira FT. Assessment of quality of care in family planning services in Jimma zone, Southwest Ethiopia. Ethiop J Health Dev. 2003;18:1–13.
5. Peabody, Taguiwalo, Robalino F. Disease control priorities in developing countries. 2nd ed; 2006.
6. Bongaarts J, Cleland J, Townsend JW, Bertrand JTGM. Family planning programs for the 21 st century family: rationale and design. New York: The Population Council; 2012. https://www.popcouncil.org/uploads/pdfs/2012_FPfor21stCentury.pdf. Accessed 25 Apr 2018.
7. Ministry of Health, Community Development, Gender, Elderly and Children (MoHCDGEC) [Tanzania Mainland], Ministry of Health (MoH) [Zanzibar], National Bureau of Statistics (NBS), Office of the Chief Government Statistician (OCGS), and ICF. Tanzania Demographic and Health Survey and Malaria Indicator Survey (TDHS-MIS) 2015–16. Dar es Salaam and Rockville: MoHCDGEC, MoH, NBS, OCGS, and ICF; 2016. https://dhsprogram.com/pubs/pdf/FR321/FR321.pdf. Accessed 25 Apr 2018.
8. United Nations, Department of Economic and Social Affairs, Population Division (2015). World Fertility Patterns 2015 – Data Booklet (ST/ESA/ SERA/370). http://www.un.org/en/development/desa/population/publications/pdf/fertility/world-fertility-patterns-2015.pdf. Accessed 25 Apr 2018.
9. Ministry of Health and Social Welfare (MoHSW). The national family planning costed implementation program 2010–2015: MoHSW; 2010. https://www.fhi360.org/sites/default/files/media/documents/national-fp-costed-implementation-plan-tanzania-main-text.pdf. Accessed 25 Apr 2018.
10. Hutchinson PL, Do M, Agha S. Measuring client satisfaction and the quality of family planning services: a comparative analysis of public and private health facilities in Tanzania, Kenya and Ghana. BMC Health Serv Res BioMed Central. 2011;11:203.
11. Williams T, Schutt-Aine J, Cuca Y. Measuring family planning service quality through client satisfaction exit interviews. Int Fam Plan Perspect. 2000;26:63–71.
12. Blanc AK, Curtis SL, Croft TN. Monitoring contraceptive continuation: links to fertility outcomes and quality of care. Stud Fam Plan. 2002;33:127–40.
13. Morris C, Bailey K. Measuring health care Quality : an overview of quality measures. Issue Breif. Family USA; 2014. http://familiesusa.org/sites/default/files/product_documents/HSIQualityMeasurement_Brief_final_web.pdf. Accessed 25 Apr 2018.
14. Donabedian A. The quality of care. How can it be assessed? 1988. Arch Pathol Lab Med. 1997;121:1145–50.
15. Derose KP, Hays RD, McCaffrey DF, Baker DW. Does physician gender affect satisfaction of men and women visiting the emergency department? J Gen Intern Med. 2001;16:218–26.
16. Bara AC, Van Den HWJA, Maarse JAM, Van DJP. Users' satisfaction with the Romanian health care system : an evaluation of recent health care reforms. Eur J Pub Health. 2002;12:39–40.
17. Chu-Weininger MYL, Balkrishnan R. Consumer satisfaction with primary care provider choice and associated trust. BMC Health Serv Res. 2006;6:139.

18. Agha S, Do M. The quality of family planning services and client satisfaction in the public and private sectors in Kenya. Int J Qual Health Care. 2009;21:87–96.
19. Kaoje U, Oche M, Isah B, Sambo M, Saad A, Raji M. Determinants of client satisfaction with family planning services in government health facilities in Sokoto, northern Nigeria. Sahel Med J Medknow Publications and Media Pvt Ltd. 2015;18:20.
20. Chavane L, Dgedge M, Bailey P, Loquiha O, Aerts M, Temmerman M. Assessing women's satisfaction with family planning services in Mozambique. J Fam Plan Reprod Heal Care. 2017;43:222–8.
21. World Health Organization (WHO). Working together for health: the world health report 2006: WHO; 2006. http://www.who.int/whr/2006/whr06_en.pdf. Accessed 25 Apr 2018.
22. Bintabara D, Nakamura K, Seino K. Determinants of facility readiness for integration of family planning with HIV testing and counseling services: evidence from the Tanzania service provision assessment survey, 2014–2015. BMC Health Serv Res. 2017;17:844.
23. Kakoko DC, Ketting E, Kamazima SR, Ruben R. Provision of family planning services in Tanzania: a comparative analysis of public and private facilities. Afr J Reprod Health. 2012;16:140–8.
24. Aldana JM, Piechulek H, Al-Sabir A. Client satisfaction and quality of health care in rural Bangladesh. Bull World Health Organ. 2001;79:512–7.
25. Wambua JM, Mbayaki R, Munyao PM, Kabue MM, Mulindi R, Change PM, et al. Client satisfaction determinants in four Kenyan slums. Int J Health Care Qual Assur. 2015;28:667–77.
26. Agwanda A, Khasakhala A, Kimani M. Assessment of Family Planning Services in Kenya: Evidence from the 2004 Kenya Service Provision Assessment Survey. Working Papers No. 4. Calverton: Macro International Inc; 2009. http://dhsprogram.com/pubs/pdf/wpk4/wpk4.pdf. Accessed 25 Apr 2018.
27. Wang WJ, Do M, Hembling J, Ametepi P. Assessing the quality of care in family planning, antenatal, and sick child services at health facilities in Kenya, Namibia, and Senegal. DHS Anal. Stud. DHS Analytical Studies No. 44. Rockville: ICF International; 2014. https://dhsprogram.com/pubs/pdf/AS44/AS44.pdf. Accessed 25 Apr 2018.
28. Pongsupap Y, Van LW. Choosing between public and private or between hospital and primary care: responsiveness, patient-centredness and prescribing patterns in outpatient consultations in Bangkok. Trop Med Int Heal. 2006;11:81–9.
29. Bitrán R. Efficiency and quality in the public and private sectors in Senegal. Health Policy Plan. 1995;10:271–83.
30. Berman P, Laura R. The role of private providers in maternal and child health and family planning services in developing countries. Heal Policy Plan. 1996;11:142–55. 14p
31. Wouters A. The cost and efficiency of public and private health care facilities in Ogun state, Nigeria. Health Econ. 1993;2:31–42.
32. Abdel-Tawab N, Roter D. The relevance of client-centered communication to family planning settings in developing countries: lessons from the Egyptian experience. Soc Sci Med. 2002;54:1357–68.
33. Tafese F, Woldie M, Megerssa B. Quality of family planning services in primary health centers of Jimma zone, Southwest Ethiopia. Ethiop J Health Sci. 2013;23:245–54.
34. Shireen A, Wang WJ, Mallick L. Quality of care in family planning services at health facilities in Senegal. DHS Analytical Studies No. 55. Rockville: ICF International; 2015. https://dhsprogram.com/pubs/pdf/AS55/AS55.pdf. Accessed 25 Apr 2018.
35. Leonard K, Masatu MC. Outpatient process quality evaluation and the Hawthorne effect. Soc Sci Med. 2006;63:2330–40.

6

Quality of IVF status registration in the Estonian Medical Birth Registry: a national record linkage study

Kärt Allvee[1], Mati Rahu[2], Kai Haldre[3], Helle Karro[4,5] and Kaja Rahu[2*]

Abstract

Background: Information regarding in vitro fertilization (IVF) as a pregnancy risk factor (yes/ no) is stored in each birth record of the Estonian Medical Birth Registry (EMBR). This study aimed to assess the validity of registration of newborns' IVF status in the EMBR.

Methods: To identify the newborns conceived by IVF, the birth records in the EMBR were compared to individual records on the embryo transfer procedures in the Estonian Health Insurance Fund (EHIF) database as a reference. Maternal age was restricted to 40 years, the age limit for IVF treatment covered by the EHIF. The embryo transfer procedures, that dated up to eight weeks before pregnancy, were additionally checked in the infertility treatment clinics. The validity of IVF status was measured by sensitivity, specificity, positive and negative predictive values (PPV and NPV). Relative risk (RR) of unrecorded IVF status among IVF mothers by socio-demographic characteristics and birth plurality was estimated using modified Poisson regression models.

Results: There were 3198 newborns identified as conceived by IVF in the EMBR in 2005–2014. Eight of them were incorrectly entered as born after IVF. The record linkage with the EHIF database revealed 1014 newborns with unrecorded IVF status in the EMBR. A total of 4204 newborns were verified as conceived by IVF, 24.1% of them were not categorized as born after IVF. The sensitivity of the IVF status registration was poor (75.9%), specificity (100.0%), PPV (99.8%) and NPV (99.3%) were high. The misclassifications were significantly more common among mothers of younger age or non-Estonians or with singleton birth.

Conclusion: Information based on mother's self-report or her antenatal chart does not accurately identify the newborn's IVF status. The lack of a specialized country-wide assisted reproductive technology register in Estonia requires routine record linkage of the EMBR, EHIF and the infertility treatment clinics' databases to obtain adequate information regarding IVF status in the EMBR. Electronic record linkages between databases would help considerably to improve the validity of data to be used in medical decision making, in research and for statistical purposes.

Keywords: Birth registry, Data quality, Embryo transfer, In vitro fertilization, Record linkage

* Correspondence: kaja.rahu@tai.ee
[2]Department of Epidemiology and Biostatistics, National Institute for Health Development, Hiiu 42, 11619 Tallinn, Estonia
Full list of author information is available at the end of the article

Plain English summary

Birth records in the Estonian Medical Birth Registry (EMBR) include information on the IVF status of newborns relying on mothers' self-report or their antenatal charts. As there is no mandate to sanction data exchange between the EMBR and infertility treatment clinics, current study aimed to assess the validity of the IVF status registration in the registry via linkage records of the EMBR and Estonian Health Insurance Fund (EHIF) reimbursement database as a reference. Solidarity based EHIF covers unlimited number of IVF cycles for all women aged 40 years or less. The embryo transfers resulting in birth were identified using the mother's personal identification number as the key. If necessary, additional verification in the infertility treatment clinics was performed. According to the EMBR data, 146,526 infants with maternal age up to 40 years were born to Estonian residents in 2005–2014. A total of 4204 newborns were verified as conceived by IVF; 1014 newborns had lacked the IVF status on the birth record. The sensitivity of the IVF status registration was poor (75.9%). The IVF status was better recorded for mothers of the older age group (35–40 years) or with a multiple birth, because they were more likely to have IVF pregnancy and were more carefully questioned. As far as Estonia lacks a specialized country-wide assisted reproductive technology register, record linkages of the EMBR, EHIF and the infertility treatment clinics' databases are requested to obtain adequate information on the IVF status of the newborns in the EMBR.

Background

The 2014 Estonian Women's Health Questionnaire Survey indicated that 15.8% of the sexually active respondents at 18–44 years of age had experienced infertility, and 13.4% of them reported the use of in vitro fertilization (IVF) to have a child [1]. The proportion of births after IVF in Estonia is similar to the European average, which ranges from 2% to 4% [2]. It is important to obtain reliable data on the IVF status of a newborn to monitor IVF pregnancy outcomes and long-term health of children conceived by IVF. As there is currently no specialized country-wide assisted reproductive technology register in Estonia, sole information regarding IVF as a pregnancy risk factor (yes/ no) (defined as embryo transfer after conventional in vitro insemination or intracytoplasmic sperm injection [3]) is stored in each birth record of the Estonian Medical Birth Registry (EMBR).

The unique personal identification numbers (PINs) of the newborn and his/ her mother are registered in the EMBR and allow for record linkage [4]. The IVF status is recorded on the birth notification form by the mothers' self-report or using her antenatal chart. As a result, omissions are common because there is no routine information exchange between the EMBR and the infertility treatment clinics. However, IVF treatment is generously covered by the Estonian Health Insurance Fund (EHIF). Therefore, majority of the IVF procedures are recorded in the reimbursement database with women's PINs [5].

The previous study that estimated effectiveness and costs of IVF treatment in Estonia using linkage of the EMBR and EHIF records, reported 15.5% fewer IVF entries in the EMBR in 2006–2011 than were based on the EHIF data. A birth in the EMBR was considered an IVF birth if the embryo transfer procedure was performed within 42 weeks before delivery [6].

Current study aimed to assess the validity of registration of newborns' IVF status in the EMBR by linking the EMBR and EHIF records.

Methods

We assessed the validity of registration of newborns' IVF status in the EMBR by comparing information about it on the records of the EMBR and of the EHIF.

The EMBR, currently under the responsibility of the National Institute of Health Development, was established in 1991 and collects data on all infants born in Estonia [4, 7]. The hospitals with a maternity unit are obliged to notify births to the EMBR. A paper birth notification form is filled in for every newborn (live or stillbirth). This form includes the name, PIN, date of birth, ethnicity, education and place of residence of the mother and the father; the mother's marital status, reproductive history, pregnancy risk factors, complications during pregnancy and delivery, labor interventions, mode of delivery and birth plurality; the newborn's PIN, date of birth, gender, gestational age, birthweight, length, condition at birth, health indicators and status by the end of the first week. In the EMBR, data from birth notifications are key-entered and electronic records are created [8].

The EHIF, founded in 2001, is the only institution in Estonia that administers the national compulsory solidarity-based health insurance system [5]. The fund covers the costs of health services provided to insured persons, who constitute 95% of the Estonian population. The EHIF maintains an electronic health insurance database that consists of reimbursement claims for medical care. The reimbursement claims are sent to the EHIF electronically, the records in the database are stored at the individual level. Each record contains the name and PIN of the patient, medical diagnosis codes, provided service codes, service provider, amount requested for reimbursement and other associated information [9]. The age limit for IVF treatment covered by the EHIF was raised from 35 to 40 years in 2005, and unlimited number of IVF cycles is subsidized since 2008 [10].

The validity of registration of newborns' IVF status in the EMBR was measured by comparing the birth records in the EMBR and the corresponding embryo transfer records in the EHIF. Thus, the EHIF was treated as a reference. Individual records of the embryo transfers in 2004–2014 (earlier data were not available) including woman's PIN, date of the procedure and name of the clinic were obtained from the EHIF database (6208 women with 15,927 embryo transfers in all five clinics providing the service) (Fig. 1). The embryo transfers resulting in birth were identified via linkage of these records to the EMBR data using the mother's PIN as the key. As the EHIF data were available since 2004 and considering the age limit for IVF treatment, we selected the birth records in the period of 2005–2014 and maternal age was restricted to 40 years (146,526 infants born to Estonian residents).

We compared the date of embryo transfer with the date of the beginning of pregnancy (calculated by subtracting gestational age from the date of birth in the EMBR). The beginning of pregnancy after IVF (comparable to that of spontaneously conceived newborns) dates 2–3 weeks prior to the date of the embryo transfer [11, 12]. Thus, all births to mothers with date of the embryo transfer procedure within the pregnancy period were categorized as births after IVF.

Whereas the reimbursement claims of the EHIF may contain inaccuracies in documenting the date of the embryo transfer procedure, additional validation of the IVF status was undertaken in the infertility treatment clinics. In site visits, we wished to ascertain that embryo transfers performed during eight weeks before the beginning of pregnancy (by EHIF data), were not related to the pregnancies under study, and these newborns were spontaneously conceived after unsuccessful IVF treatment. Repeated embryo transfers, except the last one before the pregnancy that resulted in birth, were not taken into consideration. Thus, first, a list of eligible mothers (PIN, date of embryo transfer, pregnancy period, child's date of birth, the name of the clinic) was printed out. Second, in the infertility treatment clinics, the list of these mothers was visually compared with a screen output of their clinical data. As a result, IVF and non-IVF newborns were distinguished (Fig. 1). All births notified as after IVF but without corresponding embryo transfer record in the EHIF database were compared with paper birth notifications at the archives of the EMBR.

The validity of the IVF status in the EMBR was evaluated by determining the sensitivity, specificity, positive predictive value and negative predictive value, all often used in validation of health databases [13–16]. The sensitivity shows how accurately the IVF status has been recorded in the EMBR (true-positive cases divided by true-positive plus false-negative cases). The specificity demonstrates the ability of the EMBR to record non-IVF births (true negative cases divided by true-negative plus false-positive cases). The positive predictive value indicates how likely it is that the birth after IVF in the EMBR is registered correctly (true positive cases divided by true-positive plus false-positive cases). The negative predictive value reveals how likely is the non-IVF birth correct in the EMBR (true negative cases divided by true-negative plus false-negative cases).

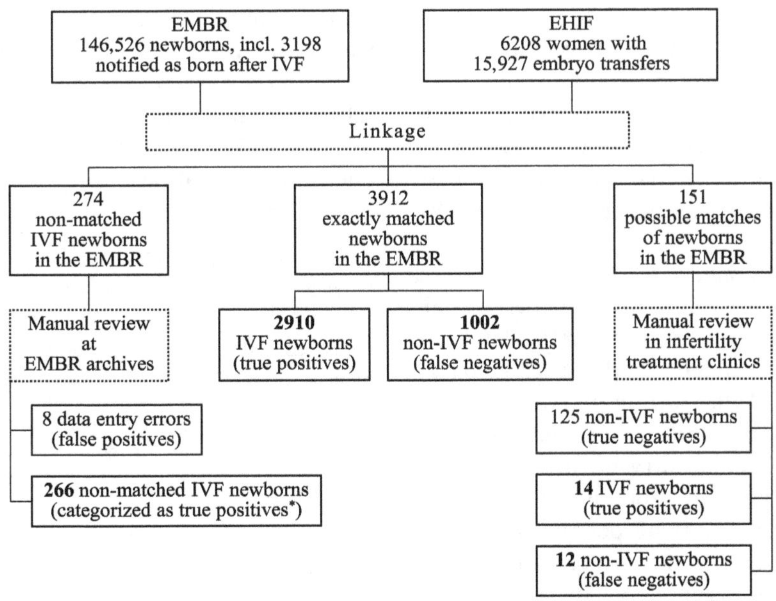

Fig. 1 Data collection process for estimation validity of IVF status registration in the Estonian Medical Birth Registry (EMBR), mothers aged ≤40 years, 2005–2014. Sum of the numbers formatted as bold gives the number of newborns conceived by IVF in the EMBR.
* Embryo transfers were not covered by the Estonian Health Insurance Fund (EHIF)

Additionally, we calculated the relative risks (prevalence proportion ratios; RR) with 95% confidence intervals (CI) of unrecorded IVF status among IVF mothers by available socio-demographic characteristics and birth plurality. Modified Poisson regression models (with a robust error variance) [17] included maternal age (< 35/ 35–40 years), education (higher/ secondary or less), ethnicity (Estonian/ non-Estonian), marital status (married/ other), and plurality (singleton/ multiple birth). Age group of 35–40 years, higher education, Estonian ethnicity, being married and multiple birth were selected as reference categories. In a separate model we tested whether the data quality on IVF status was higher if the infertility treatment and delivery occurred in the same clinic; on this occasion, 167 records with unknown data on the infertility treatment clinic were excluded.

Visual FoxPro 9.0 (Microsoft Corporation, Redmond, WA, USA) was used for database management and linkages, and Stata 14 (StataCorp LP, College Station, TX, USA) for validity calculations and statistical modeling.

Results

According to the EMBR data for 2005–2014, 3198 infants were born to mothers aged 40 years or less and identified as conceived by IVF. The record linkage with the EHIF database resulted in 3912 newborns in the EMBR with the corresponding embryo transfer record (the date of the embryo transfer procedure was within the pregnancy period), whereas 1002 of them were with unrecorded IVF status, i.e., erroneously categorized as conceived spontaneously (false negatives) (Fig. 1). Among them were 778 singletons, 230 twins and 6 triplets. From the 151 additional comparisons of birth records with the embryo transfer procedure before the beginning of pregnancy in the infertility treatment clinics, 14 newborns were verified as born after IVF (true positives) and 12 newborns notified with non-IVF status were found to be conceived by IVF (false negatives) (Fig. 1).

The record linkage revealed 274 newborns notified to be born after IVF in the EMBR with no corresponding embryo transfer record in the EHIF database. These records were examined at the EMBR paper archives and it was found that during data entry in the EMBR eight newborns have been incorrectly categorized as born after IVF (data entry errors; false positives) (Fig. 1). The rest of 266 newborns were categorized as born after IVF (true positives) as there could be a few IVF mothers who covered their treatment themselves (see Discussion). A total of 4204 infants born to 3435 mothers were verified as conceived by IVF; 1014 infants (24.1%) born to 895 mothers (26.1%) had lacked the IVF status on the birth record.

The 1014 false negative IVF entries resulted in poor sensitivity of the registration of IVF status (75.9%; 95% CI 74.6–77.2); specificity (100.0%), PPV (99.8%) and NPV (99.3%) were high (Table 1).

An unrecorded IVF status was significantly more common among mothers of younger age (< 35 years) or with non-Estonian ethnicity or with a singleton birth (Table 2). The misclassification did not depend on mother's education or marital status. We did not observe higher registration quality of IVF status if the infertility treatment and delivery occurred in the same clinic ("not the same" as reference: adjusted RR = 0.96; 95% CI 0.86–1.07).

Discussion

This study presents the results of the record linkages of the EMBR and the EHIF data to evaluate births following embryo transfer procedures. Although a decade ago the general data quality of the EMBR has been found to be acceptable [18], the currently estimated sensitivity of 75.9% of IVF status registration is worrying despite of high values of other validity measures.

Similarly, nearly a quarter of missing IVF entries was found in the Finnish Medical Birth Registry after linkage with insurance reimbursement files, drug prescriptions and IVF statistics [19]. Given that data from medical birth registries are often used to compare perinatal outcome and subsequent health of IVF babies with that of their counterparts conceived spontaneously [20–22], under-registration of IVF status biases effect measures.

The IVF status recorded on the antenatal chart is completed by the doctor or midwife at the first antenatal visit. The source of this information can be the electronic health record or self-report of the pregnant woman. In the cases where the IVF status is not mentioned on the antenatal chart, it is based on the mother's self-report after the delivery as "yes/ no" answer to the question: "Did you have IVF pregnancy?" However, the question is not always asked and the mother can refuse

Table 1 Number of IVF and non-IVF newborns in the Estonian Medical Birth Registry (EMBR) compared to the Estonian Health Insurance Fund (EHIF) data, and the IVF registration validity measures with 95% confidence intervals (CI), 2005–2014

EMBR	EHIF database (a reference)		
	IVF newborn	Non-IVF newborn	Total
IVF newborn	3190	8	3198
Non-IVF newborn	1014	142,314	143,328
Total	4204	142,322	146,526

Sensitivity (%) = 75.9 (95% CI 74.6–77.2)

Specificity (%) = 100.0 (95% CI 100.0–100.0)

Positive predictive value (%) = 99.8 (95% CI 99.5–99.9)

Negative predictive value (%) = 99.3 (95% CI 99.2–99.3)

Table 2 Relative risk (RR) with 95% confidence interval (CI) of unrecorded IVF status in the Estonian Medical Birth Registry by maternal characteristics, 2005–2014

Maternal characteristic	No. of IVF mothers		RR (95% CI)	
	Unrecorded IVF status	Total	Crude	Adjusted*
Age (years)				
< 35	587	2146	1.14 (1.02–1.29)	1.17 (1.04–1.32)
35–40	308	1289	1	1
Education				
Higher	483	1846	1	1
Secondary or less	412	1589	0.99 (0.89–1.11)	0.96 (0.86–1.08)
Ethnicity				
Estonian	627	2534	1	1
Non-Estonian	268	901	1.20 (1.06–1.36)	1.20 (1.06–1.36)
Marital status				
Married	500	1925	1	1
Other	395	1510	1.01 (0.90–1.13)	1.05 (0.93–1.18)
Plurality				
Singleton birth	778	2693	1.83 (1.54–2.19)	1.85 (1.55–2.21)
Multiple birth	117	742	1	1

*Adjusted for all other characteristics in the table

to reveal her IVF status. Additionally, if the abbreviation IVF is used, it may lead to misunderstanding. Expectedly, the IVF status was better registered among mothers aged 35–40 years, and mothers with multiple birth, because they were more likely to have IVF pregnancy and were more carefully questioned. The higher under-recording of IVF status among non-Estonians could be due to language or poor attention to the question in the clinics located in the regions with a high proportion of non-Estonians (northeastern Estonia). We found equally low-quality registration of IVF status when the birth occurred in the same clinic that performed IVF treatment, or when the birth took place in another clinic. This finding indicates that there is limited information exchange even between the departments of the same clinic. Thus, the validity of the IVF entries in the EMBR has so far relied on self-report of mothers and on the accuracy of the medical personnel when completing the antenatal chart.

However, there were 266 records of the newborns after IVF in the EMBR with no corresponding embryo transfer record in the EHIF database verifying the IVF status. We had no reason to classify them as non-IVF newborns (false positives) as their mothers could have paid for the treatment themselves because they did not have health insurance; or because of a will to have out-of-pocket service; or because they have used IVF services in other countries; or because only the limited number of IVF cycles were covered by the EHIF prior to 2008 [10]. On the other hand, we cannot deny that among newborns notified in the EMBR as spontaneously conceived could be a few newborns after IVF (false negatives). On this occasion, mothers who have had out-of-pocket service have not disclosed their IVF status. Even so, very small number of these cases would not change the results notably.

The previous linkage study [6] with somewhat different methodology (incorporating maternal age above 40 in the EMBR, not considering individual length of gestation, and without verification of an uncertain IVF status in the infertility treatment clinics) and covering shorter period, found 15.5% fewer newborns after IVF in the EMBR than were expected from the EHIF data. This estimate was much smaller than the percentage of unrecorded IVF entries in the EMBR in the current study. It should be noticed, that in the previous study, only the difference in the number of newborns after IVF based on the EHIF data and the number of newborns after IVF in the EMBR were compared not considering individual unrecorded IVF entries in the EMBR. These outcomes of the two studies would have been of the same magnitude if all newborns after IVF in the EMBR were reflected in the EHIF database. The discrepancy is explained by the number of newborns after IVF in the EMBR with no confirming record in the EHIF database.

Conclusions

It is difficult to obtain complete data for newborns' IVF status in the EMBR by exclusively relying on mother's self-reported information or her antenatal chart. As far as we do not have a specialized country-wide assisted reproductive technology database in Estonia, the routine linkages between the EMBR, the EHIF database, and data from infertility treatment clinics would be helpful. Furthermore, collecting valid data for IVF pregnancies is important due to the common use of assisted reproductive technology [23]. The increasing number of digital health databases gives better than ever possibilities for additional data quality control. Electronic record linkages between databases would help considerably to improve the validity of data to be used in medical decision making, in research and for statistical purposes.

Abbreviations

CI: confidence interval; EHIF: Estonian Health Insurance Fund; EMBR: Estonian Medical Birth Registry; IVF: in vitro fertilization; PIN: personal identification number; RR: relative risk

Acknowledgements

We acknowledge Helis Puksand from the EHIF, Tiina Loog from the East-Tallinn Central Hospital, Aivar Ehrenberg from the Tartu University Hospital, Merike Seer from the Nova Vita Clinic and Andrei Sõritsa from the Elite Clinic for their advice and assistance.

Funding

The authors had no specific funding for this study. KR and MR were salaried by the grant IUT5-1 and HK by the grant IUT34-16 from the Estonian Research Council.

Authors' contributions

HK, KA, KR and MR conceived and designed the study; KA, KH and KR prepared the data; KR and MR analyzed the data; KA, KR and MR drafted the manuscript; all authors contributed to the interpretation of findings, revised the manuscript critically and approved the final version of the manuscript.

Competing interests

The authors declare that they have no competing interests.

Author details

[1]Estonian Medical Birth Registry, National Institute for Health Development, Hiiu 42, 11619 Tallinn, Estonia. [2]Department of Epidemiology and Biostatistics, National Institute for Health Development, Hiiu 42, 11619 Tallinn, Estonia. [3]Centre for Reproductive Medicine, West Tallinn Central Hospital Women's Clinic, Sõle 23, 10614 Tallinn, Estonia. [4]Department of Obstetrics and Gynecology, Institute of Clinical Medicine, University of Tartu, L. Puusepa 8, 51014 Tartu, Estonia. [5]Tartu University Hospital's Women's Clinic, L. Puusepa 8, 51014 Tartu, Estonia.

References

1. Lippus H, Laanpere M, Part K, Ringmets I, Rahu M, Haldre K, et al. Eesti Naiste Tervis 2014: seksuaal- ja reproduktiivtervis, tervisekäitumine, hoiakud ja terviseteenuste kasutamine. Uurimisaruanne – Estonian Women's Health 2014: sexual and reproductive health, health behaviour, attitudes and use of healthcare services. Survey report. Tartu: University of Tartu; 2015. Available https://sisu.ut.ee/sites/default/files/naisteterviseuuring/files/uusestre2014_loppraport.pdf. Accessed 22 June 2018.
2. Euro-Peristat Project with SCPE and EUROCAT. European Perinatal Health Report. In: The health and care of pregnant women and babies in Europe in 2010; 2013. Available http://www.europeristat.com. Accessed 22 June 2018.
3. Zegers-Hochschild F, Adamson GD, Dyer S, Racowsky C, de Mouzon J, Sokol R, et al. The International Glossary on Infertility and Fertility Care, 2017. Hum Reprod. 2017;32:1786–801.
4. Karro H, Rahu M, Gornoi K, Baburin A. Estonian medical birth registry 1992–1995: association of risk factors with perinatal mortality. Eur J Obstet Gynecol Reprod Biol. 1998;80:151–6.
5. Lai T, Habicht T, Kahur K, Reinap M, Kiivet R, van Ginneken E. Estonia: health system review. Health Syst Transit. 2013;15:1–196.
6. Tonsiver T, Ehrenberg A, Ringmets I, Saare K, Lepik K, Kiivet RA. Kehavälise viljastamise efektiivsus ja kulud Eestis. In: Effectiveness and costs of in vitro fertilization (IVF) in Estonia. Tartu: Tartu Ülikooli tervishoiu instituut; 2013. (in Estonian).
7. Koupilova I, Rahu K, Rahu M, Karro H, Leon DA. Social determinants of birthweight and length of gestation in Estonia during the transition to democracy. Int J Epidemiol. 2000;29:118–24.
8. National Institute for Health Development. Estonian Medical Birth Registry and Estonian Abortion Registry. http://www.tai.ee/en/r-and-d/registers/estonian-medical-birth-registry-and-estonian-abortion-registry. Accessed 22 June 2018.
9. The Estonian Health Insurance Fund (EHIF). The organisation. https://www.haigekassa.ee/en/organisation. Accessed 11 June 2018.
10. Eesti Haigekassa tervishoiuteenuste loetelu. [List of healthcare services of the Estonian Health Insurance Fund.] RT I 2005, 4, 13 (in Estonian).
11. Tunón K, Eik-Nes SH, Grøttum P, von Düring V, Kahn JA. Gestational age in pregnancies conceived after in vitro fertilization: a comparison between age assessed from oocyte retrieval, crown-rump length and biparietal diameter. Ultrasound Obstet Gynecol. 2000;15:41–6.
12. Koudstaal J, Braat DDM, Bruinse HW, Naaktgeboren N, Vermeiden JPW, Visser GHA. Obstetric outcome of singleton pregnancies after IVF: a matched control study in four Dutch university hospitals. Hum Reprod. 2000;15:1819–25.
13. Feldman AL, Johansson ALV, Gatz M, Flensburg M, Petzinger GM, Widner H, et al. Accuracy and sensitivity of Parkinsonian disorder diagnoses in two Swedish national health registers. Neuroepidemiology. 2012;38:186–93.
14. McCormick N, Lacaille D, Bhole V, Avina-Zubieta JA. Validity of myocardial infarction diagnoses in administrative databases: a systematic review. PLoS One. 2014;9:e92286.
15. Thomsen MK, Njor SH, Rasmussen M, Linnemann D, Andersen B, Baatrup G, et al. Validity of data in the Danish Colorectal Cancer Screening Database. Clin Epidemiol. 2017;9:105–11.
16. Kleif J, Thygesen LC, Gögenur I. Validity of the diagnosis of appendicitis in the Danish National Patient Register. Scand J Public Health. 2018; (in press)
17. Zou G. A modified Poisson regression approach to prospective studies with binary data. Am J Epidemiol. 2004;159:702–6.
18. Vorobjov S, Rahu M, Rahu K, Karro H. Eesti Meditsiinilise Sünniregistri andmete kvaliteet. [Data quality in the Estonian Medical Birth Registry.]. Eesti Arst. 2008;87:608–14. (in Estonian)
19. Gissler M, Klemetti R, Sevón T, Hemminki E. Monitoring of IVF births outcomes in Finland: a data quality study. BMC Med Inform Decis Mak. 2004;4:3.
20. Räisänen S, Randell K, Nielsen HS, Gissler M, Kramer MR, Klemetti R, et al. Socioeconomic status affects the prevalence, but not the perinatal outcomes, of in vitro fertilization pregnancies. Hum Reprod. 2013;28:3118–25.
21. Davies MJ, Rumbold AR, Marino JL, Willson K, Giles LC, Whitrow MJ, et al. Maternal factors and the risk of birth defects after IVF and ICSI: a whole of population cohort study. BJOG. 2017;124:1537–44.
22. Delnord M, Szamotulska K, Hindori-Mohangoo AD, Blondel B, Macfarlane AJ, Dattani N, et al. Linking databases on perinatal health: a review of the literature and current practices in Europe. Eur J Pub Health. 2016;26:422–30.

7

Healthcare provider-patient communication: a qualitative study of women's perceptions during childbirth

Precious Madula[1,2*], Fatch Welcome Kalembo[2], Hong Yu[1] and Atipatsa Chiwanda Kaminga[2]

Abstract

Background: There is limited information on the impact of effective healthcare provider-patient communication on facility-based delivery in Malawi. The purpose of this study was to examine the nature of communication in the maternity ward, identify facilitators and barriers to healthcare provider-patient communication, and understand how they affect maternal healthcare.

Methods: This was a descriptive study that used qualitative data collection and analysis methods. Data were collected through face-to-face in-depth interviews using a semi-structured interview guide to collect information about women's perceptions of their communication with healthcare providers. A total of 30 in-depth interviews were conducted with women admitted for delivery in six health facilities drawn from three administrative regions in Malawi. The information collected focused on the communication that pregnant women had with healthcare providers, their perception of that communication, and the barriers to effective communication. A thematic approach was used for data analysis.

Results: The main themes that emerged regarding the nature of communication between healthcare providers and patients were: 1) good healthcare provider-patient interaction; 2) verbal abuse and lack of respect; 3) failure by healthcare providers to answer or entertain questions; 4) linguistic barriers to communication and lack of competency in non-verbal communication; and 5) discrimination due to one's status.

Conclusion: This study has revealed the existence of some communication barriers such as disrespecting and verbally abusing pregnant women, language limitations by some healthcare providers and discrimination due to one's status which are affecting maternal service delivery in some health facilities in Malawi. The study has also shown that pregnant women who are happy with the way healthcare providers communicate with them have the motivation to deliver at a health facility. There is a need, therefore, to develop an intervention that could help healthcare providers to communicate better with their patients.

Keywords: Maternal mortality, Communication, Pregnant women, Traditional birth attendants, Skilled birth attendant, Health facility

* Correspondence: preciousmadula@yahoo.co.uk
[1]School of Journalism and Information Communication, Huazhong University of Science and Technology, 1037 Luoyu, Road, Wuhan 430074, People's Republic of China
[2]Mzuzu University, Private Bag 201, Luwinga, Mzuzu 2, Malawi

Plain English summary

Effective healthcare provider-patient communication is a key element in optimal maternal service delivery. In order to build a good relationship, there is a need for healthcare providers and patients to communicate effectively. When there is positive communication between healthcare providers and women in the maternity ward, women are encouraged to utilise maternal services at a health facility. On the other hand, poor patient-healthcare provider communication results in some pregnant women deciding not to deliver at a health facility with skilled attendance in favour of delivery with a traditional birth attendant (TBA) or delivery at home, which might lead to pregnancy complications and maternal mortality. It has been reported that some healthcare providers in Malawi communicate poorly with their patients. We, therefore, conducted this study in order to examine the nature of communication in the maternity ward between healthcare providers and their patients. The study has revealed that some healthcare providers communicate poorly with pregnant women in the maternity ward. There is, therefore, a need to develop an intervention which could help healthcare providers to improve their communication to better serve women in the maternity ward.

Background

In order to build a positive relationship between healthcare providers and patients, there is a need for the existence of effective healthcare provider-patient communication. This will help to ensure that all parties involved are able to listen to each other and fully understand what is being said [1]. Effective healthcare provider-patient communication can be facilitated by healthcare provider behaviours such as establishing a positive rapport by avoiding shouting and rudeness, encouraging two-way dialogue, bridging any social gaps between healthcare providers and patients, effectively using both verbal and non-verbal communication, allowing patients ample time to tell their sickness story and exhibiting positive attitudes when talking to patients [2]. Lack of effective communication between healthcare providers and patients can result in negative health outcomes. For instance, a study in rural Zimbabwe showed that rudeness, unfriendly and abusive behaviour by nurses discouraged pregnant women from accessing maternal services at a healthy facility, a major contributor to maternal mortality and pregnancy complications [3].

Healthcare provider-patient communication is a fundamental component in effective maternal service delivery [4]. Alongside expertise, effective healthcare provider-patient communication is a prerequisite to building a therapeutic healthcare provider-patient relationship [5, 6]. Thus, a good relationship between health workers and pregnant women remains an important precursor in encouraging pregnant women to utilise maternal services at a health facility [7]. Furthermore, "where effective communication prevails between patients and healthcare providers, immediate outcomes include patient satisfaction and information recall; intermediate variables include adherence to recommendations; and long-term outcomes include changes in health status or lifestyle" [8].

Empirical data indicate that in health care settings, effective interactions between healthcare providers and patients are essential for a shared understanding of the feelings and symptoms experienced by patients as well as the goals of the provider [9]. Effective communication is particularly important in the provision of maternal services because labour and birth are vulnerable and stressful times where lapses in communication can result in health complications, failure to access health facilities for maternal services and, in worst case scenarios, maternal mortality [10, 11].

In Malawi, a number of studies have reported about poor communication between some healthcare providers and pregnant women [4, 7, 12]. Poor communication may be one of the contributing factors to maternal deaths and complications that are experienced in Malawi. According to a World Health Organisation (WHO) (2016) report, approximately 830 women die every day from preventable causes related to pregnancy and childbirth around the world [10]. Ninety-nine per cent of all maternal deaths occur in low and middle-income countries, and maternal mortality is higher (546 deaths per 100,000 livebirths) in women living in rural areas and among the poor - 511 deaths per 100,000 livebirths in urban areas and 652 deaths per 100,000 livebirths in rural areas [10]. Malawi is a low-income country where the maternal mortality rate is estimated at 439 deaths per 100, 000 births [13] and the neonatal mortality rate is 31 per 1000 live births with skilled attendance [4].The current maternal mortality rate is very high compared to the target of Sustainable Development Goal number 3 which aims to reduce the global maternal mortality ratio to less than 70 per 100,000 live births by 2030 [http://www.who.int/en/news-room/fact-sheets/detail/maternal-mortality].

WHO [http://www.who.int/en/news-room/fact-sheets/detail/maternal-mortality], asserts that in Sub-Saharan Africa and South Asia, women in rural areas do not receive adequate health care due to the low number of skilled health workers and that lack of information is one of the factors that prevent women from receiving or seeking care during pregnancy and childbirth. Better healthcare provider-patient communication could mitigate some pregnancy-related problems and complications.

Reduction of maternal mortality is a global health priority, and one way to combat maternal and pregnancy complications is by encouraging pregnant women to use maternal health services. Research that was conducted in Chikhwawa and Mangochi in southern Malawi, indicates that women are dissuaded from utilising maternal services offered by skilled healthcare providers because of rudeness, insults and disrespect by some health personnel [14, 15]. This clearly demonstrates that despite the existing policy of the Malawi Government encouraging all women to deliver in health facilities where they can be cared for by skilled attendants, not all pregnant women do. Poor attitudes and behaviours by health workers are one of the documented reasons why some women may not choose to deliver at a health facility [4]. There is a need for healthcare providers to ensure that they conduct themselves in a manner that will motivate women to utilise professional maternal health services [16]. Good communication with pregnant women could be one of the ways of persuading them to deliver at a health facility in line with the government policy. The objective of this study was therefore, to explore the nature of communication between healthcare providers and pregnant women in some hospitals in Malawi with the view to establishing whether communication is one of the reasons behind women's choice to deliver at a health facility or not.

Methods

Setting

Malawi is an African country located in Southern Africa. It is a member state of Southern African Development Community (SADC). It is bordered by Tanzania on the northern and eastern sides, Mozambique on the eastern, southern and south-western sides and Zambia on the western side. The World Bank estimated that the population of Malawi in 2016 was 18.2 million [17]. The country is divided into three administrative regions, namely Northern, Central, and Southern Regions. These regions exhibit great diversity in socio-economic, cultural, and geographical features. Each region has a city; Lilongwe in the Central Region, Blantyre in the Southern Region, and Mzuzu in the Northern Region. The population of Lilongwe is estimated at 1.2 million people. Blantyre has about 1 million people whereas Mzuzu is estimated to have a population of approximately about 300, 000 people [18, 19].

Healthcare in Malawi is primarily delivered by two sectors; the government run public sector, and the private sector, which includes the Christian Health Association of Malawi (CHAM) and other private providers [20]. The Government provides 60%, the CHAM 37%, and the other private providers the remaining 3% [20] http://www.cham.org.mw. Healthcare facilities in the country are organised into three tiers: primary, secondary, and tertiary [21]. The levels are linked through a referral system [21]. At the primary level, healthcare is provided through community-based outreach programmes, dispensaries, health posts, healthcare centres and community hospitals. The primary level facilities refer obstetric emergencies and patients requiring inpatient medical, surgical or paediatric care to secondary level facilities. Secondary level care is provided through district hospitals (for the public sector) and CHAM hospitals (for the private sector). Patients who require special care from the secondary level facilities are referred to tertiary level facilities [21]. The tertiary healthcare service is provided by four central hospitals with two in the Southern Region (Queen Elizabeth and Zomba Central Hospitals), one in the Centre (Kamuzu Central Hospital) and another in the Northern Region (Mzuzu Central Hospital) [20]. The tertiary hospital in each region caters for all primary and secondary level facilities for that particular region. Each of the three tertiary public hospitals included in this study, provides specialist referral services including obstetrics and gynaecology for their respective regions.

Data were collected from three tertiary hospitals and three private hospitals located in the three administrative regions of the country. One tertiary hospital and one private hospital were identified as research sites in each region. Although the three private hospitals are not as big as the government tertiary hospitals, they provide specialised obstetric and gynaecological care but for a fee.

Study design, and study participants

The study was a descriptive qualitative study that used a semi-structured interview guide. The qualitative research design was chosen because it was important to hear the views and experiences of pregnant women and those who had just given birth in their own words on what they feel about patient-healthcare provider communication that they had experienced in the maternity ward. We collected data through interviews with women admitted to six tertiary hospitals (three government and three CHAM hospitals also referred to as public and private health facilities respectively) drawn from three administrative regions of Malawi (Northern, Central and Southern). We conducted 30 interviews across the three regions of Malawi, with five interviews conducted per hospital. Data collection started in the Southern Region, then Central Region before winding up in the Northern Region. Saturation was reached within the first 19 interviews, but we still completed the remaining 11 interviews in order to obtain sample heterogeneity [22]. Participants were heterogenous because they were recruited from hospitals and regions that exhibit great diversity in cultural, geographical, historical, political, and religious background. Saturation level of data was considered to have been reached if there was no new information arising from the interviews [16].

The six hospitals were selected as research sites for the following reasons: 1) to obtain a deep understanding of women's perception of their communication with healthcare providers in the maternity ward given the fact that women who are admitted to these hospitals tend to have complications with their pregnancies and are likely to be engaged in deep and long conversation with healthcare providers; 2) to achieve a good representation of participants from all the three administrative regions of the country that could help to provide a deep understanding of women's perception of healthcare provider-patient communication in the maternity wards in Malawi; and 3) to compare the perception of women regarding their communication with healthcare providers between public and private healthcare systems in Malawi. Participants were recruited in the study if they were 18 years or older (the legal age to provide consent to participate in a study in Malawi); were admitted to maternity ward at the participating hospital; had given birth at the participating hospital within 5 days of the interview, regardless of their mode of delivery; and if they were able to give consent.

Data collection procedure

Following approval from the management of the hospitals, the principal researcher approached midwives working in the maternity ward to start the recruitment process. We anticipated that many women would be willing to participate in the study. However, we only needed a limited number of participants per hospital. As such, we used systematic random sampling using admission numbers to recruit study participants. Normally women admitted to the maternity ward in Malawi are given admission numbers. The first person to be admitted is assigned one, and the last person is assigned the last number according to the number of people admitted to the ward on that particular day. We recruited five women with the first five odd admission numbers per hospital. The principal researcher conducted all the interviews while the women were still admitted to the health facility. The interviews were conducted in a separate room where nobody could hear the conversation between the researcher and the participant. In addition, all interviews were conducted after working hours (after 4.30 p.m) when the women were not being seen by doctors or midwives. On average, each interview took 30–50 min to be completed. The interviews were conducted in the Malawian local language (Chichewa). During the interviews, follow-up questions using probes were asked in order to acquire deeper understanding when an explanation provided by the interviewee was unclear or ambiguous. Data were collected between February and March, 2017.

Study instrument

An interview guide was developed in Chichewa through review of literature. The guide was piloted with five maternity patients at a hospital which did not participate in the main study. The interview guide had questions that focussed on: (a) patients' communication with healthcare providers; (b) the perception of patients on their communication with their healthcare providers; and (c) barriers to effective communication between patients and healthcare providers. The principal researcher (a doctoral student) interviewed all the participants and where necessary, he asked further probing questions in line with the participants' answers in order to gain more clarity on the issue and obtain as much information as possible. All interviews were digitally recorded and transcribed verbatim.

Data analysis

A thematic analysis of the interviews was conducted to generate an understanding of how women in the maternity ward perceived their communication with healthcare providers. This was done in accordance with Braun and Clarke's [23] six steps of thematic analysis. The six steps include: 1) familiarisation with data; 2) initial coding; 3) searching for themes; 4) reviewing themes; 5) defining and naming themes; and 6) writing up the research report. Prior to data analysis, the recorded interviews were transcribed by the research team in Chichewa before being translated into English. The principal researcher verified the transcriptions by reading them while listening to the recordings and any identified errors were corrected. To ensure that no original meaning was lost in the translation process, an expert translator was involved in order to check both the recordings and transcripts. Inductive thematic analysis was employed in this study since the analysis was based on what the participants reported during the interviews. The principal researcher developed a list of codes from the transcript which were discussed with members of the research team. The research team had several meetings during which they discussed and verified if the codes were coming from the transcription. Thereafter, the research team identified extracts and themes captured by the codes.

Ethical consideration

Ethical approval for the study was granted by the National Commission for Science and Technology (Protocol PO1/17/153). A written permission to conduct the study at each of the six health facilities was also obtained from the Hospital Directors and officers responsible for research activities at each institution. All participants were informed about the purpose of the study and only participated after providing informed consent. Literate participants signed consent forms while a thumbprint was used for those who were illiterate. Since participation was voluntary, participants were free to withdraw from the study at any time without facing any penalties. All participants were assured that anonymity would be observed at all times.

Results

Demographic characteristics

Thirty in-depth interviews were conducted. The majority of participants were married ($n = 25$) and over half ($n = 16$) of participants had received secondary education or higher. There were five participants from each health facility. Table 1 provides the demographic characteristics of the participants.

Identified themes

The following themes were identified through thematic analysis: good healthcare provider-patient interaction, verbal abuse and lack of respect by healthcare providers, failure by healthcare providers to answer questions or entertain questions from clients, linguistic barriers to communication and lack of competency in non-verbal communication, attitudes of some healthcare providers, and discrimination due to one's status. The results of the study indicate that generally some women admitted to the maternity wards in both public and private hospitals had good communication with healthcare workers. The study also shows that verbal abuse and lack of respect by healthcare providers were frequently reported by the participants recruited from both types of health facilities.

Table 1 Demographic characteristics of the participants ($N = 30$)

Variable Name	Total number of participants	Percentage of participants
Name of health facility		
Public hospital in Central Region	5	16.7
Public hospital in Southern Region	5	16.7
Public hospital in Northern Region	5	16.7
Private hospital in Southern Region	5	16.7
Private hospital in Central Region	5	16.7
Private hospital in Northern Region	5	16.7
Age range		
18–25	14	47
26–40	16	53
Marital Status		
Single	4	13.3
Married	25	83.3
Widowed	1	3.3
Educational Qualification		
No formal education	8	26.7
Primary education	6	20
Secondary education	12	40
Tertiary education	4	13.3

Good healthcare provider-patient interaction

Half of the participants, from both public and private health facilities, indicated that healthcare providers were very good and treated them with warmth, sympathy and respect. They even indicated that they were very happy and impressed with the way healthcare providers were communicating with them. One participant in a post-natal ward had this to say:

> *"I have been at this hospital for two weeks now. I came here well in advance to wait for my labour. I delivered three days ago. My child has a minor complication, and that's why I am still here. Honestly, the nurses and midwives I have been dealing with here are very friendly, loving and talk to me in a good manner. Before coming here, I was told that some nurses are rude and that they shout at patients but for me all has been well, and I have been well taken care of. I am very satisfied with the relationship I am having with the nurses here. This is my first pregnancy, but next time I fall pregnant again, I will certainly come back and deliver here"* (A woman who recently delivered at a public hospital)

From the above discourse, it can clearly be seen that the participant was absolutely happy with her experience at the health facility not just because of the medical care she was given, but also because of the way the nurses and midwives interacted with and treated her. Surprisingly, some participants from private health facilities complained that their communication with healthcare providers was not good. From the outset, the lead researcher's experience was that participants in private health facilities, where fees are paid for treatment, would have mostly positive perceptions of their communication with healthcare providers. However, this was not the case. Some participants in both public and private health facilities indicated that their communication with healthcare providers was poor.

Verbal abuse and lack of respect

About half of the participants from both government and private health facilities said that some midwives and nurses abused them verbally. They indicated that this abuse was generally in the form of scolding and shouting at them. None of the participants however, did not explain why they were abused. The majority of the participants who complained about verbal abuse and lack of respect were from public health facilities. Only a few participants from private health facilities described the abuse, but their complaints showed a serious degree of verbal abuse and lack of respect. One participant in a labour ward at a private health facility had this to say:

> *"Midwives and nurses shout at us and talk to us in a rude manner. At times they talk to us in a mocking manner and use words as if we are children. And when we fail to follow instructions, they shout at us instead of just talking to us in a normal way or correcting the mistake that we have made. I really don't like such nurses, and it makes me wonder whether I do come at this hospital just to be ridiculed. One day I experienced a nasty thing. There was a pregnant woman who was in labour. She called the midwife on duty for help. Sadly, instead of the midwife coming to help she just yelled at her. My friend and I had to go and help her deliver. By the grace of God, she managed to deliver a bouncing baby boy. But I don't feel happy here. What is happening here is not good. Being a private hospital, we pay a lot of money and expect good services. Sadly we are being given a raw deal. Next time I will never come here again"* (A woman waiting to deliver at a private hospital)

It is apparent that the patient was very frustrated with the services offered, no wonder she expressed the above sentiments.

More than half of the participants from both the public and private health facilities indicated that some healthcare providers were rude, disrespectful and acted towards them and indeed talked to them as if they were children. One participant in a labour ward said this:

> *"Sometimes when they are talking to us, some nurses talk as if they are talking to kids. Whenever they give us some instruction, and we fail to act accordingly, they talk to us in a rude manner, using demeaning and derogatory words. They also look at us as if we are stupid and don't deserve their time. Their tone of talking does not even show respect, and it clearly shows that they don't care about us nor do they have respect for us. This is bad because we expect them to show a caring heart and correct us in a good manner when we make mistakes".* (A woman waiting to deliver at a private hospital)

Failure by midwives and nurses to answer some questions or entertain more questions from pregnant women

The majority of the participants in both public and private health facilities indicated that generally the nurses and midwives did not give them a chance or enough time to ask some questions about subjects or issues they do not understand concerning their pregnancy. When asked why they thought healthcare providers behaved in this way, the majority of the respondents said they suspected the healthcare providers feared the workload of being bombarded by inquisitive patients if they were generous in entertaining questions. One respondent at a public health facility said the following:

> *"Nurses do not help us when we want extra information on what they normally give us. Whenever we try to ask questions, the nurse just looks away and does not even attend to us. Sometimes the nurse pretends as if she or he did not hear our questions. So yea, it's pretty frustrating to fail to get crucial information from the experts who are supposed to attend to us and meet all our needs"* (A woman waiting to deliver at a public hospital).

Linguistic barriers to communication and lack of competency in non-verbal communication

Our analysis also revealed that language is another barrier to effective communication between some healthcare providers and pregnant women in Malawi. This is particularly true in multilingual health facilities where healthcare providers and patients speak different languages. For instance, some participants at a public health facility in Mzuzu in the Northern Region of Malawi, indicated that they would have been more comfortable if most of the healthcare providers were proficient in the region's lingua franca (Chitumbuka) even though they accepted that most of the healthcare providers communicated with them in a positive and polite manner. One participant in a post-natal ward made the following statement:

> *"The nurses at this hospital are good and talk to us in a polite manner. I only have problems with nurses who do not speak Chitumbuka because we can't communicate effectively since my Chichewa is very bad, and I can't speak English either"* (A woman who recently delivered at a public hospital).

Furthermore, the study has also revealed the problems that healthcare providers face when dealing with pregnant women who can only communicate using sign language. In this study, one of the respondents in a post-natal ward at a public health facility had speech-impairment but could hear and write. She noted that most of the healthcare providers treated her in a polite, friendly and caring manner. She also indicated that sometimes she uses her relative to translate sign language if she cannot write her responses for the healthcare providers. However, she bemoaned lack of sign language expertise by healthcare providers. She described the following:

> *"Generally, I can't say that healthcare providers mistreat me nor talk to me in an impolite or unfriendly manner. They have all been good. But my biggest concern is that all the nurses I have been interacting with do not possess any knowledge of the sign language which I use, so if I can't have a chance to write down what I want to say I don't think I can manage to communicate with them. How I wish hospitals had experts in sign language who could attend to us!"* (A woman who recently delivered at a public hospital)

Discrimination due to one's status

A few participants from the public health facilities said that some healthcare providers discriminate against patients who are poor or come from rural areas. Participants from the private health facilities did not indicate that healthcare providers were discriminatory. That was not surprising because there were fewer poor patients in facilities where patients pay in order to access health services. Those participants who talked about discrimination indicated that some healthcare providers changed the way they communicated depending on the person they were talking to. They said that healthcare providers sometimes shouted and used demeaning words when addressing poor patients and chose a more respectful way of communicating when talking to patients from urban areas. A participant who came from a rural area shared the following:

> *"The nurses here discriminate against us and have a negative attitude towards us poor people. Every time they want to talk to us, they shout and use threats like... "If you continue behaving the way you are I will not help you. You are not the only one, I deal with many people here. Do you think I have time to waste with you?" On the contrary, they do not do the same when they are talking to pregnant women from urban areas"* (A woman waiting to deliver at a government hospital).

The theme of discrimination due to one's status also dominated the interviews with illiterate women in the public hospitals. There were no illiterate participants from the private health facilities, so the theme did not emerge there. Some participants in the public health facilities felt that they were failing to understand simple instructions or very basic information because of their illiteracy and that the healthcare providers were discriminating against them by not recognising the need to help them understand. This could explain why some healthcare providers were not willing to entertain questions from some patients if they were not recognising whether patients had not understood instructions or information. One participant had this to say:

> *"I did not go to school, so sometimes I don't understand what the nurses are saying. It is even worse when the nurse mixes English and Chichewa in her discourse. Now the frustrating thing is that when I want to ask for clarification, I am shouted at and at times stopped or denied any opportunity to ask questions. This is why in my first pregnancy I decided to deliver at a TBA because there she never shouted at me. She was more caring than the nurses here who take advantage of our illiteracy"* (A woman who recently delivered at a public hospital).

Discussion

This study has explored factors that can both facilitate and inhibit effective communication between healthcare providers and women in the maternity ward. The factor that is facilitating communication between healthcare providers and patients is good interaction which entails providers treating patients with warmth, sympathy and respect. On the other hand, factors that inhibit healthcare provider-patient communication include healthcare provider's verbal abuse of women, failure by healthcare providers to take questions from maternity patients, linguistic barriers and poor quality of non-verbal communication, and discrimination due to one's status. Furthermore, the study has also revealed that both private and public hospitals in Malawi have some healthcare providers who communicate poorly with their patients.

The study identified healthcare providers' good attitude and behaviour by some healthcare providers in both private and public health facilities as one of the effective facilitators in the provider-patient communication. This study has shown that women who experienced good communication at a health facility appreciated the maternal services and were satisfied. They were even committed to returning to the same hospital facility for their next delivery. Interestingly, some respondents at a private health facility indicated that some healthcare providers had a bad attitude and communicated to them poorly. This was a surprising finding because one might expect a better quality of service in private hospitals where patients pay a fee to access healthcare services. Those participants described their lack of desire to utilise that health facility again in future. This finding is similar to previous research that indicates that good provider-patient communication is the bedrock for patient satisfaction [24–26]. The more a patient is satisfied, the more likely she will utilise maternal services, follow instructions and adhere to all treatment regimens [27].

Another finding in this study is that many healthcare providers in public health facilities and some in private health facilities disrespect patients by talking to them rudely and shouting at them. This finding is consistent with other studies in Malawi which found that some health workers are impolite, rude, and shout at patients, which consequently dissuades pregnant women from delivering at health facilities where they can be helped by a skilled birth attendant [4, 7, 14, 28–30].

In addition, this study also supports the finding of Mtotha [12] which showed that some healthcare providers are negligent in their duty of care and instead of providing support they shout at women in labour. In the current study, no participant from public health facilities complained about being neglected by healthcare providers. On the contrary, it was reported that at one private hospital a skilled health worker did not assist and shouted at a patient who was about to give birth. Such behaviour is unacceptable, could have resulted in serious complications and will likely discourage women from seeking maternal services at health facilities [7, 28–30]. Previous research has shown that delivery with the assistance of professional health providers can shorten the length of labour, lower rates of intervention such as caesarean section and instrumental deliveries, lower levels of reported pain and increase maternal satisfaction [31–34].

This study also established that some healthcare providers discriminate against patients due to social status and place of residence. Discrimination was only mentioned by pregnant women in public health facilities. This discrimination is counterproductive and is likely to discourage patients from rural areas from accessing maternal service at a health facility. Even though all participants in this study appreciated the need for a pregnant woman to access maternal service at a health facility, some participants said that they would consider seeking help from a TBA if they knew that a healthcare provider would not treat them with respect and dignity. This finding is consistent with the findings from a study that was conducted in Nigeria that indicated that discrimination due to one's ethnicity, literacy level and place of residence was contributing to the low proportion of births supervised by skilled birth attendants [35–37]. To change the current status, there is an urgent need to remove any form of discrimination by healthcare providers so that they are able to effectively communicate with their patients. Frequent supportive supervision of healthcare providers and provision of refresher courses on communication skills can also greatly help to improve healthcare provider-patient communication.

Discrimination due to one's status was also observed in the way healthcare providers communicate with illiterate patients in public health facilities. No participant from the private health facilities was illiterate in our sample. Some participants reported that they sometimes fail to grasp information from the healthcare providers due to illiteracy. Unfortunately, they said that when they tried to ask questions to better understand what was being communicated to them, some healthcare providers did not give them the opportunity to ask questions or seek clarification. This widens the information gap. It is important for healthcare providers to exercise empathy and provide information to all patients regardless of their education levels. This finding is in agreement with another study that was conducted in Mangochi, Malawi which revealed that the education gap between healthcare providers and patients was one of the barriers in accessing maternal services [7]. To address this, healthcare providers should strive to increase patients' understanding of their own health needs because there is a direct correlation between understanding and compliance. Training on how providers ought to communicate with patients could help to address this problem [38, 39]. In addition, it is the responsibility of the healthcare providers to offer patients clear and concise means to understand health information regardless of patients' education levels. Thus, communication by healthcare providers has to be designed for the average or illiterate person to understand and must be put in simple language [38].

Finally, this study has revealed that language is another barrier that is inhibiting patient- provider communication. This resonates with the findings of a study that was conducted in Canada which showed that a failure to address language barriers can result in misunderstandings, problems with informed consent, inadequate comprehension of diagnoses and treatment, dissatisfaction with care, preventable morbidity and mortality, disparities in prescriptions, test ordering and diagnostic evaluations [9]. Language barriers can inhibit a healthcare provider's ability to elicit patient symptoms, often resulting in increased use of diagnostic resources or invasive procedures, inappropriate treatment and diagnostic errors. Other studies [40–43] have also found that linguistic barriers were one of the problems affecting provider-patient communication. This barrier may be challenging to overcome due to current policies in Malawi where civil servants and other personnel are posted to any part of the country without consideration of their ability to speak the dominant languages of those areas. Kamwendo [40] has argued that posting staff according to the languages that they speak would in some cases mean that civil servants work in their home district or region, which could exacerbate regionalism and ethnic loyalties at the expense of national cohesion. Where a healthcare provider does not speak the same language as a patient, an interpreter should be employed to bridge the communication gap [40, 42, 43, 44].

The findings of this study should be interpreted with some limitations in mind. Since the interviews were conducted in Chichewa and then translated into English, the translations might have lost the original meaning in the translated language. To minimize this problem, an expert translator was involved to check both the recordings and transcripts to ensure that no original meaning was lost. Another potential limitation is the small sample of participants only attending urban hospitals which means the study is unlikely to be representative of all health facilities in Malawi. Another limitation is that there was no triangulation in this study. This study only focused on patients. Comparing information from patients and healthcare providers in order to fully understand all facets of this complex situation would have strengthened the findings. There is, therefore, a need to conduct another study that will include data from both patients and healthcare providers.

Conclusions

This study has identified some of the challenges affecting interpersonal communication between healthcare providers and pregnant women in the maternity ward in both public and private health facilities in Malawi. The study has underscored the importance of effective patient-provider communication in the provision of maternal healthcare. It is, therefore, important for the healthcare providers to ensure that they are effectively communicating with pregnant women. In all the health facilities, both public and private, healthcare providers need to have good communication skills in order to encourage as many pregnant women as possible to seek maternal services at a health facility with a skilled attendant. This is particularly critical in line with Sustainable Development Goals and WHO efforts to reduce mortality rate in low and middle-income countries. In view of the study findings, it is necessary to develop an intervention to help healthcare providers to improve their communication with patients. This intervention could entail provision of in-service training or refresher courses on communication skills to healthcare providers in order to change their behaviour towards patients. Finally, since this study only focused on urban areas and patients, there is need to conduct a large scale research study involving health facilities based in rural areas that includes healthcare providers' perceptions in order to comprehensively explore the nature of healthcare provider-patient communication in Malawi.

Abbreviations

CHAM: Christian Health Association of Malawi; NSO: National Statistical Office; TBA: Traditional birth attendant; UNSG: United Nations Sustainable Goals; WHO: World Health Organisation

Acknowledgements

The authors are greatly grateful and indebted to all participants in the study for giving their time and information during the interviews. The authors also give special thanks to all Hospital Directors and staff from the research sites for their support during data collection.

Authors' contributions

PM conceptualized the study, collected, analysed data and drafted the manuscript. HY is the Principal supervisor of the study who together with FWK and ACK critically reviewed drafts, edited and provided important intellectual content. All authors read and approved the final manuscript.

Competing interests

The authors declare that they have no competing interests.

References

1. Improving Interpersonal communication between healthcare providers and patients. Bethseda, MD: Quality Assurance Project. 1997.
2. The Joint Commission. Advancing communication, cultural competence, and patient-and family-centred care: A roadmap for hospitals. 2010. Retrieved from: http://www.jointcommission.org/assets/1/6/ARoadmapforHospitalsfinal version727.pdf. Accessed 15 Oct 2016.
3. Mathole T, Lindmark G, Majoko F, Ahlberg BM. A qualitative study of women's perspectives of antenatal care in rural area of Zimbabwe. Midwifery. 2004;20:122–32.
4. Kumbani L, Bjune G, Chirwa E, Malata A, Odland J. Why some women fail to give birth at health facilities: a qualitative study of women's perceptions of perinatal care from rural southern Malawi. Reprod Health. 2013;10:9.
5. Stewart MA. Effective physician-patient communication and health outcomes: a review. Canad Med Assoc J. 1995;152(9):1423–33.
6. Ruben BD. Communication theory and health communication practice: the more things change, the more they stay the same. Health Comm. 2016;31:1–11.
7. Seljeskog L, Sundby J, Chimango J. Factors influencing women's choice of place of delivery in rural Malawi: an explorative study. Afr J Reprod Health. 2006;10(3):66–75.
8. Harrington J, Noble LM, Newman SP. Improving patients' communication with doctors: a systematic review of intervention studies. Pat Edu Counsel. 2004;52:7–16.
9. Higginbottom GMA, Hadziabdic E, Yohani S, Paton P. Immigrant women's experiences of maternity services in Canada: a meta-ethnography midwifery. Midwifery. 2014;30(5):544–59.
10. Binder P, Borne Y, Johnsdotter S, Essen B. Shared language is essential: communication in a multi-ethnic obstetric care setting. J Health Commun. 2012;17:1171–86.
11. Degni F, Suominen S, Essen B, El Ansar W, Vehvilainen-Julkunen K. Communication and cultural issues in providing reproductive healthcare to immigrant women: healthcare providers' experiences in meeting the needs of [corrected] Somali women living in Finland. J Mino Health. 2012;14:330–43.
12. Mtotha DM. An exploratory study of government health policy with special reference to maternal mortality in Malawi. PhD Thesis, University of AZTECA (2013).
13. National Statistical Office Malawi and ICF. Malawi Demographic and Health Survey 2015-2016. Zomba, Malawi, and Rockville, Maryland, USA National Statistical Office and ICF 2017.
14. Kambala C, Morse T, Masangwi S, Mitunda P. Barriers to maternal health service use in Chikhwawa. Southern Malawi Mal Med J. 2011;23(1):1–5.
15. O'Donnell E, Utz B, Khonje D, van den Broek N. 'At the right time, in the right way, with the right resources': Perceptions of the quality of care provided during childbirth in Malawi. BMC Preg Childbir. 2014;14:248.
16. Tuckett A. Qualitative research sampling-the very real complexities. Nurse Res. 2004;12(1):47–61.
17. The World Bank. (2016). Malawi. Retrieved from https://www.google.com.au/search?q=the+world+bank_population+of+Malawi&oq=the+world+bank_population+of+Malawi&aqs=chrome..69i57j0.10460j1j8&sourceid=chrome&ie=UTF-8. Accessed 13 Mar 2017.
18. Population Reference Bureau and Malawi Government. Malawi Population Data Sheet 2012. 2012 Retrieved from https://www.prb.org/malawi-population-2012/. Accessed 4 Aug 2018.
19. National Statistical Office (NSO) of Malawi, UNICEF. Malawi, multiple indicator cluster survey (2006). Final Report. NSO and UNICEF, Lilongwe Malawi 2008.

20. World Health Organisation. Human resources for health country profile, Malawi. 2010. Retrieved from Lilongwe: http://www.who.int/workforcealliance/knowledge/resources/hrh_profile_malawi/en/. Accessed 13 Jan 2017.
21. Chirwa M. Knowledge synthesis on Malawi health system: literature review. 2013. Retrieved from Malawi: http://41.87.6.35:8080/xmlui/bitstream/handle/123456789/904/Knowledge%20synthesis%20on%20Malawi%20health%20system%20literature%20review.pdf?sequence=1. Accessed 7 Aug 2014.
22. Guest G, Bunce A, Johnson L. How many interviews are enough?: an experiment with data saturation and variability. Field Meth. 2006;18(1): 59–82. https://doi.org/10.1177/1525822X05279903.
23. Braun V, Clarke V. Using thematic analysis in psychology. Qual Research Psycho. 2006;3:77–101.
24. Mrisho M, Schellenberg JA, Mushi AK, Obrist B, Mshinda H, Tanner M. Factors affecting home delivery in rural Tanzania. Trop Med Int Health. 2007;12:862–72.
25. D'Ambruoso L, Abbey M, Hussein J. Please understand when I cry out in pain: women's accounts of maternity services during labour and delivery in Ghana. BMC Public Health. 2005;5:140.
26. Bazant ES, Koenig MA. Women's satisfaction with delivery care in Nairobi's informal settlements. Intern J Quality Health Care. 2009;21:79–86.
27. Hall JA, Roter DL, Katz BA. Meta-analysis of correlates of provider behaviour in medical encounters. Med Care. 1988;26:657–75.
28. Chadwick RJ, Cooper D, Harries J. Narratives of distress in south African public maternity settings: a qualitative study. Midwifery. 2014;30:862–8.
29. McMahon SA, George AS, Chebet JJ, Mosha IH, Mpembeni RNM, Winch PJ. Experiences of and response to disrespectful maternity care and abuse during childbirth; a qualitative study with women and men in Morogoro region. Tanzania BMC Pregnancy Childbirth. 2014;14:268.
30. Austad K, Chary A, Martinez B, Juarez M, Juarez MY, Ixen C, Rohloff P. Obstetric care navigation: a new approach to promote respectful maternity care and overcome barriers to safe motherhood. Reprod Health. 2017;14:148.
31. Scott K, Klaus P, Klaus M. The obstetrical and post-partum benefits of continuous support during childbirth. J Women's Health Gender-Based Medicine. 1999;8:1257–64.
32. Sauls D. Effects of labour support on mothers, babies, and birth outcomes. J Obstetrics, Gynecol Neonatal Nurs. 2002;31:733–41.
33. Rosen P. Supporting women in labour: analysis of different types of caregivers. J Midwifery Women's Health. 2004;49:24–31.
34. Brown H, Hofmeyr J, Nikodem C, Smith H, Garner P. Promoting childbirth companions in South Africa: a randomised pilot study. BMC Med. 2007;5:7.
35. Kifle D, Azale T, Gelaw YA, Melsew YA. Maternal health care service seeking behaviours and associated factors among women in rural Haramaya District, Eastern Ethiopia: a triangulated community-based cross-sectional study. Reprod Health. 2017;14:16.
36. Okafor II, Ogwu EO, Obi SN. Disrespect and abuse during a facility-based childbirth in a low-income country. Int J Gynecol Obstet. 2015;128:110–3.
37. Bolde MD, Bangoura A, Diallo BA, Sall O, Bolde H, Niakate AS, Vogel JP, Bohren MA. A qualitative study of women's and health providers' attitudes and acceptability of mistreatment during childbirth in health facilities in Guinea. Reprod Health. 2017;14:4.
38. Bohren M, Hunter EC, Munthe-Kaas HM, Souza JP, Vogel JP, Gulmezoglu AM. Facilitators and barriers to facility-based delivery in low- and mid-income countries: a qualitative evidence synthesis. Reprod Health. 2014;11:71.
39. Weinstock D. Deer in the headlights: improving patient literacy. J Medical Practice Manag. 2015;30(4):273–5.
40. Okonofua F, Ogu R, Agholor K, Okike O, Abdus-salam R, Gana M, Randawa A, Abe E, Durodola A, Galadanci H, The WHARC, WHO, FMOH, MNCH Implementation Study Team. Qualitative assessment of women's satisfaction with maternal health care referral hospitals in Nigeria. Reprod Health. 2017;14:44.
41. Kamwendo G. Language policy in health services: a sociolinguistics study of Malawian referral hospital: Helsinki University Printing House; 2004. Retrived on: https://helda.helsinki.fi/bitstream/handle/10138/19198/language.pdf?sequence=1/.
42. Divi C, Koss RG, Schmaltz SP, Loeb JM. Language proficiency and adverse events in U.S. hospitals: a pilot study. Intern J Quality Health Care. 2007; 19(60):60–7.
43. Arungwa OT. Effect of communication on nurse-patient relationship in National Orthopaedic Hospital, Igbobi, Lagos. WA J of Nurs. 2014;25(2):37–46.
44. Ong LML, De Haes JCJM, Hoos AM, Lammes FB. Doctor-patient communication: a review of the literature. Soc Science Med. 1995;40(7):903–18.

8

'I am always crying on the inside': a qualitative study on the implications of infertility on women's lives in urban Gambia

Susan Dierickx[1,2*], Ladan Rahbari[1,2], Chia Longman[2], Fatou Jaiteh[3,4,5] and Gily Coene[1]

Abstract

Background: There is an increasing awareness that infertility in Sub-Saharan Africa constitutes a severe social and public health problem. Few of the existing studies on infertility explicitly take into account the differences between women. However, how women experience infertility is formed by their various social positions. This research explores the implications of infertility on women's lives in urban Gambia and aims to provide an in-depth understanding of how this relates to gender and cultural norms as well as different social positions.

Methods: Qualitative data were collected through interviews (33), group discussions (13), participatory observations (14) and informal conversations (31). Purposive and snowball sampling techniques were used to identify participants. The data was analysed thematically using NVivo 11.

Results: Results showed that there was strong social pressure on urban women in The Gambia to procreate. Unable to conform to their gender role, women with infertility were confronted with financial problems, social stigma, as well as emotional and physical violence in their marriage. All women expressed feelings of trauma, stress and sadness. The intersectional approach used in this study highlighted how different positions influenced women's experiences of infertility. Urban women with a high socio-economic status had a more powerful position within their marriages and the broader community, due to their financial position, professional career and, sometimes, their educational background. In contrast, women from a lower socio-economic background were more likely to be harshly confronted with the social stigma of infertility.

Conclusion: The lives of most women with infertility in The Gambia are characterized by social suffering resulting from gender and pro-natal norms, cultural beliefs and moral concerns, cultural practices and limited access to health care. An intersectional approach is an effective tool to inform public health and social policy since it highlights how, in specific situations, certain groups are more vulnerable than others.

Keywords: Childlessness, Class, Gender, Infertility, Intersectionality, The Gambia, Social suffering, Stigma

* Correspondence: Susan.Dierickx@vub.be
[1]Centre of Expertise on Gender, Diversity and Intersectionality (RHEA), Vrije Universiteit Brussel, Pleinlaan 2, 1050 Elsene, Belgium
[2]Centre for Research on Culture and Gender, Ghent University, Rozier 44, 9000 Ghent, Belgium
Full list of author information is available at the end of the article

Plain English summary

In this study infertility is understood to be a condition where women are not able to bear children or are unable to have children following previous pregnancies.

This research explores the impact of infertility on women's lives in urban Gambia and aims to investigate its relation to the cultural rules of appropriate behaviour for men and women. It will take into account how the impact of infertility differs depending on women's personal characteristics such as their social class, educational background and religion.

Results show that there is a strong pressure from the community on urban women in The Gambia to have (many) children. Since women with infertility are unable to comply with these expectations, they face financial difficulties. Infertility also influences peoples relationships with their family-in-law, and women with infertility are also confronted with emotional and physical violence in their marriage. In addition, community members confront them with a negative attitude. All interviewed women expressed feelings of trauma, stress and sadness. The background characteristics of urban women influences the ways infertility impacts their lives. Urban women who are financially strong have a more powerful position within their marriages and the broader community, due to their financial position, professional career and, sometimes, their educational background. In contrast, poor women are more likely to be harshly confronted with a negative attitude from community members due to their infertility. Muslim respondents feared that their husband would take a co-wife.

Background

Infertility is a global reproductive health problem; the World Health Organization (WHO) estimates that 48.5 million couples worldwide are unable to conceive [1]. In Sub-Saharan Africa (SSA) many people are confronted with primary infertility (i.e. when a woman is unable to ever bear a child, either due to the inability to become pregnant or the inability to carry a pregnancy to a live birth) (1.9%) and there continues to be a high rate of secondary infertility (i.e. when a woman is unable to bear a child, either due to the inability to become pregnant or the inability to carry a pregnancy to a live birth following either a previous pregnancy or a previous ability to carry a pregnancy to a live birth) (11.6%). The very high primary and secondary infertility rates in West Africa largely result from poorly managed or untreated reproductive tract infections, including sexual transmitted infections and pregnancy-related sepsis (i.e. postpartum, post-abortion and iatrogenic infections) [2, 3]. Across SSA, access to biomedical health services directed at preventing and treating infertility remains very limited, although this is slowly changing in some countries [4]. The limited services can partly be explained by the relative absence of the topic of infertility on the international health agenda and the confined attention from national policymakers [2, 5–7]. As Harcourt [5] argues, the focus remains on controlling the population growth obscuring the rights of non-reproductive bodies in SSA.

Infertility also constitutes a social problem negatively affecting people around the world [8–11]. Previous anthropological and sociological research has indicated that, due to strong cultural norms to bear (multiple) children, women in SSA countries are often more negatively affected [7, 12–24]. In SSA societies with high levels of gender inequality, regardless of diagnosis, women are blamed for failing to bear children [2, 7, 12, 14, 20, 25–27]. Women may suffer from stigma, social isolation and ridicule within their communities [7]. Fertility problems are also a potential source of tension between partners [13, 17, 27–29]. When a marriage remains childless, some men abuse their wives, verbally or even physically [18, 29]. Women expressed feelings of anxiety, frustration, grief, lack of self-esteem and a general sense of powerlessness [17, 19, 30].

Most of the research on infertility in SSA has been focussed on the impact of infertility on the lives of rural women, and to a lesser extent on men's experiences of infertility [3, 7, 12, 16]. There is a limited amount of research on the implications of infertility for women living in urban areas [31]. Moreover, few studies on infertility in SSA explicitly consider the differences between women, seemingly assuming the homogeneity of women's lives and experiences concerning infertility [32]. However, women living in urban areas are a very heterogeneous group, belonging to different social categories (e.g. religious background, ethnicity, class and education level) [33, 34]. The implications of infertility may differ tremendously between women depending on e.g. their class, age, religion, ethnicity [35]. The concept of intersectionality provides an analytical tool to grasp the multifaceted realities of women's lives which co-exist and interact [35–38]. It allows us to understand how social categories influence the lives of women with infertility and how the intersection of these social categories may lead to different and distinct experiences of oppression and opportunity. It looks into the context-specific interactions of these social categories and the power relations underpinning inequalities.

The existing research on infertility in SSA is overwhelmingly conducted in South and Central Africa, with less attention paid to infertility in West Africa [14, 39]. Given the political, economic, cultural and social differences between these regions, there is a need to understand the implications of infertility in West Africa. This paucity of research on infertility in West Africa is also reflected in the few studies conducted in The Gambia

[2, 15]. The Gambia has a score of 0.641 on the gender inequality index indicating high levels of gender inequality [40–45]. The total fertility rate remains high in The Gambia with 5.8 live births per woman [46]. The studies reporting infertility rates in The Gambia are quite old, with a contraceptive prevalence study conducted in 1993 stating that around 2% of women at the end of their reproductive period had no children [47]. Considerably more women (11.6–15.2%) had a longer than expected time interval since their last birth. Another study found 9.8% of participants to be infertile, with secondary infertility (i.e. no pregnancy after at least 12 months of regular unprotected sexual intercourse) affecting 8.8% of all participants [24].

This qualitative study provides an in-depth understanding of the implications of infertility on women's lives in the urban communities of the West Coast region of The Gambia today and how these relate to broader gender norms and cultural practices. In order to understand the complexities of the lives of women with infertility, the analysis relies on the conceptual framework of intersectionality.

Methods

Study setting

Fieldwork was conducted between September 2017 and April 2018 in the urbanized West Coast region of The Gambia (e.g. Bakau, Brufut, Banjul, Fajikunda, Old Jeshwang, New Jeshwang). The Mandinka are the largest ethnic group in The Gambia, comprising 42% of the population, followed by the Fula (18%), the Wolof (16%), the Jola (10%) and the Serahule (9%) [48]. The pre-dominant religion in The Gambia is Islam (90%), 8% are Christian and 2% other. Polygyny is a common practice among Muslims; a study reported that 54.3% of married women live in a household with one or more co-wives [24].

Research design

This research is part of a larger anthropological research project on gender, culture and infertility in The Gambia (West Coast region) and Senegal (Casamance). This research opted for a qualitative research approach, combining interviews, group discussions and participant observation with informal conversation. Method triangulation was used to provide an in-depth understanding of the research topic and to enable the researchers to reflect on local narratives and personal stories of the participants. When respondents were fluent in English, the interview took place in English. However, in most cases conversations were carried out with the assistance of a trained translator in Mandinka or Wolof. It is unavoidable that some level of meaning was lost in translation and transcription, as personal perspectives influence the interpretation and translation process [49]. To minimize this, the translator was trained extensively for four days. The translator was familiarized with the themes and supplied with a question guide with potential questions that were translated beforehand. This allowed the first author and translator to discuss the terminology, phrasing and translation of potential questions. During data collection, attention was paid to non-verbal communication such as body language, gestures and silences.

Interviews

A total of 33 semi-structured interviews were conducted by the first author at locations where respondents felt at ease (Table 1). Most interviews were recorded but if the interviewee preferred not to be recorded or the interviewer was under the impression that it might make the respondent uncomfortable, the responses were written down in detail during or after the interview. Interviews lasted approximately one hour. The interviews were conducted with a flexible question guide. The question guide started by capturing the basic socio-demographic information, this was to help respondents feel more at ease. Then open questions were asked concerning (i) people's personal history and marriage, (ii) the impact of infertility, (iii) the relationships with partner, in-laws and community members and (iv) emotional consequences.

Group discussions

In total, 13 group discussions were conducted either when informants wanted to be interviewed together, or when the researcher wanted to collect different views on a particular topic in which case a group interview was requested. The number of participants varied between three up to nine people. Two group discussions on the topic of divorce and the position of women with infertility in urban Gambia include both male and female respondents. The other eleven group discussions on aetiological beliefs and the position of women with infertility in Gambian society were conducted with women experiencing infertility. Group discussions took place in several places including the privacy of people's homes, the offices where people were working and public spaces such as restaurants.

Participant observations

Participant observation consisted of participating in everyday activities, such as cooking and cleaning in the compound. The main author also went to the Muslim Cadi Court, attended naming ceremonies and participated in a march to increase awareness about infertility. Notes were taken whenever possible and a voice recorder was used to record findings when the situation did not allow to take notes. These observations offered the opportunity

Table 1 Overview of the interviewed respondents' socio-demographic characteristics

Interview	Education level	Main source of income	Ethnicity	Religion	Marital status	Age category[a]
1	University Gambia	Housewife	Mandinka	Muslim	Monogamous marriage	Adult
2	University abroad	Civil servant	Mandinka	Muslim	Monogamous marriage	Adult
3	University abroad	Civil servant	Mandinka	Muslim	Monogamous marriage	Adult
4	University abroad	Civil servant	Mandinka	Muslim	Monogamous marriage	Adult
5	University abroad	Civil servant	Mandinka	Muslim	Monogamous marriage	Adult
6	No education	Market vendor	Mandinka	Muslim	Polygynous marriage	Elder
7	No education	Housewife	Mandinka	Muslim	Divorced	Adult
8	University abroad	Civil servant	Mandinka	Muslim	Monogamous marriage	Adult
9	No education	Market vendor	Mandinka	Muslim	Widow	Elder
10	No education	Housewife	Fula	Muslim	Widow	Elder
11	No education	Cleaning lady	Mandinka	Muslim	Polygynous marriage	Elder
12	No education	Market vendor	Masuwanka	Muslim	Polygynous marriage	Elder
13	No education	Market vendor	Mandinka	Muslim	Polygynous marriage	Elder
14	No education	Farming	Fula	Muslim	Polygynous marriage	Adult
15	No education	Market vendor	Wolof	Muslim	Polygynous marriage	Adult
16	High school	Housewife	Wolof	Muslim	Monogamous marriage	Elder
17	No education	Market vendor	Mandinka	Muslim	Polygynous marriage	Elder
18	No education	Housewife	Mandinka	Muslim	Polygynous marriage	Adult
19	No education	Market vendor	Mandinka	Muslim	Polygynous marriage	Elder
20	No education	Housewife	Serer	Muslim	Polygynous marriage	Elder
21	Arabic school	Market vendor	Mandinka	Muslim	Polygynous marriage	Elder
22	No education	Housewife	Mandinka	Muslim	Polygynous marriage	Adult
23	Arabic school	Housewife	Mandinka	Muslim	Polygynous marriage	Adult
24	University abroad	Civil servant	Mandinka	Muslim	Monogamous marriage	Adult
25	University abroad	Civil servant	Aku	Muslim	Monogamous marriage	Adult
26	University abroad	Civil servant	Aku	Muslim	Monogamous marriage	Adult
27	University abroad	Civil servant	Aku	Muslim	Monogamous marriage	Adult
28	No education	Gardening	Mandinka	Muslim	Polygynous marriage	Elder
29	High school	Housewife	Karoninka	Muslim	Monogamous marriage	Adult
30	University Gambia	Housewife	Mandinka	Muslim	Polygynous marriage	Adult
31	College	Teacher	Aku	Christian	Monogamous marriage	Adult
32	Arabic school	Business woman	Mandinka	Muslim	Monogamous marriage	Adult
33	Arabic school	Cleaning help	Mandinka	Muslim	Monogamous marriage	Adult

[a]Adult: 18–49 years old/Elder: + 50 years old

for 31 informal conversations on relevant themes with community members and women experiencing infertility. Participant observation was important for the research project, providing a more contextualised understanding of the research questions. This method also facilitated gaining access to respondents and building trust between the researcher and participants. This was particularly important given the sensitive nature of the research topic and questions, allowing to minimize socially desirable or otherwise biased answers.

Sampling framework and method

When analysing infertility, it is important to acknowledge that standard epidemiological and demographical conceptualizations of infertility, subfertility, miscarriage and stillbirth are not always meaningful for people living in low- and middle-income countries [19, 21, 50–53]. Conceptualizations about what is natural, normal or expected in terms of fertility varies in time and over situations [18, 26, 53]. Therefore, in this study women were defined as infertile when they considered themselves as such, regardless of the duration of their fertility problems and their number of living children. In practice this meant that in our study sample, people were included who did not have children or who already had children. Purposive and snowball sampling strategies were utilized to enable maximum variation of identified participants through gradual selection processes. Critical cases (i.e. informants that presented us with important or unusual findings) were continuously included in the sample frame. These sampling techniques enhanced participants' trust and confidence in the researcher. When possible, informants were visited multiple times to increase levels of familiarity and trust between researcher and respondents to reduce bias.

Data analysis

The process of analysis began whilst still in the field, this included both process and thematic content analysis. Process analysis included self-reflectivity and discussion with the translator on methodological approaches. Thematic data analysis was an explorative, concurrent and iterative process including several stages [54]. First, incoming raw data was analysed to inform further data collection. Second, each incoming transcript was read and open codes were generated in NVivo 11 Analysis Software (QSR International Pty Ltd. Cardigan UK) (e.g. experiences with polygyny, importance of children). The third phase consisted of axial coding to create themes by grouping open codes according to their coherence after careful reading the analyses of the coded text fragments with attention to potential interrelations (examples of themes are pro-natal norm, the economic impact of infertility, the emotional impact of infertility). This served as the basis for a final code tree design. Throughout the analyses data were constantly set against findings of the existing literature. The first author received feedback from the co-authors based on analytic discussions, which informed the final interpretations. The emergent codes and themes and the relevance of women's social positions are discussed below, supported by respondents' quotes. Specific quotes were mainly chosen from interviews based on their intrinsic richness on a particular theme.

Positionality and reflexivity

The first author had resided in The Gambia prior to carrying out this research (in total 14 months over the course of three years). She was informally adopted by a local family and acquainted with culturally appropriate expressions and behaviour. Her position as a married woman was important in facilitating discussion around to marriage and fertility. Personal stories were shared by both the researchers and the participants during interviews, aiming to make the interview more intimate and reciprocal [55]. The interviewer's positionality – as a white, Western woman – made her at times an outsider which might have influenced the answers provided by the respondents [49, 56]. This twofold position as insider and outsider was helpful for some of the respondents, as it made the researcher a confidential conversation partner for those who wanted to share their stories and secrets. The emotions shared during the research made the lead researcher reflect on ethical questions of moral responsibility, injustice and powerlessness.

Ethics, consent and permission

Ethical approval for this study was received from The Gambia Government/MRC Joint Ethics Committee (SCC1562) and the ethical commission of the Vrije Universiteit Brussel (Belgium). The interviewer followed the Code of Ethics of the American Anthropological Association (AAA). People were informed about project goals, the topic and type of questions as well as their right to decline participation or to interrupt the conversation at any time. Anonymity was guaranteed and confidentiality assured. If people consented to be interviewed, during each interview participants were asked if they had any questions.

Results

Positionality of respondents

Throughout the presentation of the results, references are made to the influence of different social positions of women with infertility and the impact of relevant cultural practices where relevant. This makes it important to indicate the socio-demographic characteristics of the respondents, and how these interrelate. While some respondents of the informal conversations, interviews and group discussions were illiterate and in a more vulnerable financial position living from subsistence farming, others were highly educated with a secure job in the public sector or owned a business. In this study sample, the educational background of respondents related to women's professional career – in particular women who were educated abroad had a good job. However, there was no straightforward causality: one uneducated woman did run a successful business, while other well-educated women were stay-at-home mothers with no personal income. People born and educated in rural areas were more likely to be financially vulnerable. They also tended to have married quite young in an arranged marriage to a distant relative. In contrast, families who had been living in the urban area for several generations were more likely to have gone to school, have a stronger financial position and were less likely to be in an arranged marriage. In this study sample, people's educational and financial background was unrelated to their ethnic and religious background.

Pro-natal norm

The data showed that in order to understand the impact of infertility on women's lives, it is important to describe the pro-natal norm in Gambian society. All respondents of group discussions and interviews said married people should become parents. Observations and group discussions showed that there is a strong orientation in urban Gambia towards family life and values. An important reason given for having male children in this patrilineal society is the continuation of the family lineage. Observations indicated that the family unit was held together by complementary gender and age roles; women were responsible for the running of the household and men should be the financial providers. Considerations about the future welfare of the family were also relevant to understand the pro-natal norm. Older respondents explained that in the absence of a welfare system, more hands to work meant more revenue for the family, leading to more savings and security. In contrast, respondents who went to school expressed that they did not want to have more than four children since this implied a financial burden for the future well-being of their family. Interviewees also wanted to have some daughters because they were considered trust worthier to take care of their parents during old age. Women with infertility also explained that children are an important source of fun, pride and companionship.

Gender aspect of infertility

Married couples that remained childless were not in accordance with dominant norms prescribing them to have children. Respondents from group discussions and interviews agreed that the perceived cause of infertility is gendered. Regardless of any (biomedical) diagnosis, women are often perceived to have fertility problems. While within their communities and families most interviewed women seemed to accept their responsibility for not having children, during private interviews several interviewed women confided they found it troublesome that women were always accused of infertility.

> *'Some community members would say "she takes family planning tablets which destroys her stomach that is why she could not have children", some will say "the woman has jinnee [spirits] that is why she could not have children", but their minds would never tell them that because of the husband she cannot have children.'* (Interview 7)

The economic impact of infertility

> *'The economic impact is that you tend to spend a lot. Like me, I have spent a lot, a lot of my savings, three quarter of my savings, going to doctors, doing different tests. I do research online and buy supplements that you can use to boost your fertility. Whatever you name it, I have tried.'* (Interview 2)

Regardless of women's financial position, infertility has an economic impact on their daily lives. Muslim women without children were in vulnerable positions when their husband died. Observations at the court and interviews indicated that local interpretation of Sharia law was often followed closely when it came to inheritance, and sons received at least double the share of daughters and wives. As a result, in-laws or co-wives could expel widows without children from the compound with few resources to rely on. This is illustrated in the story shared by a Muslim adult woman with infertility in a household with a co-wife with sons living in Europe (interview 15). She explained that when her husband died, her co-wife wanted to sell her house. The woman with infertility was desperate that she would need to live on the street and pleaded so that she could stay inside the compound. This was accepted by the co-wife. However, the co-wife still did not want to cook together nor share the electricity. Since the woman had limited resources she used candlelight, until she got money from a women's savings organisation allowing her to pay her own electricity meter.

The economic position of the couple also has an impact on their health-seeking behaviour. In order to conform to dominant gender roles, initially often both partners – regardless of their financial position – would invest resources in order to find treatment. However, when this treatment-seeking did not lead to children, the financial support of the husband commonly decreased. As this quote from interview 29 indicates:

> *'You know sometimes when men spend a lot looking for health care and they didn't see any result, they will sometimes feel reluctant to pull out more money.'*

Most respondents explained that they continued to look for treatment even when their husband no longer provided financial support. Observations at the public and private clinics and interviews indicated that for women who had a salaried job, it was much easier to look for treatment independently from their husband. Not only the financial position of both partners had an impact on people's treatment seeking, education was also relevant. Educated women were more likely to look for biomedical health care:

> *'There is a lack of education and sensitization. Some of the uneducated women, you do not blame them because they do not know that they have to go and see*

the medical doctor. They do not know that infertility is not about marabouts [i.e. traditional healers].' (Interview 2)

Observations and interviews indicated that only women with infertility who were financially strong could afford to travel abroad for medical treatments that are not available in The Gambia.

Lastly, infertility also had an impact on women's daily livelihood. While our research indicated that gender roles prescribed that men should provide 'fish money' (i.e. money for the daily livelihood of the wife), in practice many women with infertility complained they did not receive fish money. This was particularly stressful for women who did not have a salaried job as an educated woman explained during a group discussion:

'Having children is also important for the economic security of women. When a woman remains childless, the husband will refuse to give his wife fish money or to provide clothes. She is chased away directly, but commonly indirectly by not providing financial support. These women will often return to the compound of their parents.'

The impact of infertility on social relationships

Differential social experiences depending on women's position

Most interviewed women experienced difficulties within their social relationships because of infertility. However, the impact of infertility on women's lives differed to some extent depending on their financial position. The interviewed women in strong financial positions often had more power to negotiate their relationships both with other community members, their family-in-law and within their marriages. Some of them supported their family-in-law financially. Their economic strength implied they could take care of themselves even when divorced. Therefore, they were less afraid that their husband would abandon them or remarry. The story told by an educated woman with infertility illustrates this: *'My husband's brother divorced from his wife after ten years of marriage because they could not have a child. The lady decided to break the marriage due to the social stigma and the in-laws. She has her work, she is educated and has her papers so why allow people to traumatize you?'* (Interview 5). Furthermore, women with a good job had the opportunity to go outside of their community to work, which allowed them to escape from the pressure to become pregnant.

Despite their stronger financial and social position, women with a salaried job also explained that they were confronted with stigma and occasionally community members would accuse them of not wanting to have children. As these women described themselves as *'desperate to have children',* these comments were experienced as painful and resulting from ignorance.

In contrast, interviewees who didn't have a well-paid job were more likely to be restricted to their traditional roles as daughters, wives and mothers and have less opportunity to escape the tensions and hurtful comments from their family-in-law and other community members.

'Sometimes people can even be saying words to you that hurt you. There is a lot of social stigma. I got married and I had my first child after five years of marriage and that one passed away [...] It took me another four years to become pregnant. Sometimes I will be sitting down, I will be hearing comments, they will be throwing words at me, but you know: people are different, we are the educated ones. We have our work and everything, you can't traumatize us, but what of the poor women in the household?' (Interview 5)

Stigmatization within the community

All interviewed women with infertility explained that gossip, jokes and rumours about infertility spread easily within communities. Women corroborated about the suffering caused by community members, being called *'barren', 'a witch'* and *'eating their own children'.* This social stigmatization can be partly explained by (i) gender norms and roles; and (ii) the perceived aetiology of female infertility. While respondents discussed several aetiological interpretations during interviews and group discussion, two of these are relevant for this discussion. First, infertility can be associated with witchcraft whereby women were accused of being witches eating their own children. Second, while premarital and extra-marital intercourse are considered immoral, infertility was associated with abortions, sexual infections and sometimes 'overdoses' of family planning injections and tablets. Despite the stigmatization of women with infertility, few of our respondents were explicitly excluded from attending social events such as naming ceremonies and weddings. When it did happen, it led to alienation, as explained during an interview:

'Yes, I used to feel shy. Some will say about me: "a woman who refuses to give birth is coming". Even if I want to eat porridge, they will say "do not touch this porridge, it is only for women who gave birth", and if there is naming ceremony, they would not inform me'. (Interview 9)

Adverse consequences for relationship with in-laws

Observations, group discussions and interviews indicated that two cultural practices increased the tensions in the relationship between women with infertility and their family-in-law. Firstly, the virilocal residence pattern, whereby the newly-wed moves in to her new marital family home. In this new home, she has to negotiate her position with her family-in-law, and having a child helped in this process. Respondents who did not live with their extended family were on both extremes of the socio-economic classes: some originated from rural areas and were renting a small house, unable to afford their own place, or they came from a high socio-economic class and could afford their own house separated from the family-in-law. Several respondents who stayed in the compound with their family-in-law were confronted with harassment and pressure by the in-laws, in particular the mother-in-law. Secondly, the bride price increased the pressure on women. Bride prices illustrated the exchange between families: the transfer or reproductive and productive capacities of a woman to her husband's family. This bride price differed between ethnic groups and families, and had to be discussed among the families involved, but it often consisted of large amounts of goods, cash or animals. An argument often made by the family-in-law is that despite the bride price, they did not get a 'good' wife in return. They encouraged the husband to marry another wife as the excerpt of interview 9 indicates:

> Respondent: *'My [previous] husband's family told my husband to divorce, or get a second wife, by then his mother and sisters where all living with me. I used to quarrel with them.'*
>
> Interviewer: 'How did your husband deal with that pressure from the family?'
>
> Respondent: *'My [previous] husband loves me so much but he used to tell me that if you do not have a child, I will marry a second wife.'*

Adverse consequences for marriage

Regardless of the type of marriage, through time, few couples were able to manage with the burden of infertility and remain supportive of each other. Many respondents suffered because of this. During a march to support couples experiencing infertility, a young woman said: *'men are very hard. They don't love you when you are faced with fertility difficulties.'* The long-term impact of infertility on marital relationships was diverse.

Firstly, some women experiencing infertility spontaneously said they were beaten by their husband because of their condition: *'I sat for so many years without having a child. When I came to bed my husband used to beat me, beat me, beat me! And he said that I am not a woman; that I cannot be pregnant.'* (Interview 19).

Secondly, during interviews women with infertility explained their fears of a divorce. A woman who was first married at the age of 14 to a 50-year-old man explained that during this period she did not even want to be pregnant and ran away several times. However, when she was in her second arranged marriage, she feared her new husband would divorce her when she did not get pregnant within the first four years of her marriage which proved to be true: *'I said to myself: "if he divorces me, where would I go? And even if I remarry, it [the infertility] is still going to be the same problem"'* (Interview 9).

Thirdly, women expressed that the lack of social and financial support is very painful. As a woman with infertility said: *'If he neglects you and you go to your people, all they would say is that "your husband loves you, if he didn't love you he would have divorced you, so go back to your husband's house and have patience. In the long run he will come back to you". That patience is very painful. When you feel that stress, it may make you lose your life because stress affects your heart'* (Interview 9). The following extract of interview 11 with a woman who lost seven children either during pregnancy or delivery indicates the suffering due to the lack of support from her husband:

> Respondent: *'If I lost my baby that is the end of my husband's support. He will not give me courage or make me active or to feel supported unless I become pregnant again.'*
>
> Interviewer: 'How did you feel at that moment?'
>
> Respondent: *'Death is the will of God but we need to share the sadness together, so it made me feel sad.'*

Fourthly, while none of the respondents talked about their personal situation, they would share gossip about both Christians and Muslims engaging in extramarital relationships. These extramarital relationships clash with gender norms for both men and women. However, in practice, (i) consequences are less severe for men since it was regarded as being in the 'nature' of men to have sexual relationships outside of the marriage and (ii) some interviewed women confessed they thought that if the husband was likely to be infertile it was better to become pregnant from a stranger than to divorce.

Lastly, many of the Muslim respondents feared their husbands would engage in polygyny, and 15 of the interviewed women were already in polygynous marriages. While men were supposed to engage in polygyny only if they had the financial means to treat all wives equally, in practice men often did not treat their wives equally leading to tensions between co-wives. When a co-wife was able to have children, for wives experiencing infertility it was a daily reminder of their own inability to have children.

Despite the marital problems many of the interviewees faced, women rarely left their unhappy marriages. Interviewees explained that marriage is an important social and cultural institution. Therefore, most of the divorced and widowed respondents re-married quite soon after losing or divorcing their husband.

Emotional impact of infertility

> *'Sometimes I face challenges. When things become difficult, sometimes I feel like crying. I would say to myself: "what if I had more than one child? It might be that when it is difficult with one child, the other child might be able to support" [...]. For me, my mother and father passed away, and the man I am married to now [her first husband died], he is an old man and financially we are both not strong, so I leave everything in the hands of God'* (Interview 15).

During some interviews, women cried discussing the financial and social problems they were confronted with in their lives. Interviewed women with infertility said they were often under stress (*neku-yaa*, lit. translated as an unsteady mind), which led to heart problems. Respondents experiencing infertility said it was the greatest grief they had in their lives and explained they felt desperate. They reported symptoms of depression ranging from extended periods of crying to isolation. This is further corroborated by the silence surrounding the topic of infertility, complicating women's ability to talk about their stress and fears. As a woman who lost seven children either during her pregnancy or delivery explained: *'Most of the time whenever I lost my child, my co-wife didn't take it as something serious or sympathized with me. That is something that affects me a lot and I feel bad'* (Interview 6). Feelings of hope, sadness and frustration were for many linked to the (sometimes) long periods (up to 20 years) of looking for health care. Expressions of sadness and loss were common among women who had salaried jobs but they explained that they found it helpful to be able to focus on their work.

Discussion

Although the authors want to warn against the victimisation of women experiencing fertility problems, it remains important to articulate the precarious situation of many of these women in urban Gambia. This study showed that motherhood is still considered an essential aspect of the adult female role, leaving the pro-natal norm unquestioned. What has changed among the urban population is the desired gender and number of children. That is (i) daughters are perceived to be trustworthy – they can be relied on during old age – and (ii) young educated urban women prefer to have less children, which enables them to support their children's education. Initially it was believed that when couples did not have children, it was the women's fault. Due to dominant unequal gender norms and roles, women had more social pressure to overcome their condition and become pregnant.

As in other SSA countries [12, 18, 20, 30], the lives of women with infertility in urban Gambia were marked by various kinds of economic, social and emotional problems. The concept of social suffering can be used to describe the impact of these various problems on women's lives. Social suffering refers to the social misery, pain and hurt people experience individually and collectively due to institutionalized inequalities and systematic discrimination [57, 58]. It is problematic that infertility is seldom recognized as a key reproductive health priority at the international and national level [5, 22, 59]. This lack of commitment stands in stark contrast with the stigmatization of women experiencing infertility in urban Gambia. This social stigma is not only related to the normative construction of women to become mothers, but also to the cultural beliefs and moral concerns about the aetiology of infertility. The social pressure to become pregnant was even more stressful as a result of cultural practices such as the bride price and virilocal residence patterns. All women experiencing infertility feared marital problems and many women reported emotional and financial neglect and abuse.

By employing an intersectional framework, this study attended to the subtle differences between women's experiences of infertility depending on their social position. An intersectional framework is rarely used within anthropological or health system research in low- and middle-income countries [36, 60, 61]. Although recently, several authors [36, 62] have stressed the advantages of an intersectional approach to understand complex social situations. In anthropological or social science research on infertility, few studies have explicitly taken into account the different social categories influencing women's lives. In urban Gambia, the manifestation and intensity of the financial, social and emotional problems differed between women with a strong financial position and women with a more vulnerable financial position. In general, the stronger economic position gave these women more resilience to deal with stigma. Being financially independent, they had a more powerful position within their marriage to negotiate relationships with their husbands and in-laws. A salaried job made women more resistant towards outside pressures by providing them an independent space outside the compound and community. Furthermore, women who were financially strong were less dependent on their husbands to look for health care and found it easier to go to private health centres or to travel abroad for IVF treatment.

This study contributes to the few earlier studies looking at the influence of social positions on the lives of women with infertility in low-and middle-income countries. Inhorn [32] was the first to discuss the importance of class differences on the stigma faced by women with infertility in urban Egypt. Women with a lower social status were more devalued, disempowered and stigmatised. Nahar & Richers [34] studied the position of women experiencing infertility in Bangladesh doing research among both poor rural woman and wealthy urban women. The main difference found was that rural childless women had more social pressure. As in these studies, also in urban Gambia, people with fewer financial resources suffer more. However, taking into account their intersectional position, including the relevance of religion, educational background and having a salaried job also influenced these women's experiences.

Conclusion

Intersectionality is an effective tool of analysis and for informing social policy since it highlights how in specific situations social positions and identities interact and influence people's behaviour. Our findings stress the urgent need for targeted services for all individuals and couples experiencing infertility in The Gambia. Infertility has negative financial implications, leads to social stigmatization, marital problems and emotional difficulties. Therefore, the capacity of the health system needs to be built not only to prevent and treat fertility problems among both women and men, but also to follow up and provide psychological and emotional support especially for women. While all women would benefit from these services, special efforts should be made to target those women who have little financial and social resources.

Abbreviations

SSA: Sub-Saharan Africa; WHO: World Health Organization

Acknowledgements

We would like to thank the fieldworker Bintou Jarju for her assistance with data collection during fieldwork as well as for transcription and translation of recorded interviews and discussions. We are most grateful to all women for their time and efforts while participating in the study and their confidence in our research. We would also like to thank Neneh Touray (Women's Bureau) and Ed Clarke (Medical Research Council Unit The Gambia at the London School of Hygiene and Tropical Medicine) for their continuous support. We would like to thank Fleur Van Bocxlaer, Liesbeth Van Den Bossche, Megan Evans and Jonas De Meulenaere for editing the text.

Funding

This research is funded by the FWO (Research Foundation-Flanders) and the Global Minds Fund Operational Grant (VLIR-Ghent University) with the support of VLIR-UOS and the Belgian Department of Development Cooperation. These institutions approved and funded the research proposal. The publication of this paper is partly financially supported by the University Foundation in Belgium.

Authors' contributions

GC and CL developed the original research project on harmful cultural practices. SD designed the study on infertility in The Gambia and Senegal. All authors contributed to the development of the data collection tools. SD performed the data collection and analysis. All authors contributed to the analytical discussion of the paper. SD carried out the literature review and wrote the paper. All authors edited and commented on the text. All authors read and approved the final manuscript.

Ethics approval and consent to participate

Ethical approval for this study was received from The Gambia Government/MRC Joint Ethics Committee (SCC1562) and the ethical commissions of the Vrije Universiteit Brussel (Belgium). The interviewer (SD) followed the Code of Ethics of the American Anthropological Association (AAA). People were informed about project goals, the topic and type of questions as well as their right to decline participation or to interrupt the conversation at any time. Anonymity was guaranteed and confidentiality assured. If people consented to be interviewed, during each interview participants were asked if they had any questions.

Competing interests

The authors declare that they have no competing interests.

Author details

[1]Centre of Expertise on Gender, Diversity and Intersectionality (RHEA), Vrije Universiteit Brussel, Pleinlaan 2, 1050 Elsene, Belgium. [2]Centre for Research on Culture and Gender, Ghent University, Rozier 44, 9000 Ghent, Belgium. [3]Medical Anthropology Unit, Department of Public Health, Institute of Tropical Medicine, Nationalestraat 155, 2000 Antwerp, Belgium. [4]Amsterdam Institute of Social Science Research, Nieuwe Achtergracht 166, 1018 Amsterdam, The Netherlands. [5]Medical Research Council Unit The Gambia at the London School of Hygiene and Tropical Medicine, Fajara, The Gambia.

References

1. Mascarenhas MN, Flaxman SR, Boerma T, Vanderpoel S, Stevens GA. National, regional, and global trends in infertility prevalence since 1990: a systematic analysis of 277 health surveys. PLoS Med. 2012;9:e1001356.
2. Inhorn MC, Patrizio P. Infertility around the globe: new thinking on gender, reproductive technologies and global movements in the 21st century. Hum Reprod Update. 2015;21:411–26.
3. Nieuwenhuis SL, Odukogbe A-T A, Theobald S, Liu X. The impact of infertility on infertile men and women in Ibadan, Oyo state, Nigeria: a qualitative study. Afr J Reprod Health. 2009;13:85–98.
4. Hörbst V. "You need someone in a grand boubou" – barriers and means to access ARTs in West Africa. Facts, views Vis ObGyn. 2012:46–52.
5. Harcourt W. Body Politics in Development. Critical Debates in Gender and Development. London & New York: Zed Books; 2009.
6. Hough CA. Loss in childbearing among Gambia's kanyalengs: using a stratified reproduction framework to expand the scope of sexual and reproductive health. Soc Sci Med. 2010;71:1757–63.
7. Ibisomi L, Mudege NN. Childlessness in Nigeria: perceptions and acceptability. Cult Health Sex. 2014;16:61–75.
8. Ceballo R, Graham ET, Hart J. Silent and infertile: an intersectional analysis of the experiences of socioeconomically diverse African American women with infertility. Psychol Women Q. 2015;39(4):1–15.
9. Daibes MA, Safadi RR, Athamneh T, Anees IF, Constantino E. 'Half a woman, half a man; that is how they make me feel': a qualitative study of rural Jordanian women's experience of infertility. Cult Health Sex. 2017;20(5):516–30.
10. Batool SS, de Visser RO. Experiences of infertility in British and Pakistani women: a cross-cultural qualitative analysis. Health Care Women Int. 2016; 37:180–96.

11. Batool SS, de Visser RO. Psychosocial and contextual determinants of health among infertile women: a cross-cultural study. Psychol Health Med. 2014; 19(6):673–9.
12. Dhont N, Van De WJ, Coene G, Gasarabwe A, Temmerman M. Mama and papa nothing: living with infertility among an urban population in Kigali, Rwanda. Hum Reprod. 2011;26:623–9.
13. Fehintola AO, Fehintola FO, Ogunlaja OA, Awotunde TO, Ogunlaja IP, Onwudiegwu U. Social meaning and consequences of infertility in Ogbomoso, Nigeria. Sudan J Med Sci. 2017;12:63.
14. Fledderjohann JJ. "Zero is not good for me": implications of infertility in Ghana. Hum Reprod. 2012;27:1383–90.
15. Hollos M, Whitehouse B. Women in limbo: life course consequences of infertility in a Nigerian community. Hum Fertil. 2014;17:188–91.
16. Tabong PT, Adongo PB. Infertility and childlessness: a qualitative study of the experiences of infertile couples in northern Ghana. BMC Pregnancy Childbirth. 2013;13. https://doi.org/10.1186/1471-2393-13-72.
17. Dyer SJ, Abrahams N, Hoffman M, Van Der SZM. 'Men leave me as I cannot have children': women's experiences with involuntary childlessness. Hum Dev Rep. 2002;17:1663–8.
18. de Kok BC. Infertility and relationships: the importance of constructions in context. Fam Relationships Soc. 2013;2:23–42.
19. Gerrits T. Social and cultural aspects of infertility in Mozambique. Patient Educ Couns. 1997;31:39–48.
20. Tabong PTN, Adongo PB. Understanding the social meaning of infertility and childbearing: a qualitative study of the perception of childbearing and childlessness in northern Ghana. PLoS One. 2013;8:e54429.
21. Van der Sijpt E. Ambiguous ambitions: on pathways, projects, and pregnancy interruptions in Cameroon. Amsterdam: Universiteit van Amsterdam; 2011.
22. Inhorn MC, Van Balen F. Infertility around the Globe. New Thinking on Childlessness, Gender and Reproductive Technologies. London: University of California Press; 2002.
23. Inhorn MC. Interpreting infertility: medical anthropological perspectives: Introduction. Soc Sci Med. 1994;39:459–61.
24. Walraven G, Scherf C, West B, Ekpo G, Paine K, Coleman R, Bailey R, Morison L. The burden of reproductive-organ disease in rural women in the Gambia, West Africa. Lancet. 2001;14:1161–7.
25. Dyer SJ, Abrahams N, Mokoena NE, van der Spuy ZM. "You are a man because you have children": experiences, reproductive health knowledge and treatment-seeking behaviour among men suffering from couple infertility in South Africa. Hum Reprod. 2004;19:960–7.
26. Gijsels M, Mgalla Z, Wambura L. "No child to send": context and consequences of female infertility in Northwest Tanzania. In: Boerma JT, Mgalla Z, editors. Women and infertility in sub-Saharan Africa: a multidisciplinary perspective. Amsterdam: KIT publishers; 2001. p. 204–21.
27. Donkor ES. Socio-cultural perceptions of infertility in Ghana. Afr J Nurs Midwifery. 2008;10:22–34.
28. de Kok BC. Automatically you become a polygamist': "culture" and "norms" as resources for normalization and managing accountability in talk about responses to infertility. Health (Irvine Calif). 2009;13:197–217.
29. Dhont N. Clinical , epidemiological and socio-cultural aspects of infertility in resource-poor settings. Evidence from Rwanda. Facts, views Vis ObGyn. 2011;3:77–88.
30. Donkor ES, Naab F, Kussiwaah DY. "I am anxious and desperate": psychological experiences of women with infertility in the Greater Accra region, Ghana. Fertil Res Pract. 2017;3:6.
31. Larsen U, Hollos M: The Importance of Motherhood: A study of infertility in urban Northern Tanzania.
32. Inhorn MC. Infertility and patriarchy: the cultural politics of gender and family life in Egypt. Philadelphia: University of Pennsylvania Press; 1996.
33. Hollos M, Larsen U. Motherhood in sub-Saharan Africa: the social consequences of infertility in an urban population in northern Tanzania. Cult Health Sex. 2008;10:159–73.
34. Nahar P, Richters A. Suffering of childless women in Bangladesh: the intersection of social identities of gender and class. Anthropol Med. 2011;18:327–38.
35. Withaeckx S, Coene G: 'Glad to have honour ': continuity and change in minority women's lived experience of honour. J Gend Stud. 2013;33(4):37–41.
36. Larson E, George A, Morgan R, Poteat T. 10 best resources on… intersectionality with an emphasis on low- and middle-income countries. Heal Policy Plan. 2016; 31:964–9.
37. Choo HY, Ferree MM. Practicing intersectionality in sociological research: a critical analysis of inclusions, interactions, and institutions in the study of inequalities. Sociol Theory. 2010;28:129–49.
38. Crenshaw K. Mapping the Margins: intersectionality , Identity Politics , and Violence against Women of Color. Stanford Law Rev. 1991;43(6):1241–99.
39. Sundby J. Infertility in the Gambia: traditional and modern health care. Patient Educ Couns. 1997;31:29–37.
40. Saine A: Culture and Customs of Gambia. Sante Barbara, California: ABC-CLIO, LLC; 2012.
41. Sundby J. A rollercoaster of policy shifts : global trends and reproductive health policy in the Gambia. Glob Public Health. 2014;9:894–909.
42. Tunkara-bah H. Sociocultural Factors Influencing Fertility among the Soninke Tribe in the Gambia. African Renaissance. 2016;13(1&2):31–44.
43. Perfect D. The Gambia under Yahya Jammeh: an assessment. The Round Table. 2010;99(406):53-63.
44. Chant S, Evans A. Looking for the one(S): young love and urban poverty in the Gambia. Environ Urban. 2010;22:353–69.
45. United Nations: Development Report: Gender Inequality Index [http://hdr.undp.org/en/composite/GII]. Accessed 28 Feb 2017.
46. UN Data: Gambia.
47. Sundby J, Mboge R, Sonko S. Infertility in the Gambia: frequency and health care seeking. Soc Sci Med. 1998;46:891–9.
48. O'Neill S, Clarke E, Peeters Grietens K. How to protect your new-born from neonatal death: infant feeding and medical practices in the Gambia. Womens Stud Int Forum. 2017;60:136–43.
49. Davies CA. Reflexive ethnography: a guide to researching selves and others. Oxon: Routledge; 2012.
50. de Kok BC: Constructing infertility in Malawi: management of interpersonal, normative and moral issues in talk. 2007(November).
51. Greenhalgh S. Anthropology theorizes reproduction: integrating practice, political economy, and feminist perspectives. In: Greenhalgh S, editor. Situating fertility: anthropology and demographic inquiry. Cambridge: Cambridge University Press; 1995. p. 3–28.
52. Mumtaz Z, Shahid U, Levay A. Understanding the impact of gendered roles on the experiences of infertility amongst men and women in Punjab. BMC Reprod Heal. 2013;10. https://doi.org/10.1186/1742-4755-10-3.
53. Bledsoe CH. Contingent lives: fertility, time and aging in West Africa. London: The University of Chicago Press; 2002.
54. Creswell JW. Qualitative inquiry and research design: choosing among five traditions. Qual Health Res. 1998;403
55. Smith JA, Flower P, Larkin M. Interpretative phenomenological analysis: theory, method and research. Thousand Oaks: SAGE Publications; 2009.
56. Scheyvens R, Storey D. Introduction. In: Scheyvens R, Storey D, editors. Development fieldwork. A practical guide. London: SAGE Publications; 2006. p. 1–15.
57. Bourdieu P. The Weight of the World: Social Suffering in Contemporary Society. Stanford (California): Stanford University Press; 1999.
58. Kleinman A, Das V, Lock MM. Social suffering. Berkeley: University of California Press; 1997.
59. Ombelet W. Global access to infertility care in developing countries: a case of human rights. equity and social justice. 2012;3(4):7–16.
60. Logie CH, LI J, Tharao W, Loutfy MR. HIV, gender, race, sexual orientation, and sex work: a qualitative study of intersectional stigma experienced by HIV-positive women in Ontario, Canada. PLoS Med. 2011;8:e1001124.
61. Sen G, Iyer A, Mukherjee C. A methodology to analyse the intersections of social inequalities in health. J Hum Dev Capab. 2014;10:397–415.
62. Gueta K. A qualitative study of barriers and facilitators in treating drug use among Israeli mothers: an intersectional perspective. Soc Sci Med. 2017;187: 155–63.

9

Health and sustainable development; strengthening peri-operative care in low income countries to improve maternal and neonatal outcomes

Isabella Epiu[1,2*], Josaphat Byamugisha[3], Andrew Kwikiriza[4] and Meg Amy Autry[5]

Abstract

Background: Uganda is far from meeting the sustainable development goals on maternal and neonatal mortality with a maternal mortality ratio of 383/100,000 live births, and 33% of the women gave birth by 18 years. The neonatal mortality ratio was 29/1000 live births and 96 stillbirths occur every day due to placental abruption, and/or eclampsia – preeclampsia and other unkown causes. These deaths could be reduced with access to timely safe surgery and safe anaesthesia if the Comprehensive Emergency Obstetric and Newborn Care services (CEmONC), and appropriate intensive care post operatively were implemented. A 2013 multi-national survey by Epiu et al. showed that, the Safe Surgical Checklist was not available for use at main referral hospitals in East Africa. We, therefore, set out to further assess 64 government and private hospitals in Uganda for the availability and usage of the WHO Checklists, and investigate the post-operative care of paturients; to advocate for CEmONC implementation in similarly burdened low income countries.

Methods: The cross-sectional survey was conducted at 64 government and private hospitals in Uganda using preset questionnaires.

Results: We surveyed 41% of all hospitals in Uganda: 100% of the government regional referral hospitals, 16% of government district hospitals and 33% of all private hospitals. Only 22/64 (34.38%: 95% CI = 23.56–47.09) used the WHO Safe Surgical Checklist. Additionally, only 6% of the government hospitals and 14% not-for profit hospitals had access to Intensive Care Unit (ICU) services for postoperative care compared to 57% of the private hospitals.

Conclusions: There is urgent need to make WHO checklists available and operationalized. Strengthening peri-operative care in obstetrics would decrease maternal and neonatal morbidity and move closer to the goal of safe motherhood working towards Universal Health Care.

Keywords: Maternal health, Universal health care, SDGs, Patient safety, Health systems, Health policy, Health financing, Global surgery, Safe anaesthesia

* Correspondence: HSIEpiu@gmail.com; isabellaepiu@gmail.com
[1]NIH Fogarty Global Health Fellow, University of California Global Health Institute, San Francisco, CA, USA
[2]Health Solutions International, P.O.Box 2336, Kampala, Uganda
Full list of author information is available at the end of the article

Plain English summary

The 2015 Lancet Commission on Global Surgery reports that although remarkable gains have been made in global health in the past 25 years mortality and morbidity from common conditions needing surgery have grown in the world's poorest regions. They estimate that 5 billion people lack access to safe, affordable surgical and anaesthetic care. Only 12% of the specialist surgical workforce practice in Africa and Asia, where a third of the world's population lives. It is this inequality and the lack of access to safe surgical interventions in low- and middle-income countries (LMICs), that leads to unacceptable rates of morbidity and mortality.

Surgery and anaesthesia have long been neglected in global health work with the focus on communicable diseases. However, the recent World Health Assembly emphasized universal care for all, including strengthening of surgery and anaesthesia.

It is reported that 40% of maternal deaths could be averted with access to cesarean sections; therefore strengthening peri-operative surgical care in obstetrics would improve maternal and neonatal outcomes working toward the milestone of safe motherhood.

In conclusion, we believe that strengthening peri-operative care in obstetrics would decrease maternal and neonatal morbidity and move closer to the goal of safe motherhood working towards Universal Health Coverage.

Background

Current estimates of 300,000 maternal deaths every year from pregnancy-related causes translates into a global maternal mortality ratio (MMR) of 216 deaths per 100,000 live births in 2015, a 37% reduction since 2000 [1]. Achieving the Sustainable Development Goals target of less than 70 maternal deaths per 100,000 live births by 2030 requires a global annual rate of reduction of at least 7.5%, more than double the rate achieved between 2000 and 2015 [1].

The potential for improvements in maternal and neonatal health outcomes with increased facility utilization in these countries is undermined by a lack of appropriate and timely treatment [2]. Providing antenatal care during pregnancy and skilled care during childbirth, as well as care and support in the weeks after childbirth can prevent most maternal and neonatal deaths [1]. As part of the continuum of care, safe surgery and safe anaesthesia are essential components of the comprehensive obstetric care package. Implementing timely and appropriate evidence-based practices during the peri-operative and immediate postoperative period can improve maternal and fetal health.

The main agenda in implementation of the Sustainable Development Goals by 2030 was to transform the world in 15 years building peaceful, inclusive societies as a foundation to free humanity from poverty, and ensure health and well being for all. Of the more than 130 million births occurring each year, there's an estimated 2.6 million stillbirths, and another 2.7 million newborn death within the first 28 days of birth. The majority of these deaths occur in low-resource settings, often lacking skilled birth attendants. At least half of all stillbirths occurred in the intrapartum period [3]. In 2015, 1,700,000 babies were born in Uganda among young women aged 20–24, (33% gave birth by age 18) [4]. The Maternal Mortality in was 383/100,000 live births, with neonatal mortality of 29/1000 live births and 96 stillbirths occurring every day [5], due to placental abruption, and/or eclampsia – pre-eclampsia and other unkown causes. The major causes of maternal death are amenable to emergency surgical treatment, including hemorrhage (18%), [6] obstructed labor (8%) [6], unsafe abortion (18%) [6], in addition to uterine rupture, genital tract trauma, retained placenta, and ectopic pregnancy. These maternal and neonatal deaths could be prevented with access to timely safe surgery and safe anaesthesia by adequately implementing the Comprehensive Emergency Obstetric and Newborn Care services, and appropriate intensive care post operatively.

Anesthetic providers are also integral to the resuscitation and management of critically ill pregnant and postpartum women including sepsis and preeclampsia/eclampsia, responsible for 9% and 12% of maternal deaths, respectively [6].

In a study aimed at establishing the factors affecting maternal mortality in Uganda, investigating whether the number of antenatal Care visits, maternal education, age, area and region of residence had any effect on maternal mortality.

found mothers who make fewer or no ANC visits had a higher likelihood of death, both for themselves and their babies, than those who had more visits. It was also found that, mothers living in rural areas, compared to those in urban areas, are more likely to die due to pregnancy or related conditions [https://www.ajol.info/index.php/ajer/article/view/136040].

Acknowledging the complexity around childbirth an and the importance of surgical and anesthesia access in decreasing maternal and neonatal morbidity and mortality the, the World Health Organisation introduced the safe surgical and more recently the safe childbirth checklists [2, 7] as a means of improving the safety around the world; following reports that surgery may account for 40% of all hospital adverse events [8]. Furthermore, the World Health Organization (WHO) recommends that countries should achieve cesarean delivery (C-section) rates of 10% at a population level, to achieve reductions in maternal and newborn mortality rates [9].

Growing evidence has supported promotion of the use of checklists in several areas of healthcare with evidence of improved surgical outcomes [10–12]. In a multinational study involving eight hospitals from diverse economic settings, checklist implementation reduced death rate following surgery by approximately 50% [4]. All sites had a reduction in major postoperative complications, significantly at three sites, one in a high-income location and two in lower-income locations [4]. This is in-line with WHO pilot study that confirmed the conclusions of a number of earlier studies indicating that preoperative team introductions and briefings and postoperative debriefings contribute to improved surgical processes and outcomes [13].

Our group published data regarding availability of the WHO Safe Surgical Checklists in main referral hospitals throughout the East African region and reported 25% usage for obstetric patients [14]. Despite initial results demonstrating that properly implemented surgical checklists can make a substantial difference to patient safety; the implementation has not been straightforward. The reasons for this are varied and complex but include inconsistent leadership, lack of flexibility, and teamwork requirements [15].

The maternal mortality in Uganda is 343/ 100,000 live births [16] with 73% facility deliveries reported in the last 5 years [17]. Six percent of the live births were delivered by cesarean section with a cesarean section rate in urban areas at 11% and rural areas at 5% [18]; and there is currently no national policy regarding the use of the WHO checklist [14]. The WHO checklist was first introduced within the obstetric department at Mbarara Regional Referral Hospital in 2011 as part of a program to improve maternal care. This center has 15,000 deliveries per year. Here, checklist-training sessions were conducted over a five-month period by a visiting anaesthetist; but use of the checklist was not sustained after the volunteer left the hospital [15]. The main barriers identified were: the lack of clarity about responsibilities; lack of leadership and support from higher-level staff; no trained nurse to assist; and not enough time to complete the checklist [https://onlinelibrary.wiley.com/doi/full/10.1111/anae.13226].

We therefore sought to obtain data at the district level where most maternity care occurs, by assessing government and private hospitals in Uganda for the availability and usage of the WHO Safe Surgical Checklists and postoperative care of these patients.

Methods

The cross-sectional survey was conducted in Uganda from September 2014 to August 2015. A total of 64 hospitals across Uganda were selected based on the criteria that they provided obstetric anaesthesia At least 15 hospitals from each region; East, West, North and Central were included:- 13 regional referral, 21 general (district), 7 private for profit and 7 private not for profit hospitals across the country. Our study represents 41% of all the hospitals in the country and 100% of the government regional referral hospitals, 15% of government general (district) hospitals and 33% of all private hospitals in Uganda. This included 26% of private for profit and 37% of the private non-for profit hospitals.

As published in by Epiu et al.** survey tool to evaluate compliance to the World Federation of Societies' of Anaesthesiologists (WFSA) international guidelines for safe anaesthesia was developed [19]. These included quantitative and qualitative data on pre-operative assessment of patients, staffing and continuous monitoring intra-operatively and post-operatively. In this report we have included the peri-operative components on the use of the WHO Safe surgical Checklist, and documented the postoperative care of the parturient. I.E and trained research assistants interviewed on anaesthetist at each hospital, the hospital director and using a checklist assessed the theatre and recovery areas.

We purposefully selected all 14 regional referral hospitals as they are tertiary centres and serve as the surgical referral hospitals for lower health centres. We also randomly selected hospitals from other types of hospitals present in Uganda to include general (government district hospitals), private for profit and private not for profit hospitals.

With the help of a statistician, data was subsequently cleaned and coded into Epidata version 3.1. Range. Consistency and Validity checks were built in to minimize errors. Data was exported and analyzed using STATA version 14 (Statcorp, College Station, Texas, USA).

Ethical approval was obtained from Makerere University School of Medicine Research and Ethics Committee (SOMREC) REC REF No 2014–133, the appropriate participating hospitals, and the Uganda National Council for Science and Technology. Informed consent was obtained from all individuals participating in the study.

Results

Only 22/64 (34.38%: 95% CI = 23.56–47.09) used the WHO Safe surgical checklist, and Table 1 highlights its per facility. The difference between the WHO Checklist usage in government and private hospitals was not statistically significant ($p = 0.081$) Lack of availability of the checklist was the reason given for why the WHO Safe surgical checklist was not used, Fig. 1.

Post operatively the patients were cared for in a recovery area in 20/64 (33%) of the hospitals. Although 88% stated that they ensured the patients were pain free; only 7.8% of the anesthetists revisited the patients 48 h later for pain review. Only 9/64 of the health facilities (14%, *P*-Value 0.002) had intensive care unit services available for postoperative care of critical parturients requiring close monitoring, Table 1. Of these, access to ICU services for parturients post-operatively were mainly available in private hospitals (57%), Table 1.

Table 1 Use of the WHO Safe surgical checklist intraoperative, post operative care and monitoring, and availability of ICU Services

Variable	Health facility type N (%)			Chi square *p*-value
	Government *N* = 34	Private *N* = 7	Not for profit *N* = 23	
Use of surgical checklist				
Yes	11 (32.35)	5 (71.43)	6 (26.09)	
No	23 (67.65)	2 (28.57)	17 (73.91)	0.081
Patients taken care of postoperatively in recovery				
Yes	9 (29.03)	5 (71.43)	6 (27.27)	
No	22 (70.97)	2 (28.57)	16 (72.73)	0.075
Postoperative pain review				
24 h	30 (88.24)	5 (71.43)	21 (95.45)	
48 h	3 (8.82)	1 (14.29)	1 (4.55)	
> 48 h	1 (2.94)	1 (14.29)	0	0.345
Basic monitoring ICU services available				
Yes	2 (6.06)[a]	4 (57.14)	3 (13.64)[a]	
No	31 (93.94)	3 (42.86)	19 (86.36)	0.002

[a]missing one

Most private hospitals had an organized post anaesthesia care unit sometimes with a dedicated member of staff monitoring the patients, compared to improvised spaces or corridors in the other hospitals. Additionally, only 6% of the government hospitals and 14% not-for profit hospitals had access to ICU services for postoperative care compared to 57% of the private hospitals.

Discussion

Safe anaesthesia and safe surgery are indispensable components of emergency comprehensive obstetric healthcare. To address the complexities around childbirth the WHO has introduced the safe surgical and safe childbirth checklists. This cross-sectional survey at 64 hospitals provided data on peri-operative use of the WHO Safe Surgical Checklist and postoperative care for the obstetric patients in Uganda.

Seventy-one percent of the private hospitals used the safe surgical checklist, which demonstrates a disparity in delivery of care between the rich who can pay out of pocket, insured patients and poor patients who cannot afford the high quality services. The use of the safe surgical checklist in government hospitals was 32%, which can possibly be attributed to lack of resources and/or shortage of personnel for implementation. Generally there was no significant difference in proportions among the health facilities – meaning that almost all facilities didn't use the surgical checklist because they were not available. The response "It is not available" is perhaps a reflection of the culture and attitudes in these hospitals rather than an indication of the actual inavailability, similar to our published data from the multi-national East Africa survey [14]. This response may reflect a lack of enthusiasm for checklist use because it can actually

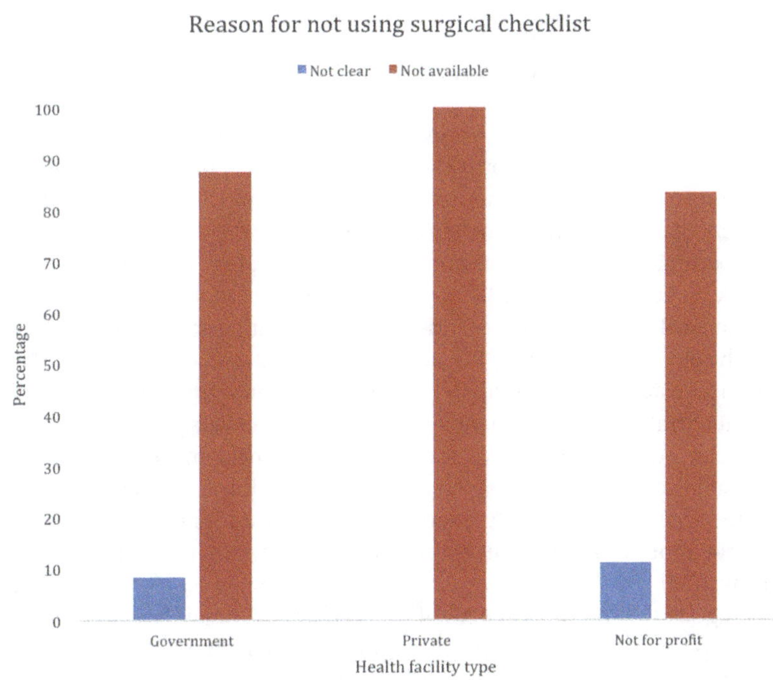

Fig. 1 Reason why WHO safe surgical checklist was not used at the 64 Hospitals in Uganda. Note: *p*-value = 0.989 (No differences in proportions among the health facilities – meaning that almost all facilities didn't use the surgical check list because they were not available)

be accessed online. However, future research may be required on motivations for use and access to internet in various settings. In addition, more training may be needed with providers on where to locate the checklist online. Other challenges of access, like availability to internet can be addressed by regularly providing printed copies to surgical centers.

From our study private facilities also provided more postoperative care compared to the government and not for profit hospitals. An ICU requires an intensivist and specialized ICU nursing team, which is a big challenge in a country that has very few specialists relative to the growing population. A 7-year retrospective audit from 2003 to 2009 by Kwizera et al. estimated that there were 33 ICU beds in the whole country for a population of 33 million people in Uganda, representing 0.1 ICU beds/ 100,000 population. Head injuries were a common reason for ICU admission and associated with the highest mortality rates in this audit and 23/33 ICU beds in the whole country were at private hospitals [18]. This limitation is further compounded by a well-documented dearth of anaesthesiologists- a critical human resource for intensive care units [20, 21].

The private hospitals provide ICU service, potentially requiring catastrophic out of pocket financial expenses for those who do not have insurance. Uganda has a large population that is below the poverty line and most patients cannot afford the expense of a private hospitals resulting in an overwhelming number of patients in the government hospital which is then compounded by other factors like understaffing eventually affecting the quality of services given to patients. This data presents significant barriers to achieving Universal Health Care particularly in accessing safe surgery and safe anaesthesia, an essential component of the comprehensive emergency obstetric and neonatal care. Similarly, Wall et al. state that intrapartum-related neonatal deaths can be substantially reduced by improving the quality of services for all childbirths that occur in health facilities, identifying and addressing the missed opportunities to provide effective interventions to those who seek facility-based care [22].

Bringing about a change in health policy on a worldwide basis by guaranteeing health and well-being for all age groups – the crux of the Sustainable Development Goal, is easier said than done. Strategic health financing is one the key aspects that can push this objective forward, along with considerable efforts by the global health workforce. If measures are to be properly exercised regarding global health, around 18 million extra health workers are needed by 2030.

Data form 2005 to 2015 suggests that more than 40% of countries have less than one physician per 1000 people and around half have fewer than three nurses or midwives per 1000 people. If the situation isn't rectified, the circumstances might become worse due to an increased rate of migration of qualified health professionals to high income countries. Without targeted interventions, the situation in some of these countries could be further exacerbated by increased labour migration of trained health personnel towards high-income countries with greater demand and compensation, thereby further undermining already vulnerable health systems [23].

It isn't all bad news though as the Lancet Commission on surgery reports that quality of health care has improved globally in the last 25 years, but the progress is inconsistent. Unfortunately morbidity and morality from common condition requiring surgery have spiked in the poorest of places. Almost 5 billion are yet to be provided access to affordable and safe anesthesia and surgical care when required. Steps should be undertaken to remove the disparity of access in certain regions as well [24]. Sub-Saharan Africa, North Africa and Middle East have a population of 1305 million with a total surgical burden of 73 million Cases per 100,000 population, there is a total estimated unmet need of 38,871,266 surgical cases [25, 26]. In addition, within those countries, as our study demonstrates, there is a disparity of access to evidence based interventions with poor women suffering greater burden.

To address this gap in surgery, the Lancet Commission recommends a work force density of 20 Surgeons Obstetricians and Anaesthetists per 100,000 population, with 5 per 100,000 population as anaesthetists in each country. Our research demonstrated the profound lack of safe anaesthesia in East Africa with delays in performing cesarean deliveries when needed due to lack of anaesthetists, lack of equipment and emergency drugs, shortage of blood supply, and a failed referral system. In a previous publication, we found that for a population of 142.9 million in the East African Community, there were only 237 anesthesiologists, with a workforce density of 0.08 in Uganda, 0.39 in Kenya, 0.05 in Tanzania, 0.13 in Rwanda, and 0.02 in Burundi per 100,000 population in each country [27].

To achieve the sustainable development goals of 2030, it is imperative to operationalize more medical schools and professional colleges in the region and train more doctors equipping them with essential skills in surgery and anaesthesia. We must implement the evidence based international guidelines for safer outcomes including WHO Checklists.

While The Lancet Commission focuses on increasing surgical volume; in low to middle income countries the value of these surgical procedures needs to be closely considered. Highly cost effective procedures that are affordable for the community should be implemented.

There are many larger discussions to be had regarding health care in sub-Saharan Africa to include infrastructure building to improve roads and transportation for quicker access to critical surgical procedures. Healthcare financing is also an essential discussion where millions of families are one disease away from poverty following catastrophic out of pocket medical payments. The shortage of ICU services in government facilities forces patients to pay out of pocket in private facilities. It is time we develop modeled health approaches to bridge the gap in domestic health financing in low and middle-income countries. If communities are able to pay for clean pumped and/or piped water, and electricity, how much more to contribute to a collective pool for better health services?

Conclusions

Surgery and anaesthesia have long been neglected in global health work with the focus on communicable diseases. However, the recent World Health Assembly emphasized universal care for all, including strengthening of surgery and anaesthesia. Increasing access to quality cesarean sections and obstetric safe anaesthesia would improve maternal and neonatal outcomes working toward the milestone of safe motherhood. Now is the time to re-configure the global health target to specifically address these health disparities in low-income countries; developing health leadership, mentorship, strengthening health systems, designing and implementing local and international policies in order to achieve equity in health care.

Abbreviations

ICU: Intensive Care Unit; LMICs: Low-and middle-income countries; MMR: Maternal mortality ratio; WHO: World Health Organisation

Acknowledgements

Special thanks to the Rockefeller Foundation for Dr. Epiu's Practitioner Residence 2018 at Bellagio Center where initial drafts of this manuscript was written and edited.

Funding

This study was sponsored by the National Institutes of Health; (NIH Research Training Grant Number #R25TW009343) during the corresponding author' 2014/2015 Post-doctoral Fellowship in Global Health with UCGHI.

Author's contributions

IE was the principal investigator, designed the research, sought ethical approval, conducted the interviews, entered the results and wrote the report. AK participated in data collection and writing the report. JB, AMA participated in analyzing the data and writing the report. All authors read and approved the final manuscript.

Competing interests

The authors declare that they have no competing interests.

Author details

[1]NIH Fogarty Global Health Fellow, University of California Global Health Institute, San Francisco, CA, USA. [2]Health Solutions International, P.O.Box 2336, Kampala, Uganda. [3]Makerere University, Kampala, Uganda. [4]Mbarara University, Mbarara, Uganda. [5]University of California San Francisco, CA, USA.

References

1. UN Statistics https://unstats.un.org/sdgs/report/2017/goal-03/. Accessed Oct 2018.
2. Metin Gülmezoglu A, Lawrie TA. Impact of training on emergency resuscitation skills: Impact on Millennium Development Goals (MDGs) 4 and 5. Best Pract Res Clin Obstet Gynaecol. 2015;29(Issue 8):1119–25 ISSN 1521-6934.
3. WHO. Media center, Maternal mortality fact sheet N°348, 2014.
4. Uganda Demographic and Health Survey 2011 via the DHS Program STATcompiler. (http://www.statcompiler.com). Accessed Oct 2018.
5. Lawn JE, Blencowe H, Waiswa P, for Lancet Ending Preventable Stillbirths Series study group with The Lancet Stillbirth Epidemiology investigator group, et al. Stillbirths: rates, risk factors, and acceleration towards 2030. Lancet. 2016; published online Jan 18. https://doi.org/10.1016/S0140; 6736(15):00837-5.
6. Graham W, Woodd S, Byass P, et al. Diversity and divergence: the dynamic burden of poor maternal health. Lancet. 2016;388:2164–75.
7. Spector JM, et al. Improving quality of Care for Maternal and Newborn Health: prospective pilot study of the WHO safe childbirth checklist program. PLoS One. 2012;7(4):e35151.
8. Society of obstetricians and Gynaecologists of Canada (SOGC)Surgical Safety Checklist in Obstetrics and Gynaecology, https://sogc.org/wp-content/uploads/2013/04/JOGC-Jan2013-CPG286-ENG-Online.pdf. Accessed Oct 2018.
9. Department of Reproductive Health and Research World Health Organization. World Health Organization statement on caesarean section rates. 2015. Available at: http://apps.who.int/iris/bitstream/handle/10665/161442/WHO_RHR_15.02_eng.pdf;jsessionid=4E6E15479FC4C3E70B4BFD4A7511EEA9?sequence=1. Accessed Oct 2018.
10. Haynes AB, Weiser TG, Berry WR, Lipsitz SR, Breizat A-HS, Dellinger EP, et al. A surgical safety checklist to reduce morbidity and mortality in a global population. N Engl J Med. 2009;360(5):491–9.
11. Blot K, Bergs J, Vogelaers D, Blot S, Vandijck D. Prevention of central lineassociated bloodstream infections through quality improvement interventions: a systematic review and meta-analysis. Clin Infect Dis. 2014; 18(1):96–105. https://doi.org/10.1093/cid/ciu239.
12. de Vries EN, Prins HA, Crolla RM, den Outer AJ, van Andel G, van Helden SH, et al. Effect of a comprehensive surgical safety system on patient outcomes. N Engl J Med. 2010;363(20):1928–37.
13. WHO Surgical Safety Checklist Implementation http://www.who.int/patientsafety/topics/safe-surgery/checklist_implementation/en/. Accessed Oct 2018.
14. Epiu I, Tindimwebwa JVB, Mijumbi C, Ndarugirire F, Twagirumugabe T, Lugazia ER, et al. Working towards safer surgery in Africa; a survey of utilization of the WHO safe surgical checklist at the main referral hospitals in East Africa. BMC Anesthesiology. 2016;16(1):60. https://www.ncbi.nlm.nih.gov/pubmed/27515450.
15. Walker IA, Reshamwalla S, Wilson IH. Surgical safety checklists: do they improve outcomes? Br J Anaesth. 2012;109:47–54 175.
16. Maternal mortality ratio, The World Bank Group https://data.worldbank.org/indicator/SH.STA.MMRT. Accessed Oct 2018.
17. Uganda Demographic hEALTH survey 2016. https://www.ubos.org/wp-content/uploads/2018/03/Uganda_DHS_2016_Report.pdf. Accessed Oct 2018.
18. Kwizera A, Dünser M, Nakibuuka J. National intensive care unit bed capacity and ICU patient characteristics in a low income country. BMC Research Notes. 2012;5(1):475.
19. Epiu I, Wabule A, Kambugu A, Mayanja-Kizza H, Tindimwebwa JVB, Dubowitz G. Key bottlenecks to the provision of safe obstetric anaesthesia in low- income countries; a cross-sectional survey of 64 hospitals in Uganda. BMC Pregnancy and Childbirth. 2017;17(1):387.
20. Gerald D, Sarah D, Kelly McQueen KA. Global anesthesia workforce crisis: a preliminary survey revealing shortages contributing to undesirable outcomes and unsafe practices. World J Surg. 2010;34(3):438–44.
21. Hodges SC, Mijumbi C, Okello M, McCormick BA, Walker IA, Wilson IH. Anaesthesia services in developing countries: defining the problems. Anaesthesia. 2007;62(1):4–11.
22. Wall SN, Lee ACC, Carlo W, Goldenberg R, Niermeyer S, Darmstadt GL, et al. Reducing Intrapartum-related neonatal deaths in low- and middle-income

23. SDG Target 25 UN Statistics https://unstats.un.org/sdgs/report/2017/goal-03/. Accessed Oct 2018.
24. John G, et al. Global surgery 2030: evidence and solutions for achieving health, welfare, and economic development Meara. Lancet. 386(9993):569–624 https://doi.org/10.1016/S0140-6736(15)60160-X.
25. Rose J, Weiser TG, Hider P, Wilson L, Gruen R, Bickler SW. Estimated need for surgery worldwide based on prevalence of diseases: a modelling study. Lancet Glob Health. 2015;3(Global Surgery special issue):S13–20.
26. Weiser TG, Haynes AB, Molina G, et al. Estimate of the global volume of surgery in 2012: an assessment supporting improved health outcomes. Lancet. 2015;385(Global Surgery special issue):S11.
27. Epiu I, Mijumbi C, Chokwe T, Lugazia E, Twagirumugabe T, Ndarugire F, et al. Challenges of anesthesia in low-and middle-income countries: a cross-sectional survey of access to safe obstetric anesthesia in East Africa. Anesth Analg. 2017;124(1):290–9.

10

Understanding barriers preventing pregnant women from starting antenatal clinic in the first trimester of pregnancy in Ntcheu District-Malawi

Chancy S. Chimatiro[1,5*], Precious Hajison[2], Effie Chipeta[3,4] and Adamson S. Muula[3,4,5]

Abstract

Background: Exploring barriers contributing to low utilization of Antenatal Care (ANC) during the first trimester of pregnancy is of national programmatic importance. We conducted an exploratory study in 2013 at Bilira Health Centre in Ntcheu district-Malawi with an aim of understanding barriers that prevent pregnant women from attending antenatal clinics in the first trimester of pregnancy.

Method: This was cross sectional exploratory study using qualitative approach. Data were collected from ANC clients, key informants, health services professionals and women of child bearing age (15–49 years) using an in-depth interviews and Focus Group Discussions (FGDs). Data were analysed manually by reading the transcriptions and memos several times inorder to be familiar with the themes emerged. The emerged themes were coded.

Results: Most of the women reported that they have a feeling of starting ANC in the early days of their pregnancies, however, they also reported several barriers ranging from cultural beliefs, social economic to service delivery barriers. On cultural barriers many women wait for marriage counselors from husband's side to give them advice before starting ANC in the process called *"Kuthimba"*. Some women hide the pregnancy in early months to avoid being bewitched. On social-economic barriers, some of the women mentioned that they don't start ANC early waiting for new clothes. Poor attitude of health workers also has an effect on ANC attendants. Most women pointed out that they started ANC late because some health workers were rude and do not observe confidentiality. Men's refusal to accompany their spouses to antenatal clinic in fear of HIV test and some by-laws which restrict women who had pregnancy outside marriage to seek an authorisation letter first from Traditional Leaders for them to start ANC at the health facility were also mentioned as contributing barriers.

Conclusion: Women should be oriented on the national guidelines on Focused ANC (FANC) which advocates for at least 4 visits. There should also be Information, Education and Communication (IEC) on ANC and interventions to deal with social-cultural issues while at the same time improving service delivery at the health facility so that ANC services can be accessible and responsive enough.

Keywords: Antenatal attendance, First trimester, Focused antenatal care, Pregnancy

* Correspondence: cchimatiro@gmail.com
[1]Department of Health Systems and Policy, School of Public Health and Family Medicine, College of Medicine, University of Malawi, Blantyre, Malawi
[5]Africa Center of Excellence in Public Health and Herbal Medicine(ACEPHEM), University of Malawi, College of Medicine, Blantyre, Malawi
Full list of author information is available at the end of the article

Plain English summary

Antenatal attendance during the first trimester is still low in most of the developing countries especially Sub-Saharan region including Malawi. First trimester of pregnancy is defined as a period within the first 3 months of pregnancy. This study was conducted inorder to find out what barriers prevent women from attending antenatal clinics (ANC) in the first trimester of pregnancy and what should be done to improve the situation.

Participants were asked to mention what they think prevent pregnant women from starting ANC in the first trimester. Key Informants Interviews (KIIs) and Focus Group Discussions (FGDs) were conducted.

In all KIIs and FGDs most of the women had positive perception on starting ANC early, however, they also reported several barriers ranging from cultural beliefs, social economic to service delivery barriers.

In conclusion, inadequate knowledge on the importance of attending ANC in the first 3 months of pregnancy was main contributing factors in most of the women. Therefore, this study recommends that Information, Education and Communication (IEC) on ANC should be prioritized among women if the trends is to be reversed.

Background

Antenatal care is the care provided to a woman from the beginning of pregnancy until the onset of labour [1]. This care often involves recording history, assessment of individual needs, advice and guidance on pregnancy and delivery, screening tests, education on self-help care during pregnancy, identification of conditions detrimental to health during pregnancy, first line management and referral if necessary [2]. Malawi's current guidelines are derived from the WHO/UNICEF report 2003, which recommended that women attend formal antenatal care services for at least 4 times during each pregnancy [3]. The visits are divided into trimesters namely first trimester, second trimester and third trimester. Ideally the first visit should be within 12 weeks of pregnancy but not later than 16th week of pregnancy [4]. The second visit should be within 24 to 28 weeks, the third visit shouldc be at 32 weeks and forth visit at 36 weeks of pregnancy.

Early initiation of antenatal care can be beneficial through: early identification of risk factors and provision of preventive and health promotion advice to encourage healthy lifestyles, treatment of medical conditions such as diabetes and pregnancy induced hypertension and referrals to services such as nutrition support and smoking cessation programs [5]. Some studies have reported that women who have few or inadequate visits and those who start antenatal care late than the first trimester have poorer pregnancy outcomes, such as low birth weight and pre-term birth [6, 7]. However, increasing the number of antenatal visits does not necessarily improve the outcomes of pregnancy [8] but should be responded with quality of care.

Globally about 70% of women attend antenatal visit at least once during pregnancy while in high income countries 98% of women attend antenatal visit at least once [9]. In low and middle-income countries and sub-Saharan Africa region ANC attendants is still low. Low et al. reported that only 65% and 68% of women report for at least one antenatal visit during pregnancy in low and middle-income countries and sub-Saharan region respectively [10].

Antenatal attendance during the first trimester shows good to poor coverage in different regions of the world. For example, about five out of six mothers (84%) begin antenatal care in the first trimester in the United States (US) [8]; 70% in Latin America/ Caribbean; about 68% in Middle East / North Africa region, 50% in Asia and lowest attendance in the first trimester is in Sub-Saharan region 24% [11]. Some countries have particularly low attendance; a study in Nigeria showed that only 22.8% of the women who received ANC booked in the first trimester [12]. In Kwa-Zulu- Natal, South Africa, most women (860/872; 98.6%) attended the antenatal clinic during their pregnancy of which only 72/860 (8.4%) women reported starting ANC in the first 3 months of pregnancy [13].

In Malawi, 12% of women had ANC visit in the first trimester; about 48% had their first antenatal visit between 4 and 5 months of pregnancy while 36% started at 6 and 7 months of their pregnancy [4]. And 2015–16 Malawi Demographics and Health Survey (MDHS) revealed that only 24% of women had their first ANC visit during the first trimester, 51% of women had their first ANC visit during the fourth and fifth month of pregnancy, and 2% did not receive any ANC until the eighth month or later [14]. Ideally, all pregnant women are supposed to have their first antenatal visit during the first trimester [15]. According to MDHS, 2010, there was no significant difference between urban and rural pregnant women in antenatal attendance in Malawi [4].

A study conducted to investigate factors that contribute to low antenatal attendance during the first trimester among the Sena of the lower shire in Nsanje, Malawi found that there was inadequate knowledge about the ideal time of starting ANC. Antenatal care clinics were understaffed and traditional beliefs and cultural practices were reported to affect timing for antenatal care [16]. Mgawadere F.M (Mgawadere FM: Assessing the quality of antenatal care at Lungwena health Centre in rural Malawi, unpublished) in a study assessing quality of antenatal care at Lungwena in Mangochi district, Malawi, found that pregnant women started ANC late in second and third trimester. Non-attendance to ANC during the first trimester was associated with social cultural practices such as afraid of witch craft, long distances and need for material support from family members [16]. Therefore, this current study aimed at exploring barriers preventing pregnant women from starting ANC in the first trimester of pregnancy in Ntcheu district-Malawi. Specifically, we explored perception of pregnant women towards ANC, social cultural and health service barriers that affect ANC attendance in the first trimester of pregnancy.

Methods

This was an exploratory cross sectional study using a qualitative approach. Data collection was done in 2013.

Study setting

This study was conducted in the community of Bilira Rural Health Centre in Ntcheu district. In 2010/2011 Ntcheu district registered 46,786 women who attended antenatal clinic and out of these 3462 women attended the antenatal clinic during the first trimester which represents 7.4% [17]. Bilira Health Centre had a total catchment population of 45,187 and with 58 villages. It had 11,363 women who were of reproductive age group (15–49 years).

Sampling technique

Convenient sampling was used to identify participants for in-depth interviews at the health centre. Purposive sampling technique was used to select participants for FGDs and key informants. We randomly selected twelve villages where FGDs were conducted in each village. Key informants included were health workers, traditional leaders, traditional birth attendants and religious leaders.

There were 10 pregnant women, 3 antenatal health services workers and 9 key informants that took part in depth interviews. A total of twelve FGDs categorized into 3 different age groups were conducted. The categories were as follows; four groups of women of ages between 15 and 24 years, another four groups of 25–34 years and last four groups of 35–44 years of age. Each FGD had minimum of eight participants and maximum of twelve participants. In total there were 126 participants in FGDs. The maximum study participants was reached at by looking at saturation of responses.

Data collection

In-depth interviews were conducted using open ended questions. The main thematic areas explored were on knowledge and motivations about ANC attendance, perception towards starting ANC early, Social-cultural practices, Social-economic factors and factors associated with access to ANC services. In both interviews and FGDs, digital recorders were used to collect data in the local language (Chichewa).

Data management

The proceedings of the interviews were listened to several times before transcribing the data in Chichewa which was later translated in English. Data was analysed manually by reading the transcriptions several times inorder to be familiar with it and explore the themes emerged from transcriptions and memos. The emerged themes were given appropriate codes. The codes were being assigned under the main theme it supported.

The main ideas from each participant concerning ANC were isolated and assigned under the theme in which it supported. The ideas were analysed to come up with final findings of the study.

Ethical considerations

The study protocol was reviewed and approved by the College of Medicine Research and Ethics Committee (COMREC) to ensure that ethical issues had been addressed under research approval No SP1212102. Permissions to carry out the study were obtained from District Health Office (DHO) and the District Commissioner (DC) for Ntcheu and Traditional Leaders around Bilira Health Centre.

Results

A total of 22 in-depth interviews and twelve FGDs were conducted. We grouped the results in the following themes; knowledge on ANC attendance, perception towards early ANC attendance, social-cultural practices, social-economic factors and factors related to access of service delivery.

Knowledge and motivations on starting ANC early

Through in depth interviews with ANC clients, Key Informants and FGDs, we found that most women had knowledge on time of starting ANC. Their understanding was that it is important to start ANC during the first trimester. We also found that most women understood benefits of starting ANC early such as getting early pregnant care and getting prompt treatment if someone has low blood level. Most women also understood the disadvantages of starting ANC late such as not knowing the position of the baby and also not knowing what kind of supplementary food to take.

A number of women who participated in the in-depth interviews demonstrated knowledge of starting ANC in their first trimesters but instead reported to deliberately started ANC in either second trimesters or third trimester. Two of the women said, *"I started when I was 5 months pregnant so that I can reduce number of visits of attending ANC before I deliver,"* (ID No 6) (ID NO 10).

Perception towards early ANC attendance

There was overall positive perception among women towards starting ANC early. The study found that most of the women were not starting ANC early because their partners refused to accompany them as they were afraid of being tested for HIV. Some woman reported in separate FGDs, saying *"men were the main barriers to starting ANC early in fear of HIV test"* (FGD No 2, Client ID No 8) (ID No 5, RESPO No 6).

Social-cultural practices

Authorisation from husband's side

In both FGDs and in depth interviews, participants were asked about cultural practices in the area. We found that many women wait for marriage counselors from husband's side to come and give them advice before starting ANC in the process called "**Kuthimba**". A woman said, *"Some of us don't start ANC early as we are supposed to wait for marriage counselor from man's side to come and give us some advises"* (ID No 6, FGD 4). Another woman said, *"it is our usual practice here to inform elders from man's side to come and give advise to the woman especially when it is her first pregnancy"* (ID No 9, key informant).

Beliefs regarding witch craft

We found that hiding the pregnancy in early months to avoid being witched was contributing to low ANC attendance during the first trimester. A Key informant said, *"I think most women here don't start ANC early because they normally try to hide the pregnancy in its early stages to avoid being witched"* (ID No 5). Another woman said during FGDs 6, *"elderly women give some of us traditional medicine that protects the pregnancy from being be witched and advise you to wait for the pregnancy to grow before starting ANC"* (ID No 3).

Social-economic barriers

Economic status

We found that social-economic factors have an effect on the time for starting ANC as many of women don't start ANC early waiting for new clothes. This is so due to poor socio-economic status (poverty) of most families in the area. Many women do not start ANC earlywaiting for their husbands to buy them new clothes in order to attend ANCin newly and nice looking clothes. A woman said, *"When one is pregnant she normally waits for the husband to buy new clothes so that she can start ANC in new and nice looking clothes"* (ID NO 8, in depth interviews).

The opinions of the FGD participants and KIIs were very similar on the dilemma that arises between the need to provide for the family versus the need to start ANC. This study showed that business had an effect on decision to start ANC early. Some women preferred going for business rather than starting ANC when they had less than 5 months pregnancy inorder to provide for their families. This signifies that social-economic is indeed another factor affecting decision to start ANC early. Another respondent said, *"If you have millet and it is a market day while you are also supposed to go for ANC, it is better to go to the market and sell millet so that you can have something to feed your family"* (ID No3, FGG 2).

We found that farming has little effect on starting ANC early. This is so as most of the women said that farming cannot prevent someone from starting ANC early because there are several months in the year for farming and ANC schedule is once a month. A woman said, *"I cannot fail to start ANC early because of farming as ANC schedule is only once a months while farming is our daily work for several months"* (ID NO 7, in-depth interviews).

Access to services

Long distances from home to the facility have effects on the decision to start ANC early. Some women reported to travel more than 7 km (often by foot) in order to access ANC services. This prevents women for starting ANC early in the first trimester. A woman said, *"I cannot start ANC early because I come from very far from the clinic, I do not want to have many visits and get tired before delivery"* (ID NO 7, in depth interviews). Another participant had this to say, *"When I think of distance from home to here I always get discouraged to start off"* (ID NO 6, in depth interviews at the facility).

Male involvement

We found that many women do no start ANC early if their husbands are away or refuse to accompany them. Women may also not initiate ANC if they do not have a spouse. In this study area, there was a by-law which advocates that every woman should attend ANC clinic with her spouse during the first visit. This was being reinforced by traditional leaders around the area. If women go to the health facility without their partners they are not attended to as a result most women do not start ANC early. We also found that if the woman has no partners, she is supposed to get an authorisation letter from the traditional leader in order to access ANC services at the health facility otherwise, she cannot be attended to.

A woman said during one of the FGDs, *"if my husband has refused to accompany me, then I cannot go to start ANC alone because I know that I will not be attended to"* (ID No 3).

Another woman said, *"I started ANC when I was five months pregnant as I was waiting for my husband who was away by then"* (ID No 1).

Another woman said, *"if you are pregnant outside marriage then you are supposed to go and get an authorisation letter from village headman for you to be allowed to start ANC"* (FGD 5, RESPO NO 7).

Attitude of health workers

During both FGDs and in depth interviews we found that poor attitude of health workers towards clients has an effect on decision to start ANC early. We found that some health workers at the facility rarely observed confidentiality. A woman said during one of the FGDs, *"there is a certain nurse there who even reveals what you have worn inside your wrapper (Chitenje)"* (ID No 6, FGD 5).

Another Key informant said, *"I have been receiving complaints from women concerning the way they are being handled at the clinic, in fact some of the providers are rude to our women"* (ID No 9).

Waiting time

Study participants reported that, there was long waiting time for the ANC women to access services at the facility due to integration of the service with family planning. This claim was confirmed by the study team during the key informant interviews with pregnant women at the facility as they were waiting for the ANC clinic to start.

It was reported that health workers were prioritizing family planning clients before starting attending to ANC clients. A woman said during an in-depth interview, *"I always come for ANC early so that I can be assisted and go back on time, however, nurses give priority to those who have come for family planning first than us, as a result we usually go back home very late"* (ID No 9 for ANC Clients).

Discussion

Having adequate knowledge about optimal time for starting ANC, its benefits and the downside associated with starting ANC late may not assure that women can start ANC early. Most women reported to have started ANC late with an aim of reducing number of visits before delivery. Similarly, another study done in Nsanje reported that some women started ANC late because they wanted to reduce number of visits so that they should not get tired before delivering [16].

Cultural practices have a role in determining time for starting ANC. We established that some women do not start ANC early as they wait for marriage counselors or their mother in-laws to come and give them advice especially if it is the first pregnancy. This leads to the pregnancy being kept secret until it reaches 3 to 4 months old. These findings have been noted elsewhere. Studies done in Nsanje and Nepal reported that women wait for their mother in-laws to either give them advise or make decision for them to start ANC [16, 18].

The belief that witchcraft could impact (early) pregnancy was reported to prevent women form starting ANC early as most women were influenced to hide the pregnancy and also took traditional medicine to protect the pregnancy in its early stages. These findings support what was reported in another study in Nsanje that most women were afraid to be bewitched if people discovered that they were pregnancy especially during early stages of pregnancy [16].

Socio-economic factors also assist in the decision to start ANC early. We found that some women do not start ANC early because they demand new clothes from their husbands. This was also reported in other studies done in South Africa and Nigeria where women were reported to start ANC late because they needed to find money for transport and new clothes [19, 20]. The finding of the studies shows that socio-economic status may be associated with the decision to seek health services especially on time to start ANC.

Some women are involved in small scale businesses in order to feed their families. Our study noticed that there was competing interest in decision making whether to go for business or ANC. This activity affects the decision to start ANC early as most women prefer going for business so that they can get money to buy new clothes for ANC. Similarly this was also reported in another study done in Blantyre, Malawi, which reported that some men failed to participate in accompanying their wives because of work or business obligations [21].

In addition, we report that long waiting time has also negative impact in decision to start ANC early. In another study done in Benin, they reported that waiting time was one of the determinants of low utilization of ANC during the first trimester [22].

Long distances from health facilities limit access to health care when required. This study agrees with other studies done elsewhere which reported about long distances from homes to the health facility as a barrier to access medical care [23–25].

Male involvement plays important role in encouraging women to start ANC early as some women do not start ANC early because their husbands refuses to accompany them. This has been also reported in other studies [19, 26]. Poor attitude of the health workers prevents some women from starting ANC early. Disrespectful care has been reported in different settings and impact negatively on the quality of services [21, 27, 28]. This is the strongest predictor about how responsive service delivery is to those who need them as reported by another study done Sweden about women's expectations on ANC services [29].

Conclusion

Although women may have positive perceptions towards starting ANC early, they are prevented from doing so due to various barriers. These barriers range from socio-cultural factors to service delivery factors.

We recommend that public facilities should put clients at the centre of health services by providing good quality care with respect. Therefore, a well-functioning health work-force is the one that is responsive to the needs of its users or customers. As such health systems managers should train health workers on customer care so that they can change their attitude towards women who attend ANC. This will make pregnant women not to be scared to go for ANC.

We also recommend that traditional leaders, being custodians of custom, should come up with deliberate by-laws which can help in addressing some social-cultural practices so that women should start ANC early. Policy makers should ensure that there is enough IEC materials to sensitize women on the need to start ANC early. Women empowerment through education should be enhanced so that they can make independent and reasonable decisions concerning their health and that of their unborn baby. Availability of mobile clinics with integrated services, which include ANC, should be encouraged at all level especially in hard to reach areas inorder to reduce distance covered by pregnant women to access ANC services from health facility.

Abbreviations

ACEPHEM: Africa Centre of Excellence in Public Health and Herbal Medicine; ANC: Antenatal Care; COMREC: College of Medicine Research and Ethics Committee; CRH: Centre for Reproductive Health; DC: District Commissioner; DHO: District Health Officer; FANC: Focused Antenatal Care; FGDs: Focus Group Discussions; ID: Identification No; IEC: Information, Education and Communication; KIIs: Key Informant Interviews; MDHS: Malawi Demographics and Health Survey; RESPO: Respondent; UNICEF: United Nations International Children Education Fund; WHO: World Health Organisation

Acknowledgements

We acknowledge the following people; Patrick Kavaya and Moles Nguluwe for conceptualisation of the study, data collection and data analysis.

Authors' contributions

CSC planned the study, developed study methods, developed the analysis plan, analysed the data and drafted the manuscript. PH developed and checked the manuscript. EC and ASM supervised the planning, development of the methods, analysis plan, and data analysis and contributed and supervised the manuscript writing. All authors have read and agreed to the final version of this manuscript and have equally contributed to its content. All authors read and approved the final manuscript.

Consent for publication

All participants consented for peer review and the publication of the study results.

Competing interests

The authors declare that they have no competing interests.

Author details

[1]Department of Health Systems and Policy, School of Public Health and Family Medicine, College of Medicine, University of Malawi, Blantyre, Malawi. [2]PreLuHa consult, Namiwawa Street, Newroard location, PO BOX 703, Zomba, Malawi. [3]Department of Public Health, School of Public Health and Family Medicine, College of Medicine, University of Malawi, Blantyre, Malawi. [4]Centre for Reproductive Health (CRH), University of Malawi, College of Medicine, Blantyre, Malawi. [5]Africa Center of Excellence in Public Health and Herbal Medicine(ACEPHEM), University of Malawi, College of Medicine, Blantyre, Malawi.

References

1. Van Der Spuy J, Antony J. Hand book of Obstretrics and gynacology. New York: Oxford University Press; 2002.
2. WHO. Health service coverage statistics, antenatal care coverage (percentage). 2006.
3. WHO. Antenatal care in developing countries: premises, Achievements and missed opportunities. 2003.
4. National Statistical Office and ICF Macro. Malawi Demographics and Health Survey 2010. 2010.
5. McComick JE. Siegel M. prenatal care, effectiveness and implementation. London: Cambridge University press; 2001.
6. da Fonseca CR, Strufaldi MW, de Carvalho LR, Puccini RF. Adequacy of antenatal care and its relationship with low birth weight in Botucatu, São Paulo, Brazil: a case-control study. BMC Pregnancy Childbirth. 2014;14:255.
7. Bhaskar RK, Deo KK, Neupane U, et al. A case control study on risk factors associated with low birth weight babies in Eastern Nepal. Inter J Paediatr. 2015;2015(Article ID 807373):7 https://doi.org/10.1155/2015/807373.
8. Low P, Paterson J, Wouldes T, Carter S, Williams M, Percival T. Factors affecting antenatal care attendance by mothers of Pacific infants living in New Zealand. 2005.
9. Nikiéma B, Beninguisse G, Haggerty JL. Providing information on pregnancy complications during antenatal visits: unmet educational needs in sub-Saharan Africa. Health Policy Plan. 2009;24(5):367–76.
10. National Center for Health Statistics Health, United States, 2005 With Chartbook on Trends in the Health of Americans Hyattsville, Maryland; 2005.
11. Abou-Zahr CL, Wardlaw TM, World Health Organization. Antenatal care in developing countries: promises, achievements and missed opportunities: an analysis of trends, levels and differentials, 1990–2001. 2003.
12. Galadanci H, Ejembi C, Iliyasu Z, Alagh B, Umar U. Maternal health in northern Nigeria—a far cry from ideal. BJOG: Inter J Obstet Gynecol. 2007; 114(4):448–52.
13. Horwood C, Haskins L, Vermaak K, Phakathi S, Subbaye R, Doherty T. Prevention of mother to child transmission of HIV (PMTCT) programme in KwaZulu-Natal, South Africa: an evaluation of PMTCT implementation and integration into routine maternal, child and women's health services. Tropical Med Int Health. 2010;15(9):992–9.
14. National Statistical Office (NSO) [Malawi] and ICF. Malawi Demographic and Health Survey 2015–16. 2017.
15. Lincetto O, Mothebesoane-Anoh S, Gomez P, Munjanja S. Antenatal care. Opportunities for Africa's newborns: Practical data, policy and programmatic support for new born care in Africa; 2006. p. 55–62.
16. Chitimbe E. Determinants of utilization of antenatal health care services by pregnant women during the first trimester in Nsanje. 2006.
17. MOH. Ntcheu District Health Management Information System. 2011.
18. Dhakal S, Van Teijlingen ER, Stephens J, Dhakal KB, Simkhada P, Raja EA, et al. Antenatal care among women in rural Nepal: a community-based study. Online J Rural Nurs Health Care. 2011;11(2):76–87.
19. Tshabalala MF. Utilization of antenatal care (ANC) and PMTCT services in East Ekurhuleni SUB. 1984.
20. Abimbola JM, Makanjuola AT, Ganiyu SA, Babatunde UMM, Adekunle DK, Olatayo AA. Pattern of utilization of ante-natal and delivery services in a semi-urban community of north-Central Nigeria. Afr Health Sci. 2016;16(4):962–71.
21. Nyondo AL, Chimwaza AF, Muula AS. Stakeholders' perceptions on factors influencing male involvement in prevention of mother to child transmission of HIV services in Blantyre, Malawi. BMC Public Health. 2014;14(1):691.
22. Edgard-Marius O, Charles SJ, Jacques S, Justine GC, Virginie MA, Ibrahim MA, et al. Determinants of low antenatal care services utilization during the first trimester of pregnancy in southern Benin rural setting. Univers J Public Health. 2015;3(5):220–8.
23. Ikamari LD. Maternal health care utilisation in Teso District. Afr Health Sci. 2004;11(1):21–32.
24. Magadi MA, Madise NJ, Rodrigues RN. Frequency and timing of antenatal care in Kenya: explaining the variations between women of different communities. SocSciMed. 2000;51(4):551–61.
25. Worku EB, Woldesenbet SA. Factors that influence teenage antenatal care utilization in John Taolo Gaetsewe (JTG) district of northern Cape Province, South Africa: underscoring the need for tackling social determinants of health. Int J MCH AIDS. 2016;5(2):134.
26. Kawungezi PC, AkiiBua D, Aleni C, Chitayi M, Niwaha A, Kazibwe A, et al. Attendance and utilization of antenatal care (ANC) services: multi-center study in upcountry areas of Uganda. Open JPrevMed. 2015;5(3):132–42.

27. Pell C, Meñaca A, Were F, Afrah NA, Chatio S, Manda-Taylor L, et al. Factors affecting antenatal care attendance: results from qualitative studies in Ghana, Kenya and Malawi. PLoS One. 2013;8(1):e53747.
28. Buchi S, Cignacco E, Luthi D, Spirig R. Needs and expectations of Tamil women attending an antenatal care department at a Swiss university hospital. Pflege. 2006;19(5):295–302.
29. Hildingsson I, Waldenström U, Rådestad I. Women's expectations on antenatal care as assessed in early pregnancy: number of visits, continuity of caregiver and general content. Acta ObstetGynecolScand. 2002;81(2):118–25.

Essential newborn care practices and associated factors among home delivered mothers in Damot pulasa Woreda, southern Ethiopia

Tesfaye Yitna Chichiabellu[1*], Baze Mekonnen[2], Feleke Hailemichael Astawesegn[3], Birhanu Wondimeneh Demissie[4] and Antehun Alemayehu Anjulo[5]

Abstract

Background: Globally 3.1 million children die each year in their neonatal period (first 28 days of life) according to World Health Organization (WHO) 2011 report. Half of these surprisingly occur within the first 24 h of delivery and 75% occur in the early neonatal period.

Methods: A community based cross-sectional study design was carried out from March 2016 to April, 2016 in Damot Pulasa district, Wolaita zone, Southern Ethiopia to assess selected essential newborn care practices and associated factors among home delivered mothers in Damot pulasa district. Data were entered into Epi Info version 3.5.1 and exported to SPSS version 20 software for analysis. Multiple logistic analyses were done to control possible confounding variable. A *P*-value less than 0.05 was taken as a significant association.

Result: The study showed that the prevalence of essential newborn care practice was 24%. Multivariate logistic regression analysis revealed that variables like ANC visit (AOR =0.213,*P* = 0.015,CI = 0.102–0.446),PNC visit (AOR = 0.209, *P* = 0.00,CI = 0.110–0.399), advice about essential newborn care practice (AOR =0.114,*P* = 0.0001, CI = 0.058–0.221),urban areas women (AOR =2,*P* = 0.042, CI = 1.024–3.693), planned pregnancy (AOR = 7, P = 0.00, CI =3.732–11.813), and knowledge about newborn danger signs (AOR = 0.277, *P* = 0.006, CI = 0.110–0.697) were the independent predictors of ENBC practices.

Conclusion: Generally, coverage of essential newborn care practices was low. ANC visit, advice about ENBC, PNC visit, residence, planned pregnancy and knowledge about newborn danger signs were predictors of essential newborn care practice in the study area. Therefore, Health facilities should enhance linkage with health posts to increase ANC and PNC service utilization. Health extension workers should also promote and give health education about pre-lacteal feeding, early bathing, planned pregnancy, newborn danger signs and application of materials on the newborn stump.

Keywords: Essential newborn care practice, Newborn

* Correspondence: yefaste2005@gmail.com
[1]Department of Nursing, College of Health Science and Medicine, Wolaita Sodo University, P.O.Box: 138, Wolaita Sodo, Ethiopia
Full list of author information is available at the end of the article

Plain English summary

Though many efforts had been made to overcome newborn mortality in Sub-Saharan Africa, it is continued to be great public health problems. Essential newborn care is a comprehensive strategy designed to improve the health of newborns through interventions before conception, during pregnancy, at and soon after birth, and in the postnatal period. Data associated with socio-demographic variables, maternal health services utilization, knowledge, counseling from a health worker, source of information, and traditional practices were collected. Even though majority of the women used boiled blade to cut the cord and tied with threads, application of butter on the umbilical stump practiced by most of the women. In addition to low coverage of initiation of breast feeding within one hour and giving colostrum, the majority, of the women in this study gave pre-lacteals. Bathing of the newborn after 24 h was practiced by the majority of the women. The level of coverage of essential newborn care practices in the district was generally low. The associated factors of essential newborn care practice were; ANC visit, advice about ENBC, PNC visit, residence, planned pregnancy and knowledge about newborn danger.

In conclusions; Health facilities should enhance linkage with health postse to increase antenatal and postnatal care service utilization. Health extension workers should also promote and give health education about pre-lacteal feeding, early bathing, planned pregnancy, newborn danger signs and application of materials on the newborn stump.

Background

Globally 3.1 million children die each year in their neonatal period (first 28 days of life) according to World Health Organization (WHO) 2011 report. Half of these surprisingly occur within the first 24 h of delivery and 75% occur in the early neonatal period (0 to 6 days after delivery) because of preterm births, severe infections and birth asphyxia [1]. Though many efforts had been made to overcome newborn mortality in Sub-Saharan Africa, it is continued to be great public health problems. Every year 2.9 million babies die during the neonatal period [2]; it is also the time of greatest risk for stillbirths and maternal deaths [3].

One of the targets of the MDG was a two-thirds reduction in infant and child mortality by 2015; it was intended to achieve by involving skilled birth attendants, increasing immunization coverage against six vaccine preventable diseases, improving the status of women through education, and enhancing women participation in the labor force [4].

Globally, around 40 million mothers give birth at home per year without any trained health worker. Factors like lack of good quality care during labor and birth; socio-economic aspects of poverty; poor health status of women; lack of autonomy and decision making authority; and illiteracy to health system related factors like poor antenatal and obstetric care; absence of trained birth attendant; inadequate referral system; lack of transportation facilities; poor linkages between health centers and communities favored the morbidities and mortalities of pregnant women, perinatal and neonate [5]. In Ethiopia, according to Ethiopia Mini Demographic Health Survey 2014 report, only 15% of births take place at a health institution, 40% of women receive Antenatal Care (ANC) from a skilled provider, and 12% of women receive a postnatal care (PNC) within the first two days of birth [6]. This favors neonatal morbidity and mortality rates to be high in Ethiopia; around 122,000 newborns die every year and the neonatal mortality rate is 37 per 1000 live births [7, 8].

WHO recommended Essential Newborn Care (ENBC) practices to reduce the risk of the main causes of neonatal deaths in both community and facility deliveries [8]. ENBC is a comprehensive strategy designed to improve the health of newborns through interventions before conception, during pregnancy, at and soon after birth, and in the postnatal period [9].ENBC practices, as recommended by WHO, include drying (wiping) and wrapping the newborn immediately after birth, initiating skin-to-skin contact, dry cord care (not applying any potentially harmful substance to the umbilical cord), immediate initiation of breastfeeding and delayed bathing (for at least 6 h) [10].

Ethiopia government has been striving to achieve the 3rd Sustainable Development Goal (SDG3) which is to ensure healthy lives and promote well-being for all, at all ages [11]. However, the neonatal mortality rates in Damot pulasa is still remained higher than the national level; it is 38 per 1, 000 live births [12]. Thus, new innovative strategies must be developed for safe home deliveries including essential neonatal care in order to change the practice at the household level, besides devising means of proper care of the neonate in domestic settings and ensuring proper referral of those neonates who cannot be managed at home [13]. A study showed that home-based counseling strategy using volunteers and designed for scale-up can improve newborn care behaviors in rural communities [14].

Traditional Birth Attendants (TBAs), relatives, neighbors and other aged women from the community who lack the requisite knowledge of safe delivery and newborn care practices; Meanwhile, their intervention to support mothers who give birth at home is inevitable. This may increase maternal and newborn morbidity and mortality among home delivered mothers. Traditional practice like pre-lacteal feeding, avoiding of first milk and application of material on the newborn stump was practiced by the majority of study participant in the study area. Therefore, improving newborn survival is a major priority in child health today and the government sets universal sustainable development goals which state to end preventable deaths of newborns and under-five children by 2030. Therefore, this study aimed to assess selected essential newborn care practices and associated factors among home delivered mothers in Damot pulasa district.

Methods and materials

Study area

A community based cross-sectional study design was conducted from March 2016 to April 2016 in Damot Pulasa district, Wolaita zone, Southern Ethiopia. Damot Pulasa located at 365 Km from Addis Ababa, the capital city of Ethiopia. The population of the district was estimated to be 130,515 with an estimated number of women of reproductive age group 30,818 which is 23.6% of the total population. The town has an urban kebele and 22 rural kebeles, in terms of health facilities; there are 5 governmental health centers, 8 private clinics, 1 private pharmacy, 1 drug vender and 1urban and 22 rural health posts.

Populations

The study population was randomly selected women of reproductive age group who had given birth at home in the past one year in Damot Pulasa district which encompasses 450 women who participated in the study. Those mothers who had given live birth at home within one year preceding the data collection date included in the study. The source population was list of households who had women's in the reproductive age and who had given birth at home in Damot pulasa district.

Sample size determination

The required sample size was determined by using single population proportion formula by taking 23% of expected prevalence for essential newborn care practice [8], assuming 5% margin of error and 95% confidence level, design effect of 1.5 and 10% for non-response rate. The calculated sample size was 450.

Sampling technique and procedures

Cluster multi-stage sampling technique was employed for the Selection of the sampling units. In the district, there are 22 rural and an urban kebeles. From 22 rural kebeles10 were selected by simple random sampling. The total sample size was allocated for each selected kebeles proportionally to the number of households within each kebele. Then systematic sampling technique was used to select a household where participant exist. The index case was selected and interviewed using lottery method when more than one eligible respondent present in a house.

Data collection tools and procedures

Data associated with socio-demographic variables, maternal health services utilization, knowledge, counseling from a health worker, source of information, and traditional practices were collected using interviewer administered questionnaire adapted from similar studies [8, 14, 18] (Additional file 1). The data were collected by B.Sc. nurses who are fluent speakers of the local languages.

Data processing and analysis

Data was checked visually for completeness, and then coded and entered in to Epi Info version 3.5.1 and exported in to Statistical Program Social Science (SPSS) version 20 software for analysis. Binary and multiple logistic regressions were run to assess the associations of various factors with essential newborn care practice. The results were presented in the form of tables, figures and summary statistics. A *P*-value less than 0.05 was taken as a significant association.

Results

Socio-demographiccharacterstics

In this study, a total of 450 women have participated and the response rate was 100%. In terms of religion, majority of the respondents were protestant, which accounts 238 (52.9%) and 434 (96.4%) were Wolaita in ethnicity. One hundred ninety-five (43.3%) were illiterate and 310 (68.9%) were housewife. With regard to marital status and place of residence, 444 (98.7%) were married and 393 (87.3%) were rural dweller (Table 1).

Maternal health services

A total of 364 (80.9%) of respondents belonged to the age group 19–41 years and the mean age of respondents was 30.8 (± 4.05). Majority of the study subjects conceived their last baby unintentionally, which accounts 383 (85.1%). Thirty two (7.1%) received at least one ANC visit. From all mothers, 363 (80.7%) prepared themselves for birth. From the total study subjects, 120 (26.7%) utilized PNC service and from these mothers, 35 (29%) utilized the service within 7-41 days (Table 2).

Health service availability

Concerning health service availability, 318 (70.7%) mothers had health facilities (health post)in the nearby site. Home delivered mothers mentioned the following reasons why they gave birth at home; Two hundred eighty-three (62.9%) "Not seriously ill", 247 (54.9%) "Had TBAs", 126 (28%) "Unwelcoming of health workers approach" and 123 (27.3%) "An experience of safe home delivery before" Moreover, the majority of women

Table 1 Socio-demographic characteristics of the respondent in Damot pulasa district, Wolaita Zone, Southern Ethiopia, 2016

Variable	Frequency ($n = 450$)	Percentage (%)
Religion		
Protestant	238	52.9
Catholic	124	27.6
Orthodox	76	16.9
Muslim	12	2.7
Educational status		
No education	195	43.3
Primary level	175	38.9
Secondary level	67	14.9
Higher education	13	2.9
Ethnic group		
Wolaita	434	96.4
Gammo	8	1.8
Amhara	7	1.6
Gurage	1	.2
Occupation		
Housewife	310	68.9
Farmer	13	2.9
Merchant/Trade	100	22.2
Daily labor	27	6.0
Marital status		
Married	444	98.7
Widowed	6	1.3
Residence		
Urban	57	12.7
Rural	393	87.3
Age at current pregnancy		
< 20 years	2	0.4
20–34 years	364	80.9
34–49 years	84	18.7
Planned pregnancy		
Yes	67	14.9
No	383	85.1
Parity		
1	44	12.8
2–4	194	56.6
>=5	105	30.6

participated in this study, 356 (79.1%) decided to deliver at home by themselves (Table 3) (Fig. 1).

Knowledge of the respondents

From the total study subjects, 417 (92.7%) of the women had information about newborn care. Among 415 (92.2%) women who had information about when to start breastfeeding, 141 (34%) mothers started breastfeeding within the first one hour of birth. From all mothers, 390 (86.7%) of them had knowledge about colostrum and 262 (67%) mothers mentioned the importance of colostrum. Four hundred six (90.2%) of women told that it is possible to expose the neonate for morning sunlight; In addition to this, 432 (96%) of women mentioned that, exposing the neonate for vaccination has no problem (Table 4) (Figs. 2 and 3).

Table 2 Maternal health services of respondents, in Damot pulasa district, Wolaita Zone, Southern, Ethiopia, 2016

Variable	Frequency (n = 450)	Percentage (%)
Receive ANC		
Yes	32	7.1
No	418	92.9
Number of ANC visit		
Once	13	40.6
Twice	10	31.25
Three times	6	18.75
Four times	3	9.4
Advice about ENBC		
Yes	32	7.1
No	418	92.9
Preparation for delivery		
Yes	363	80.7
No	87	19.3
Receive PNC		
Yes	120	26.7
No	330	73.3
Time for frequency of PNC		
Less than 4 h	12	10
4–23 h	20	16.7
1–2 days	27	22.5
3–6 days	26	21
7–41 days	35	29

Newborn care practice of the respondent

From all mothers, 408 (90.7%) remembered where they positioned the neonate immediately after delivery. Of all mothers, 259 (63.5%) put their newborn baby on their abdomen immediately after delivery (Table 5).

Safe cord cutting

Almost all mothers, 434 (96.4%) used boiled new razor blade in order to cut their newborn baby and 288 (64%) study subjects applied butter on the cord after the cord was cut.

Table 3 Health service utilization of respondents, in Damot pulasa district, Wolaita Zone, Southern Ethiopia, 2016

Variable	Frequency (n = 450)	Percentage (%)
Availability of HF		
Yes	450	100
Type of HF		
Health post	318	70.7
Health center	132	29.3
HF provide delivery		
Yes	227	50.4
No	179	39.8
I don't know	44	9.8
Decision for place of birth		
Self	356	79.1
Husband	77	17.1
Relatives	17	3.8

Initiation of early exclusive breastfeeding

From the total study subjects, 206 (45.8%) initiated breastfeeding within an hour of birth. From the total of 224 (49.8%) women who gave pre-lacteals, 218 (97.3%) gave water and 6 (2.7%) gave butter. Two hundred twenty three (49.6%) of the respondents gave first milk to the newborn and 247 (54.9%) mothers fed their breast greater than or equal to eight times.

Thermal care (bathing time)

From all mothers, 362 (80.4%) mothers dried/wrapped the newborn baby. Of whom 190 (52.2%) dried/wrapped the newborn before delivery of the placenta. One hundred sixty-six (45.6%) mothers used a pre-prepared towel to dry/wrap up the newborn. About 294 (65.3%) of them bathed the newborn after 24 h. The majority of study subjects, 249 (55.3%) mothers made skin to skin contact of mother and newborn.

The prevalence of essential newborn care practices

The prevalence of cord cutting, initiation of breastfeeding and thermal care practices were studied in this study. This study revealed that the prevalence of cord cutting, initiation of breastfeeding and thermal care practices were 434 (96.4%), 206 (45.8%) and 294 (65.3%) respectively (Fig. 4).

Associated factors of essential newborn care practices

In order to determine the association of independent variables with essential newborn care practices both bivariate and multivariate analysis were used. Variables that showed association with the outcome variables in the bivariate analysis were selected for multivariate analysis.

Crude analysis revealed that variables like ANC visit (COR 0.213, 95% CI: 0.102–0.446), advice about ENBC (COR 0.166, 95% CI: 0.078–0.354), PNC visit (COR0.135,95% CI:0.083–0.217), place of residence (COR2.244, 95% CI:1.251–4.025), planned pregnancy (COR 6.863, 95% CI: 3.943–11.943), birth preparedness (COR 3.511, 95% CI: 1.635–7.541), knowledge about newborn danger signs (COR 5.276, 95% CI: 2.232–12.471), and knowledge about newborn care (COR 1.892, 95% CI: 1.223–2.928) were felt to be the key predictors of essential

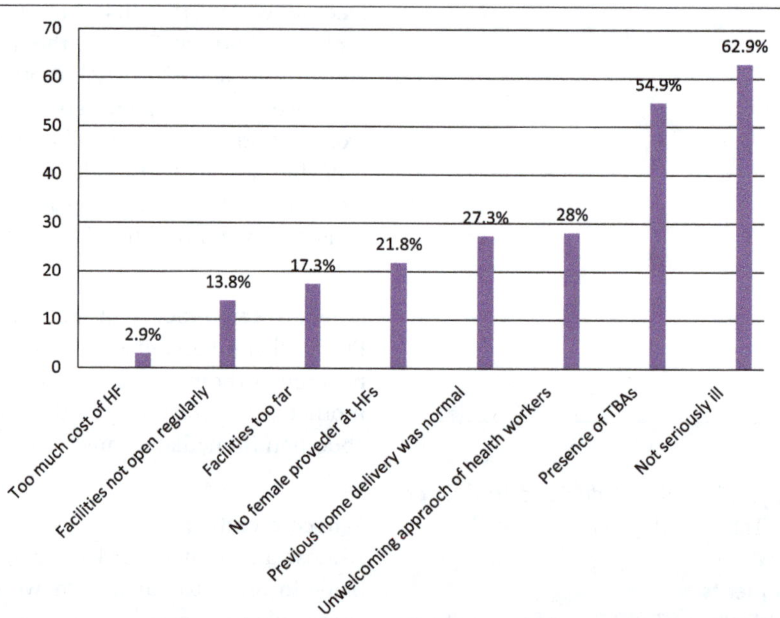

Fig. 1 Reasons of women not delivered at health facilities, in Damot pulasa district, Wolaita Zone, Southern Ethiopia, 2016

Table 4 Knowledge of the respondents, in Damot pulasa district, Wolaita Zone, Southern Ethiopia, 2016

Variable	Frequency (n = 450)	Percentage (%)
Information on newborn care		
Yes	417	92.7
No	33	7.3
Information to start breastfeeding		
Yes	415	92.2
No	35	7.8
Time to start breastfeeding		
First one hour	141	34.0
After one hour	274	66.0
Knowledge on first milk		
Yes	390	86.7
No	60	13.3
Advantage of first milk		
Advantageous	262	67.0
Disadvantageous	129	33.0
Expose neonate for morning sunlight		
Yes	406	90.2
No	44	9.8
Expose neonate for vaccination		
Yes	432	96.0
No	18	4.0
Information when to bath the neonate		
Yes	436	96.9
No	14	3.1
Time of bathing		
First 24 h	303	69.5
After 24 h	133	30.5
Knowledge about neonatal problems		
Good knowledge	87	19.3
Poor knowledge	363	80.7

newborn care practice and were used to form multivariable logistic regression analysis (Table 6).

Multivariate logistic regression was done for variables that had statistically significant association with essential newborn care practice in crude analysis. Multivariate logistic regression analysis revealed that variables like ANC visit (AOR 0.264, 95% CI:0.090–0.773), advice about essential newborn care practice (AOR 0.114, 95% CI:0.058–0.221), PNC visit (AOR 0.209, 95% CI:0.110–0.399), place of residence (AOR 2, 95% CI:1.024–3.693), planned pregnancy (AOR 7, 95% CI:3.732–11.813), and knowledge about newborn danger signs (AOR 0.277, 95% CI:0.110–0.697) were the independent predictors of essential newborn care practice after controlling the potential confounders (Table 6).

Discussion

Generally, in this study the coverage of essential newborn care practice was low. Even though majority of the women used boiled blade to cut the cord (96.4%) and tied with threads (98.2%), application of butter on the umbilical stump (64%) of the women practiced. I n addition to low coverage of initiation of breast feeding within one hour (45.8%) and giving colostrums (49.6%),the majority, (49.8%) of the women in this study gave pre-lacteals. Bathing of the newborn after 24 h was practiced by the majority (65.3%) of the women.

The prevalence of ENBC practice was 24% which was higher than the research done in Awebel district East Gojam Zone [8] which was 23.1% but which was much lower than the study conducted in Northwest Ethiopia, Mandura district [15] which was 41%. Cord cutting was practiced by the majority 96.4% of the women, using new blade, which was much higher than the study conducted in, Nawalparasi district of Nepal (48.31%) [16], Northern Ghana which revealed 90.8% [17], Sub urban areas of western Nigeria (90.3%) [18], study conducted in Northwest Ethiopia, Mandura district was (59.8%) [15],and the study conducted in four regions of Ethiopia which was 88.3% [6], the reason for this might be good awareness and custom followed in the study area but the finding was in line with the study conducted at Awebel district, East Gojam of Ethiopia (97.6%) [8]. Majority of the study participants (98.2%) the cord was tied with thread which was higher than the study conducted in the four regions of Ethiopia (48.5%) [6], this might be due to awareness in the study community. Even though majority of the women used boiled blade to cut the cord and tied with threads, application of butter on the umbilical stump (64%) of the women practiced in the study area which is higher than the study conducted in Northern Ghana (14.4%) and the study conducted in Northwest Ethiopia Mandura district was (18.18%) [15, 17] but which was lower than the study conducted in the four regions of Ethiopia (88.3%) [6].

Initiation of breastfeeding within one hour in the study area was 45.8% which was higher than the study conducted in rural Bangladesh (40%), East Gojam of Ethiopia (41.6%). This finding was not incongruent with the study conducted in India (65%), Nepal (51.3%), Northern Ghana (80%), Eastern Uganda (50%), Western Nigeria (65.3%), four regions of Ethiopia (52.1%), Northwest Ethiopia and Southwest Ethiopia (50%) [6, 15–21] respectively. The Majority, 49.8% of the women in this study gave pre-lacteals. The finding was higher as compared to study conducted in the four regions of Ethiopia (12.4%) gave pre-lacteals [6], but lower than the study conducted in East Gojam of Ethiopia Awebel district, 11.2% gave pre-lacteals [8]. The reason might be traditional beliefs of the community. Breastfeeding of the

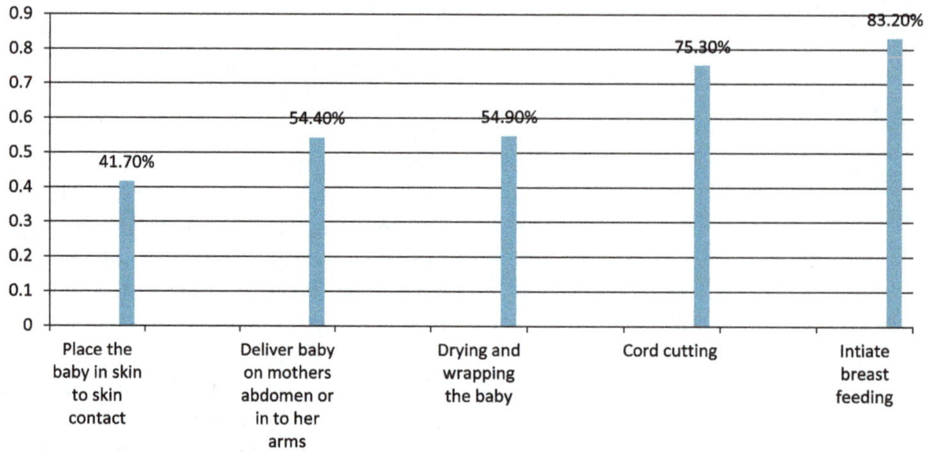

Fig. 2 Knowledge of women about ENBC practices in Damot pulasa district, Wolaita Zone, Southern Ethiopia, 2016

first milk (colostrum) was given (49.6%) of the women in the study area. This is lower than a case study of tribal women, Gujarat (63%) [22]. The reason for this was (33%) of the respondent believed that first milk was disadvantageous and from this (31%) believed that it would cause diarrhea,(60.5%) constipation and (58.9%) believed that it would decrease the growth of the newborn.

Bathing of the newborn after 24 h was practiced by the majority (65.3%) of the women in the study area which was in line with the study conducted in East Gojam of Ethiopia, Awebel district (65.6%) [8]. But this finding was lower than study conducted in Northern Ghana (93.6%), Rural Nepal (72.2%), South Sudan (99%), Easter Uganda (100%), Western Nigeria (98.2%), study conducted in four regions of Ethiopia (74.7%) [6, 16–18, 20, 23].

In this study women who didn't get ANC visit were 73.6% less likely to practiced essential newborn care practice as compared to those who initiated ANC visit (AOR =0.213,P = 0.015,CI = 0.102–0.446), which is supported by the study conducted in Northern Ghana which suggested that women who initiated ANC visit were two times more likely to practiced essential newborn care practice as compared to women who initiated ANC visit late [17]. This might be due to women who attended ANC have the chance of getting information about the components and the importance of newborn care practice from health care providers.

The finding of this study also showed that women who didn't get PNC visit early were 79% less likely practiced ENBC when compared to women who didn't get immediate PNC visit (AOR = 0.209, P = 0.00,CI = 0.110–0.399). This finding was supported by the study conducted in rural communities of Awebel district, East Gojam of Ethiopia, which stated that immediate PNC visit was statistically significant with ENBC practice of women and those women who had got immediate PNC visit after delivery were 3.2 times more likely to practice ENBC when compared with those who had not got immediate PNC after delivery [8]. This could be health extension workers

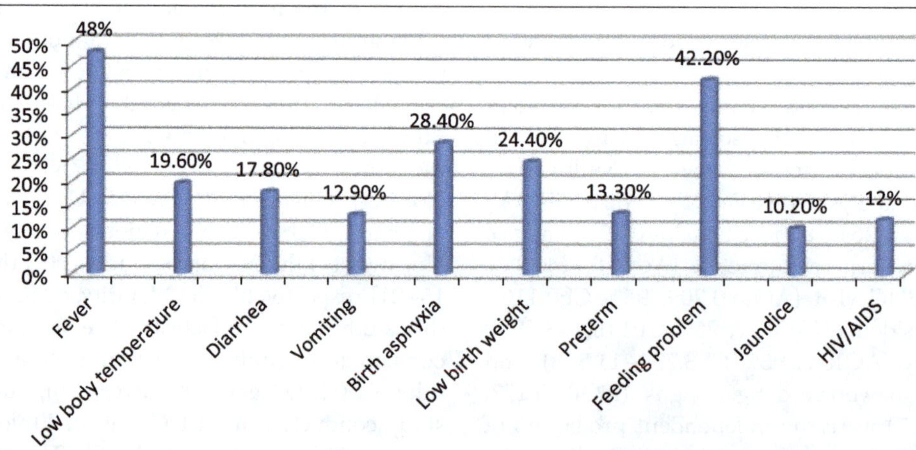

Fig. 3 Knowledge of women on newborn danger signs in Damot pulasa district, Wolaita Zone, Southern Ethiopia, 2016

Table 5 Newborn care practices of respondents, in Damot pulasa district, Wolaita Zone, Southern Ethiopia, 2016

Variable	Frequency (n = 450)	Percentage (%)
Position the neonate		
Yes	408	90.7
No	42	9.3
Place of positioning the neonate		
On the mother's abdomen	259	63.5
Near the delivery surface	86	21.1
On another bed separately	52	12.7
Transferred to father/relatives	9	2.2
I don't remember	2	.5
Dry/wrapping the neonate		
Yes	362	80.4
No	88	19.6
Time of dry/wrap the neonate		
Before delivery of placenta	190	52.2
Immediately after delivery of placenta	169	46.4
I did not remember	5	1.4
Material used for dry/wrap the neonate		
Pre-prepared towel	166	45.6
Piece of blanket/Gabi	72	19.8
Available material	126	34.6
Material used to cut the cord		
Boiled /un-boiled new razor blade	434	96.4
Used razor blade	16	3.6
Remember material used to tie the cord		
Yes	442	98.2
No	8	1.8
Material used to tie the cord		
Thread	442	100
Apply material after cord cutting		
Yes	288	64.0
No	162	36.0
Type of material applied on the cord		
Butter	288	100
Initiate exclusive breastfeeding		
Yes	226	50.2
No	224	49.8
Time of initiating exclusive breastfeeding		
First one hour	206	45.8
After one hour	244	54.2
Give pre lacteals		
Yes	224	49.8
No	226	50.2
Pre-lacteals given		

Table 5 Newborn care practices of respondents, in Damot pulasa district, Wolaita Zone, Southern Ethiopia, 2016 *(Continued)*

Variable	Frequency (n = 450)	Percentage (%)
Water	218	97.3
Butter	6	2.7
Give first milk		
Yes	223	49.6
No	227	50.4
Frequency of breastfeeding		
$<$ 8 times	203	45.1
$>=$8 times	247	54.9
Remember time of bathing		
Yes	442	98.2
No	8	1.8
Time of bathing		
First 24 h	156	34.7
After 24 h	294	65.3
Skin to skin contact		
Yes	249	55.3
No	201	44.7

and community health workers might gave proper advice about essential newborn care practice.

Those mothers who had got ENBC advice during ANC visit or other meetings were 83.4% more likely practiced ENBC practice as compared to women who did not got the advice (AOR =0.114, $P = 0.0001$, CI = 0.058–0.221). It was supported by study done, Awebel district which showed that women who had got advice about ENBC practices during monthly pregnant mothers' group meeting were 4.8 times more likely to practice ENBC as compared with those women who had not got advice about ENBC practices during monthly meeting [8]. The reason could be the health care providers could discuss about essential newborn care practice during ANC visit.

In this study, urban areas women were two times more likely practiced ENBC practice when compared to rural areas women (AOR =2, $P = 0.042$, CI = 1.024–3.693). The finding was supported by a study conducted in Mandura district which stated that women in urban areas were three times more likely to have good newborn care practices as compared to rural areas [15]. This might be due to accessibilities of health service and good knowledge secondary to better educational status of urban women when compared to rural areas women.

Those women who planned there pregnancy were seven times more likely practiced newborn care when compared to women who did not plan their pregnancy (AOR = 7, $P = 0.00$, CI =3.732–11.813). The reason for

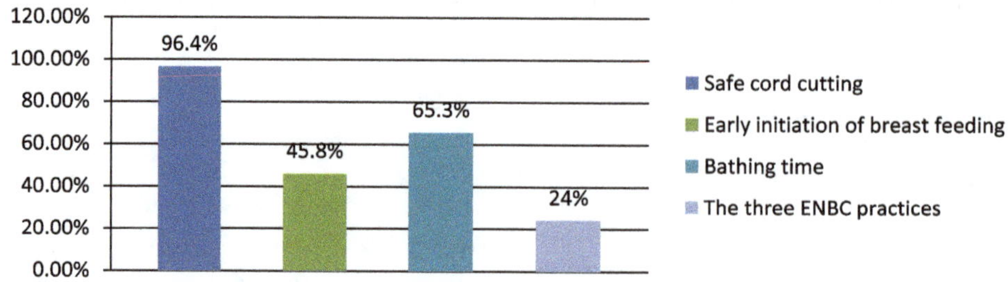

Fig. 4 Distribution of the three essential newborn care practices, in Damot pulasa district, Wolaita Zone, Southern Ethiopia, 2016

this could be women who had planned pregnancy might be more likely to use maternal and child health services.

The study showed that those women who were knowledge about newborn danger signs practiced ENBC 72% more likely when compared to women who had poor knowledge about newborn danger signs (AOR = 0.277, *P* = 0.006, CI = 0.110–0.697). This finding was supported by the study conducted in rural areas of Northern Ghana which states that women who could mention at least four danger signs of the neonates were four times more likely to give good neonatal feeding to their babies [17]. This could be most of the women in the sample may not have adequate knowledge about newborn care. This might be due to majority of the women did not get an adequate message about newborn care during antenatal care follow up. Findings in this study should be interpreted in the light of the inherent limitations of the study. Recall bias was a possibility since the women were

Table 6 Factors associated with the three essential newborn care practices by bivariate and multiple logistic analyses in Damot pulasa district, Wolaita Zone, Southern Ethiopia, 2016

Variable	ENBCP		COR	AOR
	Yes (%)	No (%)		
Receive ANC				
Yes	18	14	1	1
No	90	328	0.213(0.102–0.446)	0.264(0.090–0.773)*
Advice about ENBC				
Yes	19	13	1	1
No	61	252	0.166(0.078–0.354)	0.114(0.058–0.221)*
Receive PNC				
Yes	64	56	1	1
No	44	286	0.135(0.083–0.217)	0.209(0.110–0.399)*
Residence				
Urban	22	35	2.244(1.251–4.025)	2(1.024–3.693)*
Rural	86	307	1	1
Planned pregnancy				
Yes	40	27	6.863(3.943–11.943)	7(3.732–11.813)*
No	68	315	1	1
Birth preparedness				
Yes	8	75	3.511(1.635–7.541)	0.467(0.200–1.087)
No	100	267	1	1
Knowledge about newborn danger signs				
Good knowledge	6	102	5.276(2.232–12.471)	0.277(0.110–0.697)*
Poor knowledge	81	261	1	1
Knowledge about newborn care				
Good knowledge	49	209	1.892(1.223–2.928)	0.760(0.460–1.257)
Poor knowledge	59	133	1	1

inquired about events which occurred during a two year period. However, the questioning was focused on the most recent experiences of essential newborn care practices in order to minimize this possibility.

Conclusions

In this study, the level of coverage of essential newborn care practices in the district was generally low. Traditional practice like: pre-lacteal feeding, avoiding of first milk and application of material on the newborn stump were practiced by majority of study participant in the study area. This finding also revealed that most essential newborn interventions were not reaching the newborns. ANC visit, advice about ENBC, PNC visit, residence, planned pregnancy and knowledge about newborn danger signs were predictors of essential newborn care practice in the study area. Therefore Damot pulasa district health office should promote strong community based behavior change communication on the importance of ENBC practices to change the poor ENBC practices in the study area. Health facilities should enhance linkage with health posts to increase ANC and PNC service utilization. Health extension workers should promote and give health education about pre-lacteal feeding, early bathing, planned pregnancy, newborn dander signs and application of materials on the newborn stump.

Abbreviations

ANC: Anti Natal Care; EDHS: Ethiopian Demographic and Health Survey; ENBC: Essential Newborn Care; MDG: Millennium Development Goal; NMR: Neonatal Mortality Rate; PNC: Post Natal Care; SDG: Sustainable Development Goal; SPSS: Statistical Program Social Science

Acknowledgments

We would like to thank Addis Ababa University and Wolaita Sodo University. Our gratitude also extends to Wolaita zone health department and Damot pulasa district health office for their unreserved cooperation.

Funding

Addis Ababa University.

Authors' contributions

TY was involved in conception, designing the study, writing proposal, analysis interpretation of data and manuscript writing. BW, AA and FH were involved in designing the study, analysis, interpretation of data and manuscript writing. All authors agreed to be accountable for all aspects of the work.

Competing interest

We declared no financial, personal or professional competing interests influenced this paper.

Authors Information

[1]Lecturer in Department of Nursing, College of Health Science and Medicine, Wolaita Sodo University.
[2]Lecturer in Department of Nursing, School of nursing and midwifery, Addis Ababa University,
[3]Assistant Professor in School of Public Health, College of Medicine and Health Science, Hawassa University.
[4]Lecturer in Department of Nursing, College of Health Science and Medicine, Wolaita Sodo University.
[5]Lecturer in Department of Medical Laboratory, College of Health Science and Medicine, Wolaita Sodo University.

Ethics approval and consent to participate

Ethical clearance was obtained from Addis Ababa University College of Health Science Department of Nursing and Midwifery Institutional Review Board (IRB). Official letter was received from the department of nursing and midwifery and submitted to Damot Pulasa district Health office and letter of permission was taken from Damot pulasa district health office for each selected kebele to implement the study. Written informed consent was obtained from each respondent before the interview. The consent forms addressed issues relating to confidentiality and autonomy of the respondent during data collection.

Author details

[1]Department of Nursing, College of Health Science and Medicine, Wolaita Sodo University, P.O.Box: 138, Wolaita Sodo, Ethiopia. [2]Department of Nursing, School of nursing and midwifery, Addis Ababa University, Addis Ababa, Ethiopia. [3]School of Public Health, College of Medicine and Health Science, Hawassa University, Hawassa, Ethiopia. [4]Department of Nursing, College of Health Science and Medicine, Wolaita Sodo University, Sodo, Ethiopia. [5]Department of Medical Laboratory, College of Health Science and Medicine, Wolaita Sodo University, Sodo, Ethiopia.

References

1. WHO, PMNCH. A Global Review of the Key Interventions Related to Reproductive, Maternal, Newborn and Child Health (RMNCH). Geneva: WHO and the Partnership for Maternal Newborn & child health (PMNCH); 2011.
2. UN Inter-agency Group for Child Mortality Estimations. Levels and trends in child mortality. In: Estimates developed by the UN inter-agency Group for Child Mortality Estimation. New York: UN IGME; 2013.
3. Pattinson R, Kerber K, Buchmann E, Friberg IK, Belizan M, Lansky S, et al. Stillbirths: how can health systems deliver for mothers and babies? Lancet. 2011;377:1610–23.
4. World Health Organization: Estimates.In State of the World's Newborns. Washington, DC: Saving Newborn Lives, Save the Children/ USA; 2001:1–49.
5. Save the Children 2014. Ending newborn deaths: Ensuring every baby survives. 2014. [https://www.savethechildren.net/sites/default/files/libraries/ENDING-NEWBORN-DEATHS.pdf]. Accessed 3 Mar 2014.
6. Callaghan-koru JA, Seifu A, Tholandi M, De G-j J, Daniel E, Rawlins B, et al. Newborn care practices at home and in health facilities in 4 regions of Ethiopia. BMC Pediatr. 2013;13(198).
7. Central Statistical Agency and ICF International. Ethiopia Demographic and Health Survey 2011. Addis Ababa, and Maryland. https://dhsprogram.com/pubs/pdf/fr255/fr255.pdf. Accessed Mar 2014.
8. Kokebie T, et al. Community Based Essential Newborn Care Practices and Associated Factors among Women in the Rural Community of Awabel District. Int J Adv Sci Res. 2015;01(01):17–27.
9. Narayanan I, Rose M, Cordero D, Faillace S, Sanghvi T. Perinatal / neonatal essential newborn care. Virginia: Basics Support Institutionalizing Child Surviv Proj (BASICS II) United States Agency Int Dev Arlington; 2004.
10. WHO. Pregnancy, Childbirth, Postpartum and Newborn Care: A Guide for Essential Practice. Geneva: WHO Press World Health Organization; 2006.
11. Shiff man J. Issue attention in global health: the case of newborn survival. Lancet. 2010;375:2045–9.
12. Liu L, et al. Global, regional, and national causes of child mortality: an updated systematic analysis for 2010 with time trends since 2000. Lancet. 2012;379(9832):2151–61.
13. Central Statistical Agency. Ethiopia Mini Demographic and Health Survey. Addis Ababa; 2014.
14. Penfold S, Manzi F, Mkumbo E, Temu S, Jaribu J, D Shamba D, Mshinda H, Cousens S, Marchant T, Tanner M, SchellenbergDandSchellenberg J. Effect of home-based counselling on newborn care practices in southern Tanzania one year after implementation: a cluster-randomised controlled trial. BMC Pediatr. 2014;14:187.

15. Tegene T, Andargie G, Nega A, Yimam K. Newborn care practice and associated factors among mothers who gave birth within one year in Mandura District, Northwest Ethiopia. Clinics Mother Child Health. 2015;12: 172. https://doi.org/10.4172/2090-7214.1000172.
16. Kaphle HP, Yadav DK, Neupane N, Sharma B. Newborn care practices in rural communities of Nawalparasi District , Nepal. JHAS. 2013;3(1):35–9.
17. Saaka M, Iddrisu M. Patterns and determinants of essential newborn care practices in rural areas of northern Ghana. Int J Popul Res. 2014;(5):1–10.
18. Adelaja LM. A survey of home delivery and newborn care practices among women in a suburban area of Western Nigeria. ISRN Obstet Gynecol. 2011; 2011:9.
19. Vijayalakshmi S, Patil R, Datta SS. Community-based study on newborn care practices and its determinants in rural Pondicherry,India. J Neonatal Biol. 2014;3:158. https://doi.org/10.4172/2167-0897.1000158.
20. Waiswa P, Peterson S, Tomson G, Pariyo GW. Poor newborn care practices - a population based survey in eastern Uganda. BMC Pregnancy Childbirth. 2010;10:9.
21. Debelew GT, Afework MF, Yalew AW. Determinants and causes of neonatal mortality in Jimma zone, Southwest Ethiopia: a multilevel analysis of prospective follow up study. PLoS One. 2014;9(9):e107184. https://doi.org/ 10.1371/journal.pone.0107184.
22. Shah BD, Dwivedi LK. Newborn care practices: a case study of tribal women, Gujarat. Health. 2013;05(08):29–40.
23. Rosales AC, Hedrick JA, Cherian DT, Moore EC, Brown KM, Walumbe E. Essential newborn care in rural settings: the case of Warrap state in South Sudan. African Evaluation Journal. 2014;2(1) Art. #80, 6 pages. https://doi. org/10.4102/ aej.v2i1.80.

12

Preconception counselling for low health literate women: an exploration of determinants in the Netherlands

Mirjam P. Fransen[1*], Miriam E. Hopman[1], Laxsini Murugesu[1], Ageeth N. Rosman[2] and Sian K. Smith[3]

Abstract

Background: Women from lower socioeconomic groups tend to be at greater risk of adverse perinatal outcomes, but are less likely to participate in preconception counselling compared to higher socioeconomic groups. This could be partly because of their limited skills to assess, understand and use health related information in ways that promote and maintain good health (health literacy skills). In this study we explored determinants of participation in preconception counselling among women with low health literacy in The Netherlands.

Methods: Potential determinants of participation in preconception counselling were derived from the literature, and mapped onto a theoretical framework, which was tested for perceived relevance and completeness in an expert review ($n = 20$). The framework was used to prepare face-to-face interviews with women with low health literacy and a wish to conceive ($n = 139$). In the interviews we explored preconception counselling awareness, knowledge, considerations, subjective norms, self-efficacy, attitude, and intention. Linear regression analyses were used to test associations with intention to participate in preconception counselling.

Results: Most women (75%) were unaware of the concept of preconception counselling and the provision of counselling, even if they lived in areas where written invitations had been disseminated. Common considerations for participation were: preparation for pregnancy; perceived lack of information; and problems in a previous pregnancy. Considerations not to participate were mostly related to perceived sufficient knowledge and perceived low risk of perinatal problems. Respondents generally had a positive attitude towards participation in preconception counselling for themselves, and 41% reported that they would participate in preconception counselling.

Conclusion: Women with low health literacy were generally unaware of the concept and provision of preconception counselling, but seemed to be interested in participation. Further research should investigate how to effectively reach and inform this group about preconception counselling. This knowledge is essential for evidence-based development of interventions to increase the accessibility and understanding of preconception counselling.

Keywords: Health literacy, Preconception counselling, Theoretical framework, Determinants, Expert review

* Correspondence: m.p.fransen@amc.uva.nl
[1]Amsterdam UMC, University of Amsterdam, Department of Public Health, Public Health Research Institute, Meibergdreef 9, Amsterdam, The Netherlands
Full list of author information is available at the end of the article

Plain English summary

Women from lower socioeconomic groups are more likely to experience adverse perinatal outcomes, but less likely to participate in counselling to prepare for a healthy pregnancy (preconception counselling). These socioeconomic differences could be partly explained by women's health literacy skills, commonly referred to as the ability to access, understand and use health-related information to promote and maintain good health.). In this study we explored determinants of participation in preconception counselling among women with low health literacy in The Netherlands.

A theoretical framework was tested for perceived relevance and completeness among 20 experts, and then used to prepare face-to-face interviews with 139 women with low health literacy and a wish to conceive.

The interviews showed that most women (75%) were unaware of the concept of preconception counselling and the provision of counselling, even if they lived in areas where written invitations had been disseminated. Common considerations for participation were: preparation for pregnancy; perceived lack of information; and problems in a previous pregnancy. Considerations not to participate were mostly related to perceived sufficient knowledge and perceived low risk of perinatal problems. Respondents generally had a positive attitude towards participation in preconception counselling for themselves, and 41% reported that they would participate in preconception counselling.

In conclusion; women with low health literacy were generally unaware of the concept and provision of preconception counselling, but seemed to be interested in participation. Further research on how to effectively reach and inform this group and to encourage their intention as a catalyst for undertaking preconception counselling is essential to increase the accessibility of preconception counselling.

Background

Socioeconomic inequalities in adverse perinatal outcomes, such as preterm birth, small for gestational age, low Apgar score, congenital anomalies, and perinatal mortality have been extensively documented. These inequalities occur in both high and low income countries [1–3]. For example, in the Netherlands, fetal mortality is almost twice as high in socially deprived neighborhoods (10.4‰ versus 5.6‰ in non-deprived neighborhoods) [4].

The fact that some of these adverse outcomes are related to modifiable risk factors, such as maternal smoking, alcohol consumption, illicit drug use and inadequate medication use during pregnancy provides a potential opportunity to reduce socioeconomic inequalities through preconception care [5–7]. Preconception care is defined as a set of interventions before conception to decrease the impact of biomedical, behavioural and social risks on a woman's health, fetal development, and pregnancy outcomes [8]. By the time a woman enters prenatal care, a large part of fetal organ development has taken place [9]. Preconception care is critical for the outcome of the pregnancy, particularly for deprived groups who are more likely to adopt unhealthy behaviours before pregnancy [10]. Preconception interventions can be collective, focusing on the general public, for example by national campaigns. Interventions can also focus on women or couples that are planning a pregnancy, for example by risk assessment, screening and individual counselling [11]. In the Netherlands, individual counselling can be provided through general practices, municipal health services, or midwives and gynaecologists [8]. Preconception care has shown to be effective in improving maternal health behaviour, such as folic acid use, smoking and alcohol cessation, diabetic control and obesity prevention before pregnancy, and preventing congenital disorders [12–15]. Women with a lower socioeconomic background are at greatest risk of complications during and after pregnancy, yet they are least likely to participate in preconception screening, risk assessment and counselling [15–17]. This could be partly related to a woman's health literacy skills, commonly defined as the ability to assess, understand and use health related information in ways that promote and maintain good health [18]. Health literacy is considered to be an important variable in explaining why socioeconomic differences in health exist [19, 20]. Women with low health literacy are less likely to screen for sexually transmitted diseases, have follow-ups of abnormal test results after cervical cancer screening, and more likely to initiate prenatal care at a later stage of pregnancy [21, 22]. Little is known about the factors associated with participation in preconception counselling, particularly among women with low health literacy. Strategies are needed to improve the accessibility and effectiveness of preconception counselling.

In this study we explored determinants of participation in preconception counselling among women with low health literacy in The Netherlands. The specific objectives were:

- To gain insight into women's awareness of preconception counselling, and awareness of invitations that were used to recruit women to a pilot program in the Netherlands;
- To assess knowledge, considerations, subjective norm, self-efficacy, attitude, and intention to participate in preconception counselling or not;
- To investigate the extent to which these factors are associated with intention to participate in preconception counselling.

Methods

Aim, design and setting

We performed a cross-sectional study to explore factors that play a role in participation in preconception counselling among women with low health literacy.

The study was performed in the Netherlands between April 2014 and November 2016. The study was part of a larger project in which we developed strategies for women with low health literacy and health care providers within the Dutch pilot program 'Healthy Pregnancy for All (HP4All)'. In the HP4All program, preconception care is delivered in individual counselling that is provided by general practitioners, midwives, or youth health care providers. The HP4All program was initiated in 2011 in specific districts with perinatal mortality and morbidity above the country's average [8]. Women in the HP4All target municipalities are exposed to letters or flyers, which inform them about preconception counselling and invite them to apply if they have a wish to conceive.

Research population and recruitment

The research population consisted of 139 women with low health literacy, 72 of them were recruited from a general practice and a youth health care centre in Amsterdam that participated in the HP4All program. This means they were exposed to an invitational letter or flyer for HP4All. The other 67 women were recruited from centres that did not participate in the HP4All program (a youth health care centre, a primary school, and an intermediate vocational education school in Amsterdam, Almere, and Wageningen). This group was not actively invited for preconception counselling, but they could participate in it, as it was offered by all Dutch midwives on request.

Women that were able to communicate verbally in Dutch were personally invited to participate in the study by MH or LM in waiting rooms of the participating centres. We briefly explained the purpose of our study and then asked if they had a wish to conceive pregnancy within 5 years. Those that certainly knew that they did not want to become pregnant in the coming 5 years were excluded. Others were then asked if they had 5–10 min to participate in the Short Assessment of Health Literacy in Dutch (SAHL-D) (see below). Those that had lower health literacy according to the SAHL-D were theninvited for a personal face-to-face structured interview conducted by MH or LM at a time and location that the women preferred. We chose to conduct face-to-face interviews instead of a written or online survey, since we expected that these low health literate women would have difficulty filling in questionnaires, which would lead to unreliable results and a lower participation rate.

Theoretical framework to guide data collection

Von Wagner's framework for health literacy and health actions

The literature search and the development of the questionnaire for the structured interviews was guided by a conceptual theoretical framework (Fig. 1 Conceptual framework). This framework was based on Von Wagner's framework for health literacy and health actions, that proposes that health outcomes (e.g. preterm birth) are determined by the following actions: access and use of health care (such as preconception counselling); patient-provider interactions; and management of health and illness [23]. These actions are influenced by motivational, environmental, and volitional determinants. Motivational determinants include traditional sociocognitive constructs, such as knowledge, understanding, beliefs, and attitudes. Participation in preconception counseling could for example be influenced by knowing what the counselling involves. Volitional determinants refer to action control, for example self-efficacy, perceived barriers, and implementation skills. Self-efficacy refers to the strength of belief in own ability to complete tasks and reach goals. Implementation skills refer to planning, organizing and task-specific skills i.e. navigational skills to access preconception counselling. Motivational and volitional determinants form a symbiotic relationship with external system factors. These system factors refer to environmental determinants and could include the offer of preconception counselling or out-of-pocket costs for preconception care.

Motivational and volitional determinants are directly affected by health literacy, which in turn is influenced by epidemiological or structural determinants, such as educational attainment level and age.

Literature search

In March 2014 Medline was searched using the following search terms: social class, socioeconomic status, social*, socio-economic, low income, education*, education level, health literacy, preconception care, preconception health, preconception counsel*. Reference lists in the included papers were also scrutinized.

In accordance with the conceptual framework described above, we identified the following motivational determinants in the literature: knowledge and awareness of preconception counselling; knowledge of risk factors and preventive measures; attitude; beliefs; and expectations of preconception counselling. Practical barriers and the type of provision were identified as environmental determinants. Volitional determinants that were investigated in the studies included self-efficacy and perceived barriers to participation in preconception counselling. More information on the search and included studies is presented in Additional file 1.

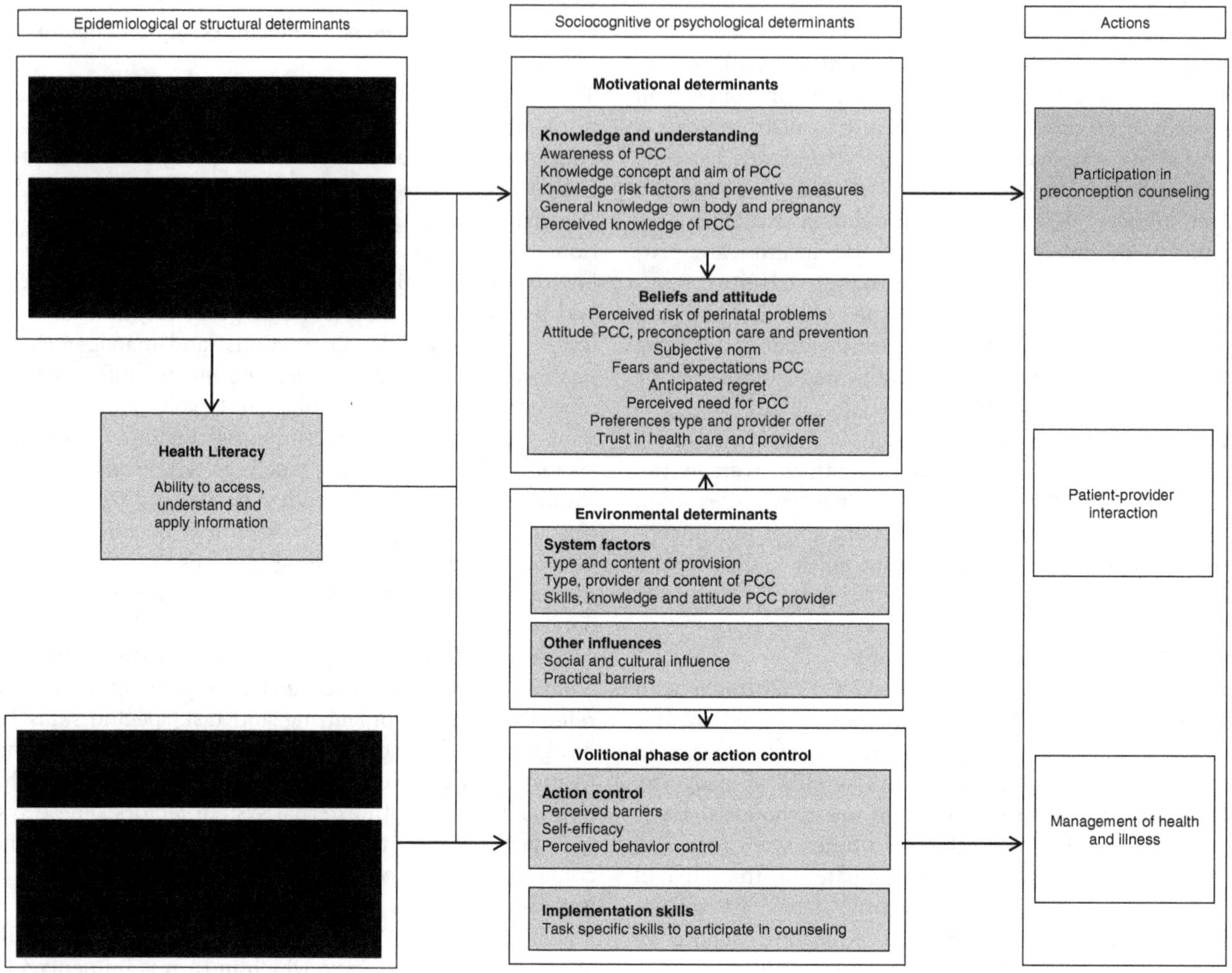

Fig. 1 Conceptual framework

Expert review

An expert review was performed to investigate whether the conceptual framework reflected the current experience and knowledge of experts, to ensure a good base for data collection. In total 31 experts were asked by email to fill in an online survey. Of those, 20 participated and filled in an online survey (response rate 64%), consisting of midwives (n = 3), researchers (n = 9), gynaecologists (n = 2), medical students (n = 2), advisors (n = 2), a nurse (n = 1), and a medical doctor (n = 1). On average, they had 15 years experience of work (range 1–35 years). The experts confirmed the determinants in the framework and suggested several important additions to complete the framework, including: skills, knowledge and attitude of health care providers (environmental determinants), and task-specific skills to participate in preconception counselling (volitional determinants).

Measures

The final framework (Fig. 1) was used to prepare data collection in face-to-face interviews. We used the following measures to assess the variables that were derived from the framework:

Health literacy was measured by the Short Assessment of Health Literacy, which was previously adapted and validated for the Dutch situation (SAHL-D) and proved to be a reliable and valid performance-based test to indicate low health literacy in the Netherlands (Cronbach's alpha = 0.77 for recognition, 0.79 for comprehension and 0.86 for the total score) [24]. Both word recognition and vocabulary are essential for reading comprehension, which is an important element of health literacy [16–18, 24]. During the SAHL-D assessment, respondents were asked to read and pronounce 33 health-related words, which was followed by a multiple choice question about the description of the words. Respondents were assigned one point for each correctly pronounced word and for each correct description. This resulted in a summary score ranging from 0 to 66 points. Following a predefined cut-off point, respondents with a score lower than 55 points were considered as low health literate and could participate in this study [24].

Educational level was based on self-report and categorized using the International Standard Classification of Education, i.e. low (level 0–2: early childhood education; primary education; lower secondary education); intermediate (level 3–5: upper secondary; post-secondary non-tertiary education; short cycle tertiary education); and high (level 6–8: bachelor's; master's; doctoral or equivalent level) [25].

Ethnic background was based on the country of birth of the respondents' parents, in accordance with Statistics Netherlands [26]. Respondents were only considered to be from Dutch ethnic background if both their parents were born in the Netherlands. The respondents were considered to be from another western background, if one parent or both parents were born in Europe, North-America, Indonesia, Japan or Oceania. Respondents were categorized as having a non-western background, if one parent or both parents were born in Turkey, Morocco, Surinam, Netherlands Antilles, Aruba, Africa, Asia (excluding Indonesia and Japan) or Latin-America. If both parents were born in different foreign countries, the mother was the identifier used for ethnicity [26].

To classify *relationship status* respondents were asked whether they were in a relationship or married and, if so, whether they were living together with their partner.

Wish to conceive was assessed by asking whether the respondent contemplated pregnancy and in which time frame. Options were 'in the next two years', 'in two to five years' or 'yes, but not sure within which time frame'.

Perinatal experiences were evaluated by asking respondents whether they had been pregnant before, and if so, whether they had ever experienced unplanned pregnancy (answer options 'yes' of 'no') or problems during a previous pregnancy (answer options 'yes' of 'no'). The interpretation of experienced problems could encompass feeling uncomfortable and vomiting during the first trimester of pregnancy up to fetal mortality. The interpretation was led by the respondents, because it was used as an evaluation of experiences that could influence women's choice to participate in counselling and not as a risk assessment.

Awareness of preconception counselling was assessed by the question: "Have you heard about preconception counselling?" and "If so, who told you about it?" or "If so, where did you hear or read about it?". Answers were categorized within predefined sources of information, such as 'general practitioner' or 'newspaper'. Awareness of the written invitation for preconception counselling was defined as having noticed any written invitation (letter or a flyer).

Considerations to participate in preconception counselling were assessed by 33 statements on considerations that we derived from the conceptual framework (Fig. 1). For each consideration we asked if this would be a reason to participate or not (answer options 'yes' of 'no'). For eight considerations (e.g. medication use or chronic illness) we assessed the specific denominator by asking if this situation accounted for the respondent (e.g. 'Do you have a long term illness, disease or disability' (such as high blood pressure or diabetes)'?').

Knowledge on risk factors for a healthy pregnancy was assessed by six statements that were developed by Temel et al.: pregnancies within a short interval are good for the baby's health; smoking adversely affects fertility; being underweight or overweight adversely affects fertility; sexually transmitted disease must be treated before pregnancy; all medications from drugstores are safe and can be used during pregnancy; the best moment to start with folic-acid supplementation is when you get pregnant. Response options consisted of 'true', 'false' or 'I do not know' [27]. Answers to the statements were scored as either correct or incorrect (including 'I do not know').

Attitude towards preconception counselling was measured by a scale of six items (Cronbach's $\alpha = 0.77$). Respondents were asked to rate preconception counselling for themselves as good versus bad, comforting versus scary, important versus unimportant, pleasant versus unpleasant, useful versus useless and embarrassing versus something to be proud of. The scale ranged from 6 to 30. For analysis, the total score was divided by the amount of items, which was 6 .

Intention to participate in preconception counselling was assessed by asking respondents to rate the likelihood of their participation to preconception counselling before their (next) pregnancy on a 5 point Likert scale ranging from one 'extremely unlikely' to five 'extremely likely'.

Self-efficacy was assessed by the statement "I will be able to participate in preconception counselling, if I would like to go" and rated on a similar scale (1 = strongly disagree; 5 = strongly agree).

Subjective norm (the perceived social pressure to engage or not to engage in a behaviour) was measured in relation to three categories of important others; friends, family and partner. Respondents were asked for each of the three categories what they assume important others think they should do (– 2 = certainly not participate; + 2 = certainly participate). Then we asked for each assumption whether this would influence their decision to participate (− 2 = not at all; + 2 = very much). After testing internal reliability in our population, we decided to divide subjective norm into two scales: subjective norm related to friends and family members (summary scores ranging from − 20 to + 20) and subjective norm related to their partner (summary scores ranging from − 10 to + 10).

Statistical analyses

Descriptive statistics were used to summarize background characteristics, awareness, considerations, attitude and intention. Educational and ethnic differences in mean knowledge, mean attitude, and mean intention were analysed by analysis of variance (ANOVA), we did not correct for other variables in this ANOVA, since the primary aim was to assess differences in background variables (educational level and ethnic background). We performed linear regression analyses to test associations with intention to participate in preconception counselling. In the regression analyses we adjusted for potential confounders (educational level and, ethnic background). The covariate was considered as a confounder and left in the model, when it changed the variation in score by 10% or more. We imputed the value of the missing data ('99') and included it in the regression analyses, so the sample size will not be reduced. The required sample size for this analysis was based on a power analyses that showed that we would be able to detect a true difference between groups with a low and higher intention to participate in preconception counselling with probability (power) 0,8. The Type I error probability associated with this test of the null hypothesis that the population means of these two groups are equal is 0,05.

Results

Background characteristics study population and awareness

A total of 226 women met the inclusion criteria, 87 (38%) did not participate in the interview since they were uninterested in the topic, or perceived the interview to be too personal or too long (response rate 62%). Characteristics of the respondents (n = 139) are presented in Table 1. Most respondents had a non-Dutch ethnic background (61%; 45% non-Western and 16% Western, had an intermediate educational level (58%)and lived together with a partner (64%). In total 111 respondents (80%) had been pregnant before, 50% of them reported to have problems during earlier pregnancies, 49% have had an unplanned pregnancy.

We included 72 respondents from areas where invitation materials for preconception counselling were disseminated in the HP4All program, 35 of them were recruited in a general practice that disseminated a written invitation by mail, 37 respondents were recruited from a youth health care service where flyers were placed in the waiting room (n = 17) or personally handed over (n = 20). The other 67 women were included from areas where invitation materials were not standardly provided.

Table 1 further shows that 35 out of 139 respondents (25%) reported that they have heard about preconception counselling before the interview. Of the 72 women that were recruited from the centres that participated in the HP4All program, 22 (31%) were aware of preconception counselling. Of the 67 women that were recruited from other centres, 13 (19%) were aware of preconception counselling.Chi-square tests showed that this difference in awareness was not statistically significant ($p >$ 0.05).

Of the 35 women that were recruited in general practices that send out written invitations within HP4All, 11 (31%) remembered receiving the written invitation. Only 1 out of 37 respondents (3%) remembered having received a flyer. Even respondents that were handed over the flyer personally (n = 20), did not remember that they received information on preconception counselling. Women that were aware of preconception counselling were slightly less likely to participate in preconception counselling (B-0.22; CI-0.72-0.28).

Considerations (not) to participate in preconception counselling

Around half of all women (51%) considered participating in preconception counselling because they wanted to prepare for pregnancy (Table 2). This was positively associated with intention to participate (B 1.43; CI 1.06–1.79) (Table 4). Other important considerations for participation were 'I want information about fertility' (31%), 'I have a high risk of perinatal problems' (29%), and 'I want to have control over pregnancy' (29%). For 58% of the 61 women that experienced problems in previous pregnancy (e.g. high blood pressure, nausea, preterm birth), these problems would be a reason to participate in preconception counselling. For 52% of the 33 chronically ill women, their disease would be a reason to participate in counselling. Answers to the open-ended question did not provide other significant categories of considerations.

Most frequently mentioned considerations not to participate in preconception counselling in the total population were: 'I already have sufficient knowledge' (25%), 'I am not interested in counselling in general' (22%), and 'I have a low risk of perinatal problems' (17%). Perceived sufficient knowledge and risk perception were negatively associated with intention to participate (Table 4).

In the subgroup of women that had a previous pregnancy (n = 110), 42% would not want to participate in

Table 1 Background characteristics ($n = 139$)

	Mean (SD; range)	N (%)
Age (years)	29.6 (5.6; 18–42)	
Educational level		
Low		10 (7)
Intermediate		81 (58)
High		48 (35)
Ethnic background		
Dutch		54 (39)
Other western (non-Dutch)		23 (16)
Non-western		62 (45)
Health literacy score (SAHL-D)	35 (13; 9–53)	
Relationship status		
Married/Living together with partner		90 (64)
Single/Not living together with partner		50 (36)
Previous pregnancy		
Was pregnant before		111 (80)
Ever had an unplanned pregnancy		54 (49)
Ever had problems in pregnancy		61 (50)
Wish to conceive		
Yes, in next 2 years		41 (30)
Yes, in 2–5 years		61 (44)
Yes, not sure in how many years		37 (26)
Aware of preconception counselling		35 (25)
Subjective norm to participate in preconception counselling[a]		
Subjective norm family/friends (– 8.00–9.00)	−1.72 (3.80; – 8 – 9)	
Subjective norm partner (– 4–5)	0.19 (2.63; – 4 – 5)	

[a]Subjective norm family/friends not applicable to 4 women; subjective norm partner not applicable to 30 women

counselling, because they had been pregnant before. In answer to the open-ended question, 27% of all respondents mentioned that they would not participate, since they already had sufficient knowledge, 14% mentioned that they would not participate since they preferred another source of information, such as the internet.

Determinants to participate in preconception counselling

Figure 2 (Knowledge risk factors) shows the correct and incorrect answers per knowledge item. Lowest scores were obtained for the items ‘Pregnancies within short interval are good for baby's health’ (63% scored correctly) and ‘Smoking adversely affects fertility’ (65% scored correctly). Highest scores were found for ‘All medications from drugstores are safe and can be used during pregnancy’ (91% scored correctly) and the item ‘Sexually transmitted disease must be treated before pregnancy’ (92% scored correctly). In total 75% of the women scored correctly on the item on body weight, this was 74% for the item on folic acid use.

Table 3 shows total knowledge score (scale 1–6) per educational and ethnic group. Women with a higher educational level scored significantly higher on knowledge than others. Women with a non-Western ethnic background scored significantly lower than women with a Western or Dutch ethnic background. Knowledge was negatively associated with intention (Table 4).

Respondents generally had a positive attitude towards participation in preconception counselling for themselves (mean 3.96; scale 1–5; SD 0.58) (Table 3). Mean intention to participate was 3.05 (scale 1–5; SD 1.30), 41% of the respondents reported that they would participate in preconception counselling, 42% would not participate, 17% would perhaps participate. We did not find any significant differences in attitude or intention between educational or ethnic groups.

Mean self-efficacy was 4.19 (scale 1–5; SD 0.64), meaning that respondents generally felt that they were able to participate in preconception counselling if they wanted to (Table 3). Women from non-Western ethnic background scored significantly lower (mean 3.97; SD

Table 2 Considerations whether or not to participate in preconception counselling (*n* = 139)

Consideration to participate	N (%)	Consideration not to participate	N (%)	Total N
I want to prepare for pregnancy	71 (51)	I already have sufficient knowledge	34 (25)	139
I want information on fertility	43 (31)	I am not interested in counseling in general	30 (22)	139
I have a high risk of perinatal problems	40 (29)	I have a low risk of perinatal problems	23 (17)	139
I want to have control over pregnancy	40 (29)	I am not interested in preconception counseling	17 (12)	139
		I already received info from family and friends	14 (10)	139
I experienced problems in previous pregnancy	35 (58)			61
I have a chronic illness	17 (52)			33
I never received info from GP/Midwife	48 (43)			113
There are hereditary diseases in my family	15 (33)			45
I use medication	9 (30)			30
I ever experienced unplanned pregnancy	14 (26)			52
I have been pregnant before	26 (23)	I have been pregnant before	47 (42)	110 *
I received info from GP/midwife	10 (11)	I already received info from GP/midwife	9 (20)	92

*=number of missing variables

0.63) on self-efficacy than women from Dutch ethnic background (mean 4.42; SD 0.60). Higher self-efficacy was positively associated with intention (Table 4).

Subjective norm whether or not to participate in counselling was generally weak. Subjective partner norm was 0.15 (range – 4 -5; SD 2.62), meaning that most women slightly expected that their partner would like them to participate in counselling and that they found his/her opinion slightly important. Women generally perceived a weak subjective norm not to participate in preconception care from family or friends (– 1.76; range – 8-9; SD 3.79). Both subjective norms (partner and family/friends) were positively associated with intention (Table 4).

Discussion

This study shows that women with low health literacy were generally unaware of the concept and the provision of preconception counselling, but have a positive attitude towards participation in preconception counselling. Intention was quite positive as well, 41% of the respondents reported that they would participate in preconception counselling, 17% would perhaps participate. Most common reasons for participation were to prepare for pregnancy and to gain information about fertility. Considerations not to participate were mostly related to perceived sufficient knowledge, lack of interest in counselling in general, and perceived low risk of perinatal problems. Women generally felt confident to participate in preconception counselling if they wanted to. Subjective norm whether or not to participate was weak. Women from a non-Dutch ethnic background scored significantly lower on knowledge of preconception care and self-efficacy to participate in it.

Only 25% of our respondents had ever heard of preconception counselling. Unawareness is considered to be an important determinant of participation in preconception counselling [28]. We do not exactly know why women in our sample had such a low awareness, even if they lived in an area where invitations for counselling were distributed. In our interviews women explained

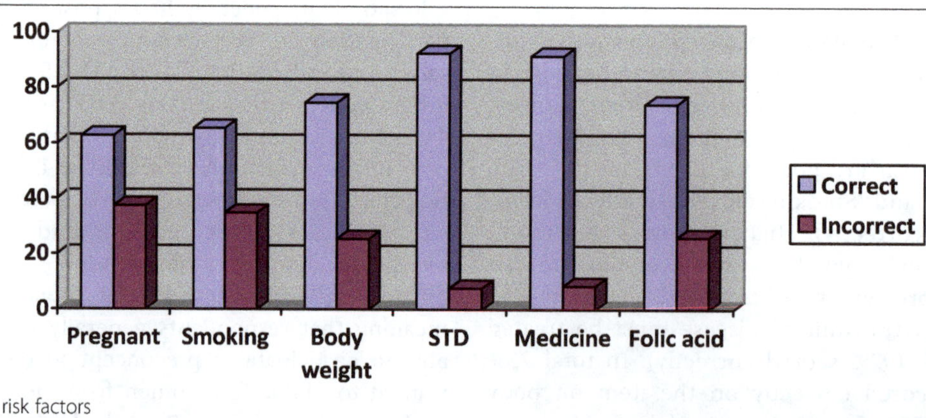

Fig. 2 Knowledge risk factors

Table 3 Knowledge, attitude, self-efficacy and intention preconception counselling (mean;SD)

	Knowledge risk factors (1–6)	Attitude (1–5)	Self-efficacy (1–5)	Intention (1–5)
Total population (*n* = 139)	4.61 (1.25)	3.96 (0.58)	4.19 (0.64)	3.05 (1.30)
Educational level				
Low (*n* = 10)	3.70 (1.49)[1]	3.75 (0.56)	3.80 (0.63)	3.60 (1.71)
Intermediate (*n* = 81)	4.38 (1.18)[2]	3.99 (0.62)	4.26 (0.61)	3.14 (1.27)
High (*n* = 48)	5.17 (1.04)[1 2]	3.96 (0.54)	4.21 (0.59)	2.79 (1.24)
Ethnic background				
Dutch (*n* = 54)	5.00 (1.06)[3]	4.03 (0.65)	4.42 (0.60)[3]	2.80 (1.12)
Other Western (*n* = 23)	5.00 (1.49)[4]	3.93 (0.62)	4.27 (0.55)	3.13 (1.42)
Non-Western (*n* = 62)	4.17 (1.18)[3 4]	3.91 (0.51)	3.97 (0.63)[3]	3.24 (1.39)

23 missings on knowledge
3 missings on attitude
3 missings on self-efficacy
[1]Difference between low and high educational level ($p < 0.05$)
[2]Difference between intermediate and high educational level ($p < 0.05$)
[3]Difference between Dutch and Non-Western ethnic group ($p < 0.05$)
[4]Difference between Western and Non-Western ethnic group ($p < 0.05$)

that they could not remember having seen any letter or flyer. They may not have been exposed to the invitational letter, for example because they did not live on the address that they were registered at their general practice, they might have not opened their mail, or perhaps they did not read the letter because it was too much text for them. As for the flyer, perhaps it was not appealing enough, they did not see the flyer, or simply forgot about it. Unawareness could be related to individual factors such as low health literacy, but could also be affected by factors at provider level. Kransdorf et al. for example reported that young women in college did not discuss reproductive life planning or preconception health with their providers, despite expressing interest in doing so [29]. A qualitative study in Italy found a lack of awareness of preconception health and care, not only among women of childbearing age, but also among midwives, medical doctors and nurses [30].

Although women in our sample were unaware of the concept of preconception counselling, they generally had knowledge on risk factors for a healthy pregnancy. Each item had over 60% of correct scores. Our findings are comparable to the findings of Temel et al. that used the same knowledge items in a study among women in a deprived area in Rotterdam, the Netherlands [27]. They also found that women had poorest knowledge about the adverse effects of smoking on fertility, and that knowledge was lowest among women with a low educational level and a non-Western background. Percentages of correct answers were slightly lower in their sample.

Table 4 Association between determinants and intention to participate in preconception counselling (*n* = 139)

	B (95% CI)	Adjusted B (95% CI)
Awareness (ref unaware)	−0.17 (− 0.67–0.33)	−0.22 (− 0.72–0.28)[a]
Knowledge risk factors (scale 1–6)	−0.15 (− 0.35–0.05)	−0.03 (− 0.25–0.19)[b]
Attitude (scale 1–5)	0.90 (0.55–1.25)	
Self-efficacy (scale 1–5)	− 0.03 (− 0.40–0.34)	0.09 (− 0.29–0.47)[a]
Subjective norm		
Family/friends	0.13 (0.07–0.18)	
Partner	0.22 (0.14–0.30)	
Considerations to participate (ref: no consideration)		
Preparation for pregnancy	1.43(1.06–1.79)	
Perceived lack of information	1.07 (0.54–1.60)	
Problems previous pregnancy	1.01 (0.51–1.51)	
Considerations not to participate (ref: no consideration)		
Perceived sufficient knowledge	−0.30 (−0.49 - -0.12)	
Perceived low risk	−0.48 (− 0.63- -0.29)	−0.53 (− 0.72—0.34)[a]

[a] adjusted for ethnic background [b]adjusted for ethnic background and education

We do not know if this was related to lower health literacy levels, since they were not measured in their study. Conrood's study among a low-income, Mexican American population also found that knowledge on preconception health was high overall, but lower than knowledge among women with a higher economic status in the same region [31].

We found that low health literate women had a positive attitude towards participation in preconception counselling, and that 41% stated that they would like to participate in it. Conrood et al. also found that 43% of the women with a low socioeconomic background in the US was interested to participate in preconception counselling. These levels of interest were similar to those of a higher economic status in the same region [31]. We also did not find any educational or ethnic differences in intention in our group, this might be related to the fact that all our respondents had low health literacy. Temel et al. did find socioeconomic differences in intention to attend preconception counselling [32]. Those with a lower socioeconomic background had a higher intention to participate. However, Temel et al. did not measure intention to personally participate, but an overall attitude towards preconception care, measured by the statement 'A woman who wishes to become pregnant should consult a GP or midwife before she tries to become pregnant'.

In contrast to most other studies, women in our study reported more considerations in favour of counselling, than considerations against counselling [28]. An important reason to participate, besides preparing well for pregnancy, was to have information on fertility. In their systematic review Poels et al. found that "believing in the benefits" and "availability of preconception counselling" were the most frequently identified facilitators for counselling use. Considerations against counselling did not seem to differ that much from those that were found in studies among women in the general population. Poels et al. also found that "Not (fully) planning pregnancy", "perceived absence of risks", "lack of awareness", and " adverse pregnancy experiences" were the most frequently identified barriers to participate in preconception counselling [28].

We found weak subjective norms regarding participation in counselling. This is not in coherence with other studies, but this discrepancy may be related to differences in measurement [27, 31]. For example, in focus group interviews Afro- American women explained how social factors influenced participation in preconception counselling, but they were not quantified [31]. Temel et al. quantitatively assessed subjective norm and also found that partners were the most important social influence in deciding whether or not to participate in counselling. However, they only assessed perceived importance of the opinion of important others, and not what respondents thought others would advise them to do [27]. Most of our respondents also rated their partner's norm to be important, but the second component of subjective norm (perceived partner's opinion on participation) was mostly scored as neutral, resulting in a weak subjective norm to participate.

Almost half of the respondents (49%) in our study have had at least one unplanned pregnancy. This is far above the national prevalence of 20% unplanned pregnancies in the Netherlands [33]. Previous studies also indicated that women with low health literacy more often have unplanned pregnancies than others [22]. This suggests that the current concept of preconception care is limited for women with low health literacy and confirms the importance of reaching this group of women on time.

This study has several strengths and limitations. A strength of this study is that it provides insight in women's considerations and other factors that could play a role in participation in preconception care. We used the SAHL-D to include women with low health literacy. This performance-based test is frequently used by others and validated in the Dutch context [24]. However, it only measures skills to read and understand and not more advanced skills like appraising or applying information, or context specific skills that are needed to participate in preconception counselling. We only included women with low health literacy. This enabled us to collect data for intervention development for this specific population, but meant we did not have a higher health literacy group to compare our findings with. More than half of our study population lived in an area where invitations for preconception care were sent out, this potentially could have led to bias in our outcome measures. However, only 17% of the women remembered that they received an invitation. Awareness of preconception care and knowledge of risk factors did not significantly differ between women who did not receive an invitation. We performed structured face-to-face interviews to increase our response and to ensure reliable data collection. Although we emphasized our neutral role as researchers, it could be possible that women provided social desirable answers. Another limitation is that the time frame chosen for 'wish to conceive' was quit broad (within 5 years). We chose this time frame to exclude women that certainly knew that they did not want to become pregnant in the coming 5 years, and to include those that have a certain interest in the topic (and may become pregnant, either planned or unplanned in the future). A last limitation is that 38% of the women that met the inclusion criteria did not participate in the study. This could have led to sampling bias, and an underestimation of our findings, since low interest in the topic was one of the reasons for them not to participate in the study.

Conclusions

Women with low health literacy are generally unaware of the concept and provision of preconception counselling, but seem to be interested in participation. This study emphasises the need for recruitment strategies that are tailored to their skills and daily lives. These strategies should raise awareness of the concept of preconception health and preconception care, and explain the benefits and importance of it. Strategies should be applied in time and to all individuals, not just women that are planning a pregnancy. Our findings raise questions about the conditions and efficacy of general advertisement for this group. Entertainment education strategies, applied games, or new media offer promising perspectives to raise awareness. Other options are to provide counselling opportunistically e.g. during other health care visits. Further research should investigate to what extent such strategies are feasible and effective for individuals with low as well as those with adequate health literacy levels.

Abbreviations

ANOVA: Analyses of variance; HP4All: Healthy Pregnancy for All; SAHL-D: Short Assessment of Health Literacy in Dutch

Acknowledgements

We would like to thank Juliette Santing for her contribution to the review of literature.

This manuscript is dedicated to the memory of Prof. Dr. M.L. Essink-Bot. She unexpectedly passed away on the 9th of May 2016.

Funding

This study was funded by ZonMW, The Netherlands Organization for Health Research and Development. (Project title: "Effective preconception care for women with low health literacy" project code 209040006).

Authors' contributions

MF designed the study and obtained funding for it. She performed the literature search and expert review, supervised MH and LM in quantitative data collection, analysis and interpretation. She wrote the manuscript. ME collected, analysed and interpreted the data (literature review, expert review and quantitative data collection) and was involved in drafting and revising the manuscript. LM collected, analysed and interpreted the data (quantitative data collection) and was involved in drafting and revising the manuscript. AR contributed to the data collection, analysis and interpretation (expert review and quantitative data collection) and was involved in drafting and revising the manuscript. SS contributed to the interpretation of the data and the design of the manuscript, and was involved in drafting and revising the manuscript for important intellectual content. All authors read and approved the final manuscript.

Competing interests

The authors declare that they have no competing interests.

Author details

[1]Amsterdam UMC, University of Amsterdam, Department of Public Health, Public Health Research Institute, Meibergdreef 9, Amsterdam, The Netherlands. [2]Rotterdam University of Applied Sciences, School for Healthcare Studies, Department of Master Physician Assistant Midwifery, Rochussenstraat 198, 3015, EK, Rotterdam, The Netherlands. [3]The University of New South Wales, Psychosocial Research Group, Prince of Wales Clinical School, Faculty of Medicine, Lowy Research Centre, Sydney, NSW 2052, Australia.

References

1. Agyemang C, Vrijkotte TG, Droomers M, van der Wal MF, Bonsel GJ, Stronks K. The effect of neighbourhood income and deprivation on pregnancy outcomes in Amsterdam, the Netherlands. J Epidemiol Community Health. 2009;63:755–60.
2. Auger N, Giraud J, Daniel M. The joint influence of area income, income inequality, and immigrant density on adverse birth outcomes: a population-based study. BMC Public Health. 2009;9:237.
3. Poeran J, Maas AF, Birnie E, Denktas S, Steegers EA, Bonsel GJ. Social deprivation and adverse perinatal outcomes among Western and non-Western pregnant women in a Dutch urban population. Soc Sci Med. 2013;83:42–9.
4. de Graaf JP, Schutte JM, Poeran JJ, van RJ, Bonsel GJ, Steegers EA. Regional differences in Dutch maternal mortality. BJOG. 2012;119:582–8.
5. Adegboye AR, Rossner S, Neovius M, Lourenco PM, Linne Y. Relationships between prenatal smoking cessation, gestational weight gain and maternal lifestyle characteristics. Women Birth. 2010;23:29–35.
6. Jaddoe VW, Bakker R, Hofman A, Mackenbach JP, Moll HA, Steegers EA, et al. Moderate alcohol consumption during pregnancy and the risk of low birth weight and preterm birth. The generation R study. Ann Epidemiol. 2007;17:834–40.
7. Nordstrom-Klee B, Delaney-Black V, Covington C, Ager J, Sokol R. Growth from birth onwards of children prenatally exposed to drugs: a literature review. Neurotoxicol Teratol. 2002;24:481–8.
8. Denktas S, Poeran J, van Voorst SF, Vos AA, de Jong-Potjer LC, Waelput AJ, et al. Design and outline of the healthy pregnancy 4 all study. BMC Pregnancy Childbirth. 2014;14:253.
9. Saravelos SH,Regan L. The importance of preconception counseling and early pregnancy monitoring. Semin Reprod Med. 2011;29:557–68.
10. de Graaf JP, Steegers EA, Bonsel GJ. Inequalities in perinatal and maternal health. Curr Opin Obstet Gynecol. 2013;25:98–108.
11. Fowler, JR JB. Preconception Counseling. [Updated 2017 Oct 8]. 2017 [cited 2018; available from: https://www.ncbi.nlm.nih.gov/books/NBK441880/.
12. de Smit DJ, Weinreich SS, Cornel MC. Effects of a simple educational intervention in well-baby clinics on women's knowledge about and intake of folic acid supplements in the periconceptional period: a controlled trial. Public Health Nutr. 2015;18:1119–26.
13. Williams L, Zapata LB, D'Angelo DV, Harrison L, Morrow B. Associations between preconception counseling and maternal behaviors before and during pregnancy. Matern Child Health J. 2012;16:1854–61.
14. Shannon GD, Alberg C, Nacul L, Pashayan N. Preconception healthcare and congenital disorders: systematic review of the effectiveness of preconception care programs in the prevention of congenital disorders. Matern Child Health J. 2014;18:1354–79.
15. Czeizel AE. Ten years of experience in periconceptional care. Eur J Obstet Gynecol Reprod Biol. 1999;84:43–9.
16. Elsinga J, Elsinga J, Van der Pal-de Bruin KM, Le Cessie S, de Jong-Potjer LC, Verloove-Vanhorick SP, Assendelft WJ. Preconception counselling initiated by general practitioners in the Netherlands: reaching couples contemplating pregnancy [ISRCTN53942912]. BMC Fam Pract. 2006;7:41.
17. Valle S, Pezzotti P, Floridia M, Pellegrini MG, Bernardi S, Puro V, et al. Percentage and determinants of missed HIV testing in pregnancy: a survey of women delivering in the Lazio region, Italy. AIDS Care. 2014;26:899–906.
18. Nutbeam D. The evolving concept of health literacy. Soc Sci Med. 2008; 67:2072–8.
19. Ratzan SC, Parker RM. In: Zorn M, Selden CR, Ratzan SC, Parker RM, editors. Intoduction, in National Library of Medicine Current Bibliographies in Medicine: Health Literacy. Bethesda, MD: National Institutes of Health, U.S. Department of Health and Human Services; 2000.
20. Sorensen K, Van den Broucke S, Fullam J, Doyle G, Pelikan J, Slonska Z, et al. Health literacy and public health: a systematic review and integration of definitions and models. BMC Public Health. 2012;12:80.

21. Berkman ND, Sheridan SL, Donahue KE, Halpern DJ, Crotty K. Low health literacy and health outcomes: an updated systematic review. Ann Intern Med. 2011;155:97–107.
22. Kilfoyle KA, Vitko M, O'Conor R, Bailey SC. Health literacy and Women's reproductive health: a systematic review. J Women's Health (Larchmt). 2016; 25:1237–55.
23. Von W, Steptoe A, Wolf MS, Wardle J. Health literacy and health actions: a review and a framework from health psychology. Health Educ Behav. 2009; 36:860–77.
24. Pander Maat H, Essink-Bot ML, Leenaars KE, Fransen MP. A short assessment of health literacy (SAHL) in the Netherlands. BMC Public Health. 2014;14:990.
25. Statistics UIf. ISCED: International standard classification of education. 2014 2014; Available from: http://www.uis.unesco.org/Education/Pages/international-standard-classification-of-education.aspx.
26. Statistics Netherlands. Themes: Ethnic background. 2014 2014 [cited 2014 12/17/2014]; Available from: https://www.cbs.nl/nl-nl/corporate/2016/43/termen-allochtoon-en-autochtoon-herzien.
27. Temel S, Birnie E, Sonneveld HM, Voorham AJ, Bonsel GJ, Steegers EA, et al. Determinants of the intention of preconception care use: lessons from a multi-ethnic urban population in the Netherlands. Int J Public Health. 2013;58:295–304.
28. Poels M, Koster MP, Boeije HR, Franx A, van Stel HF. Why do women not use preconception care? A systematic review on barriers and facilitators. Obstet Gynecol Surv. 2016;71:603–12.
29. Kransdorf LN, Raghu TS, Kling JM, David PS, Vegunta S, Knatz J, et al. Reproductive life planning: a cross-sectional study of what college students know and believe. Matern Child Health J. 2016;20:1161–9.
30. Bortolus R, Oprandi NC, Rech Morassutti F, Marchetto L, Filippini F, Agricola E, et al. Why women do not ask for information on preconception health? A qualitative study. BMC Pregnancy Childbirth. 2017;17:5.
31. Coonrod DV, Bruce NC, Malcolm TD, Drachman D, Frey KA. Knowledge and attitudes regarding preconception care in a predominantly low-income Mexican American population. Am J Obstet Gynecol. 2009;200:686–7.
32. Temel S, Erdem O, Voorham TA, Bonsel GJ, Steegers EA, Denktas S. Knowledge on preconceptional folic acid supplementation and intention to seek for preconception care among men and women in an urban city: a population-based cross-sectional study. BMC Pregnancy Childbirth. 2015;15:340.
33. Picavet C. Zwangerschap en anticonceptie in Nederland [pregnancy and contraceptin in the Netherlands]. Tijdschrift voor Seksuologie. 2012;36:121–8.

13

Prevalence of adverse birth outcome and associated factors among women who delivered in Hawassa town governmental health institutions, south Ethiopia, in 2017

Berhan Tsegaye* and Andargachew Kassa

Abstract

Background: Most pregnancies are unplanned in Ethiopia. This is due to ignorance of the types and efficacy of each method of contraception they are associated with vast and unpredictable complications. Most of the time, these complications result in adverse birth outcomes. Information about prevalence of adverse birth outcome and it's factors are relevant for designing, and initiating and intervening programs to decrease these undesirable out comes.

Objective: To assess prevalence of adverse birth outcome and associated factors among women who delivered in Hawassa town governmental health institutions, south Ethiopia, in 2017.

Method: We conducted institutional based cross sectional study among 580 pregnant women from december1–30/2017, by multistage systematic random sampling method in governmental health institution in Hawassa town. Data were collected through structured pre-tested, close ended and interview administered questionnaire in their post-partum period. Collected data was entered in Epi-info version 7 and analyzed using SPSS. Odds ratio with 95% confidence interval on multivariable logistic regression was computed and *P*-value< 0.05 considered as significance.

Result: From a total of 580 respondents 106(18.3%) respondent's had child related adverse birth outcome. Previous History of child related adverse pregnancy outcome 4.2 (95%,CI = 2.5–6.9), Attend at list one antenatal care visit 2.3 (95%CI = 1.1–4.3), Own cat in the house 2.2 (95%,CI = 1.3–3.7), Had any chronic disease/s 2.1(95%,CI = 1.1–4.8), Age of the mother (from 35 to 45 Years) 2.3(95%,CI = 1.1–4.8), Poor participants' Knowledge on preconception care 3 (95%CI = 1.4–1.6) were significant predictor of adverse birth outcome in this study .

Conclusion and recommendation: Prevalence of adverse birth outcome was found to be significant in the current study. Presence of Previous History of adverse pregnancy outcome, on ante-natal attendance, presence of cat in the house, presence of chronic disease/s, younger mother and Poor Knowledge of preconception care were significant predictor of adverse pregnancy outcome. Therefore it is better to give more attention on expanding preconception and antenatal care. Creating awareness about family planning methods type and efficacy for women of reproductive health is mandatory. Services, increasing health education on personal hygiene vaccination of cats. Moreover, early detecting and treatment of chronic disease.

Keywords: Adverse birth outcome, Women, Hawassa town, 2017

* Correspondence: birieman67@gmail.com
Department of Midwifery, College of Medicine and Health Sciences, Hawassa University, P.O. Box 1560, Hawassa, Ethiopia

Plain English summary

Most pregnancy and childbirth is a joyful experience. But it sometimes end up in adverse birth outcome which disrupt the family condition leading to high individual and social costs. Adverse birth outcome in current study includes pregnancy loss/miscarriage, congenital anomaly or birth defect, preterm baby, low birth weight, perinatal death, macrosomia and intrauterine growth restriction. Most risk factors contributing to adverse birth outcome are amenable to modification. These poor reproductive life planning, substance use, abnormal pre-gestational BMI, irrational medication use, exposure to environmental toxin and contaminants, underlying chronic pre-gestational diseases, anemia and folic acid deficiency, poor regular exercise and physical activity, and presence of stress are included.

The current study use a multistage systematic random sampling technique to select the study participants. Data was collected using a validated structured pre-tested interviewer-administered questionnaire. From a total of 580 respondents 106 (18.3%) respondents had child related adverse birth outcome. Previous history of child-related adverse birth outcome, nonattendance to antenatal care owning cat in the house, having any chronic diseases, being in the age group from, and having poor knowledge about preconception care were found to be significant predictor of child-related adverse birth outcome. In conclusion: Overall prevalence of child-related abnormal birth outcome was found to be significant. Almost all predictors found as significant predictors of abnormal birth outcome are all preconception risk factors. Focusing on prevention and management of preconception risk factors through the provision of preconception care along with early engagement in maternity care continuums is highly advised.

Background

Adverse birth outcome is a critical health issue in developing countries like Ethiopia. It resulted in many bad consequences neonatal and infant morbidity and mortality. Globally, 15 million babies are born too prematurely each year. More than a million of them die immediately after birth; many other suffer from lifelong physical, neurological, or educational disabilities [1].

According to Ethiopian Demographic and Health Survey in 2016, there was high rate of perinatal mortality. Thirty-three death per 1000 live birth was reported. It was associated with increased maternal age, primi-parity, pregnancy interval of less than 15 months and urban residence [2].

Neonatal mortality has shown less improvement than under five mortality in Ethiopia. A modeled data, indicate that Ethiopia reduced its under five mortality rate to 64/1000 live birth in 2013. It is a 69% reduction since 1990 [3]. The amazing fact here is that almost half of neonatal mortality can be prevented through tetanus toxoid vaccine, clean and skilled care at the birth, newborn resuscitation, exclusive breastfeeding, clean umbilical cord care, and management of infections in the newborns [4].

Increased number of intrauterine growth restriction is caused by low pregnancy body mass index, low short maternal stature and gestational weight. This finally leads to many low birth weight neonates in developing countries [5]. A study conducted in northern Ethiopia indicates that there were 63 deaths per 1000 live births. Among these deaths two thirds (34%) were attributable to prematurity and 21 (31%) deaths are caused by asphyxia [6].

Adverse pregnancy outcome generally increase with age. A study conducted in Nigeria, 2012 indicated that perinatal mortality, intrauterine fetal death, and neonatal death increased with age [7]. As evidenced by many research findings, adverse pregnancy outcomes had both child and maternal short term and long term undesirable effects. A study conducted in North West Ethiopia, 2016 showed that Low birth weight and preterm delivery increased the risk of asthma at age of 7 [8]. A study conducted in Nepal, 2013 showed that birth order of the child, with which wantedness is inextricably linked, has more powerful and pervasive effects, with first-born and second-born children being much less likely to show adverse effects [8]. Experiencing intimate partner violence during pregnancy has been associated with women's increased risk of antepartum hemorrhage, and perinatal death. [9] A study conducted in Boricha district of Sidama zone, southern Ethiopia,2014, indicates that having had a neonatal, infant and/or child deaths was associated with symptoms of depression at 14-year follow-up [10].

The achievement of sustainable development goal is highly associated with declining of neonatal death. Though, there are studies on the various forms of adverse birth outcomes particularly in developing countries and few part of Ethiopia, there is limited data on the overall adverse birth outcome at country level specifically at Hawassa town governmental health institution. Therefore, the aim of this study is to determine the prevalence and associated factor of adverse birth outcomes among women who give birth in Governmental health institution in Hawassa town.

Methods and materials

Study area and period

Hawassa city administration is a capital city of southern nation nationality people region and located 275 km South from Addis Ababa. Hawassa city in which 359,358 people are living according to city's Health Department Estimation in 2017, has been structured by 7 urban sub-cities collectively have 21 kebeles and 1 Rural sub-city includes 11 kebeles. The city has 83 public and private health institutions. In detail, these are one public referral and teaching hospital, one public general hospital, four private primary hospitals, 9 Public Health Centers, 17 Public Health Posts and 51 Private Clinics.

There are about a total of 852 health professionals working in the randomly selected PHIs of the city. Together with about 600 health professionals working in Hawassa University Comprehensive Specialized Hospital, the number reached1452.

Hawassa University Comprehensive Specialized Hospital is the largest hospital in southern Ethiopia with more than 300 beds which renders service to both the people in the region and other people coming from the neighboring region. The hospital was established in 2004/05, provides specialized services and comprehensive health services (prevention, treatment and research). The outpatient department consists of 17 rooms and inpatient service consists of five main departments. The average number of patients flow at the outpatient department is more than 200 people per day. The Hawassa University Comprehensive Specialized Hospital and Adare General Hospital are the only public health hospitals providing comprehensive essential obstetric care in the City. The remaining nine PHC are giving Basic essential obstetric care. In the past 6 months of the year 2009, there were a total of 4780 deliveries reported from Hawassa University Comprehensive Specialized Hospital (2073), Adare General public health officer (2022), Adare primary health care (313), Millennium primary health care (311), and Tilte primary health care (61).

Study variables

The dependent variable was the 'overall adverse birth outcomes '. Whereas, the independent variables tested in this study included factors grouped into five categories. The first category includes socio-demographic factors such as age, parity, educational status, religion, occupation, partner's occupation, residence, and family size. The next category is the mother's current obstetric condition. This obstetric condition includes parity, gravidity, antenatal care attendance, gestation, pregnancy complication, birth order, and mother's age at current pregnancy.

The third category is the presence of pre-existing medical conditions. This included conditions such as diabetes mellitus, hypertension, cardiac disease, HIV/AIDS, anemia, malaria, and oral health status. The preconception risk factors occurring before pregnancy such as the woman's pregnancy intention, psychoactive substance use, coffee consumption, pre-gestational BMI, periodontal disease, medication use, previous history of, the use of traditional medicine, environmental exposure, pre-gestational disease, preconception folic acid supplementation use status, presence of external stressors, familial/genetic history, medical insurance status, physical abuse, women's preconception health/care knowledge, inter-pregnancy interval, regular exercise, and uptake of preconception counseling. The last or fifth category is health facility-related factors. This included factors such as availability of health facility, distance, and cost of service.

Operational definition

'Adverse birth outcome" in this study implies the presence of at least one or more of the following conditions in the current pregnancies. These include fetal loss/miscarriage, low birth weight, congenital anomaly, and preterm labour. Thus, if the mothers admitted to the labour ward gave birth to a baby with a congenital anomaly, low birth weight, preterm labour, small for gestational age, perinatal death, macrosomia then the these were labeled as "mothers with a child-related adverse birth outcome. Those who gave normal live birth, without the above mentioned abnormal birth outcome , were labeled as "mothers with normal child related pregnancy outcome".

Perinatal mortality: Is defined as deaths inside uterus (Macerated and fresh stillbirths) and early neonatal deaths (first week of life).Perinatal mortality rate is the sum of both of them per 1000 total deliveries [11].

Miscarriage: Is the natural death of an embryo or fetus before it is able to survive independently [12].

Low birth weight: The weight of the newborn < 2.5 kg [13].

Preterm labour: Preterm labor is defined as regular contractions of the uterus resulting in changes in the cervix that start before 37 weeks of pregnancy [14].

Macrosomia: Macrosomia is defined as birth-weight over 4000 g irrespective of gestational age [15].

Congenital anomaly: A congenital anomaly defined as any abnormality of physical structure found at birth or during the first few weeks of life; or any irreversible condition exiting in a child before birth in which there is sufficient deviation in the usual number, size, shape, location of any part, organ, cell to warrant its designation as abnormal [16, 17].

Sample size and sampling procedures

At first stage, out of the 11 public health institutions, five public health institutions were selected using simple random sampling technique. At the second stage, we applied a systematic random sampling method to identify and include all the study participants. The calculated sampling interval (K) was 1.2. Based on the finding we consecutively recruited the study subject's i.e. using SRS up until the minimum sample size obtained. This is in accord with the assumption that deliveries in nature happened randomly. The samples were taken proportionate to the number of expected deliveries from each selected PHIs. All participants included in the study were all consented verbally to participate in the study. Excluded out of the study were mothers with a twin pregnancy.

Study design and population

A cross-sectional study was conducted among women giving birth in public health institution of Hawassa City Administration. The source populations were all pregnant women living in the Hawassa City Administration. Whereas, the study population were those laboring mothers who attended the randomly selected public health institutions for delivery service during the study period.

This study applied a multistage sampling technique to identify a total of 580 study participants.

The sample size required for this study was determined using the formula for estimating single population proportion. Since there is no research (as per the investigators best systematic literature search) no published article reported the overall prevalence of abnormal birth outcome, and also the proportion of client's attitude towards preconception care. Thus a prevalence value of 0.5 was assumed to calculate the minimum sample size. On the basis of this assumption the minimum possible sample size (n) sufficient enough to meet objectives of the study. The sample size determination considered the following assumptions. This included a 95% confidence interval (CI), a margin of error ($\alpha = 0.05$), population correction factor, a design effect of 2 and 10% non-response rate.

Data collection and analysis

The principal investigator developed the instrument used in this study by referring to various literatures. The instrument is developed based on the objectives of the study. It was primarily designed to measure all the variables listed in the preceding two paragraphs. The instrument was a validated interviewer-administered questionnaire. The instrument was first developed in English and translated into Amharic and then back to English to check the accuracy. Before the actual data collection, the questionnaire was tested on 10% of health care providers working in Public health Institutions of a nearby town called Shashemene.

Every woman who came to deliver in the selected primary health institutions during the data collection period was all interviewed. In addition to the interview, the data collectors abstracted clinical data by reviewing the mother and the babies' medical records. They also measured and confirmed the baby's birth weight, and conducted selected examinations for which they get additional training. The Data was collected by 5 BSC female midwives and 5 BSC female nurses after one-day Training about informed consent, techniques of interviewing, data collection procedures, and different sections of the questionnaire. Two health officers were assigned as Supervisors for the data collectors.

Overall supervision also made by the Principal Investigators. All collected questionnaires were rechecked for completeness and coded. Then these data were entered and cleaned using SPSS version 20 for analysis. Bivariable and multivariable logistic regression was employed to identify an association between the independent predictors and the outcome variable i.e. "child-related adverse birth outcome". Those factors found with their *P*-value ≤0.20 in the bi-variable logistic regression model were fitted into the multivariable logistic regression model to control the effect of confounding variables. Multivariable analysis using standard logistic regression technique was done to evaluate the independent effect of each covariate on 'child-related adverse birth outcome ' by controlling the effect of others. Variable having *P*-value of less than 0.05 in the multivariable logistic regression analysis was considered as significantly associated factors of 'child-related adverse birth outcome '. The adjusted odds ratios with the 95% Confidence Intervals (CI) were reported. Before the actual logistic regression analysis was done, the necessary assumption of logistic regression model was checked by using Hosmer-Lemeshow test of goodness of fit which has a chi-square distribution. For further analysis, descriptive statistics like frequencies and cross tabulation were performed. Tables and bar chart were used to present the findings of the study.

Result

Socio-demographic characteristics

From a total of 580 women delivered at governmental health institutions in Hawassa town, all participated fully in this study making a response rate of 100%. The mean age of respondents is 25.63 + 4.9 years. Majorities 492(84.6%) were in the age range of 20–34 years. Most of the study participants 560(96.6%) were married. More than half, 325(56%), of participants attended in elementary education. Whereas, only few (8.3%) attended college or university level education.

Most of the study participants (68.8%) were housewives and the greater proportion (78.6%) had a family size less than five person per a household. From the total of 580 study participants, most 375(64.7%) of the study participants were living in urban (Table 1). Almost equal number of respondent's partner (50.5%) use family planing methods (see Table 2).

Maternal related adverse pregnancy outcome

Pregnancy induced hpertension which account(4.3%) is the observed predominant maernal related adverse outcome (Fig. 1).

Prevalence of adverse pregnancy outcomes

The current study reveal that 472(81.3%) births are normal live births, while the remaining 108(18.6%) births were births with child related adverse birth outcomes. The current study identified 7 types of abnormal birth outcome. Out of which 67 (11.6%) was low birth weight and the perinatal death was 16(2.7%). The magnitude of congenital anomaly was 6(1%). The study also identified two types of abnormal birth outcome among 33 (5%) of the newborns (Table 3).

Predictors of overall adverse pregnancy outcomes identified

This study identified six statistically significant predictors of adverse pregnancy outcomes related to the child. The chance of developing an abnormal birth outcome among mothers with a previous history of child-related abnormal birth outcomes was by four times higher than those mothers who didn't have the history (AOR = 4.2, 95% CI: 2.5–6.9). Compared to mothers within the age range 20–34 years, those mothers within the age range 35–45 had two-fold higher odds of giving birth to a baby with APO than those mothers who aged 20–34 years (AOR = 2.3, 95% CI: 1.1–4.2). Non attendance to antenatal care, in contrast to attending at least one ANC, showed an increased odd of APO (AOR = 2.2, 95% CI: 1.1–4.3). The likely hood of giving a baby with an adverse pregnancy outcome was by two times higher among those mothers owned a cat in their house (AOR = 2.2, 95% CI: 1.3–3.7) and those who had any chronic diseases(AOR = 2.2, 95% CI: 1.1–4.8). The analysis also revealed that the odds of giving birth to a baby with APO are by three-fold higher among mother with poor preconception care/health knowledge than those with good preconception care/health knowledge (AOR = 3.0, 95% CI: 1.4–6.6) (Tables 3 and 4).

Discussion

This study aimed to assess the overall prevalence of abnormal birth outcome and preconception risk factors contributing to child-related abnormal birth outcome among deliveries attended in primary health institutions of Hawassa. All women approached to be included in the study attended the study. This makes the response rate 100%. The overall prevalence of adverse birth outcome in the current study was found to be 18.6% (95%CI = 0.3–38.6%). Whereas, the types and proportions of the specific abnormal birth outcome identified in this study were; low birth weight 67(11.6%),

Table 1 Socio-demographic characteristics women in postpartum period in Hawassa university referral hospital, southern Ethiopia, 2017(n = 580)

Variables	Categories	N	Percent (%)
AGE	< 20	45	7.8
	20–34	492	84.6
	35–49	43	7.4
Religion	protestant	293	50.5
	Orthodox	157	27.1
	Muslim	87	15
	catholic	8	1.4
	others	13	2.2
Marital status	Married	560	96.6
	Single	20	3.4
Ethnicity	sidama	232	40
	Amhara	42	7.2
	Gurauge	46	7.9
	Oromo	115	19.8
	wolayta	106	18.3
	silte	39	6.8
educational status	no formal education	110	19
	Primary education (1–8 grade)	325	56
	Secondary education (9–12 grade)	97	16.7
	Tertiary (college or university)	48	8.3
Women's occupation	housewife	399	68.8
	private business	87	15
	daily worker	14	2.4
	salaried employed	61	10.5
	Student	19	3.3
Husband occupation	Farmer	153	26.4
	Daily worker	41	7.1
	private business	237	40.9
	salaried employed	124	21.4
	Student	3	0.5
	others	22	3.8
Monthly income	< 1000 ETB	174	30
	1001–2000 ETB	119	20
	2001–3675 ETB	142	25
	> 3675 ETB	145	24
Total family size	< 5	456	78.6
	5–6	89	15.3
	> 6	35	6
residence	urban	375	64.7
	rural	150	25.9
	peri-urban	55	9.4

keyETB = ethiopian birr(1US$ = 27ETB)

Table 2 Reproductive characteristics of women in postpartum period in Hawassa university referral hospital, southern Ethiopia, 2017($n = 580$)

Variables	Categories	Frequency	Percent
Did you or your partner use FP?	Yes	293	50.5
	No	287	49.5
what type of FP do you use? ($n = 293$)	coc	38	6.6
	Depo	189	32.6
	Implanon	23	4
	iucd	34	5.9
	Natural	8	1.4
	no FP	287	49.5
Do you plan this pregnancy?	Yes	520	89.7
	no	60	10.3
Gestational age of the current pregnancy?	preterm	58	10
	term	519	89.5
	post term	3	0.5
Did the mother had at least 1 ANC visit?	yes	521	89.8
	no	59	10.2
mode of delivery	SVD	461	9.5
	instrumental	11	1.9
	CS	108	18.6
sex of the current baby?	male	330	56.9
	female	250	43.1
future pregnancy intention	up to 6moth	1	0.2
	7–12 months	2	0.3
	13–24 months	9	1.6
	25–36 months	8	1.4
	after 3 years	132	22.8
	undecided	375	64.7
	I don't want any more	531	9.1

KEY=FP family planning, *IUCD* intrauterine contraceptive device, *SVD* spontaneous vertex delivery, *CS* cesarean section

Table 3 Magnitudes and types of adverse pregnancy outcome related to the child among deliveries attended in public health institutions of Hawassa, Southern Ethiopia 2017

S.N	List of adverse pregnancy outcomes		Frequency	Percent
1	Perinatal death	No	564	97.2
		Yes	16	2.7
		Total	580	100.0
3	Preterm baby or birth (PB)	No	559	96.4
		Yes	21	3.6
		Total	580	100.0
4	Congenital anomaly	No	574	99.0
		Yes	6	1.0
		Total	580	100.0
5	Macrosomia	No	517	89.13
		Yes	63	10.86
		Total	580	100.0
6	IUGR	No	577	99.5
		Yes	3	.5
		Total	580	100.0
7	Low Birth Weight	No	513	88.4
		Yes	67	11.6
		Total	580	100.0
8	Number of APOs observed in a new birth	No APO observed	474	81.7
		Only 1 APO observed	73	12.6
		Two (2) types of APO observed	33	5.7
		Total	580	100.0
9	Over all APO related to the child	No APO	474	81.7
		APO	106	18.3
		Total	580	100.0

KEY
LBW low birth weight

macrosomia 26(4.5%), preterm birth 21(3.6%), congenital anomaly 6(1.0%), intrauterine growth restriction 3(0.5%), and perinatal death 16 (2.7%).

The magnitude of abnormal birth outcome in the current study is significant. Compared to other similar study findings reported from Ethiopia [18, 19], the prevalence of the overall abnormal birth outcome identified in this study is low. The possible explanation for this discrepancy may be attributable to socioeconomic variations and the difference in the quality of maternal health service. In addition the variation with regard to nutritional and cultural practices may also contribute to the observed differences.

Moreover, since most of the current study participants were urban residence their level of knowledge and utilization of health service might be the other reason to the observed lower abnormal birth outcome. Except for the mother's non-attendance to ante natal care, all of the five predictors identified in the current studies are preconception risk factors contributing to the development of child-related abnormal birth outcome. Similar to two studies in Gondar [18]and Dessie [20], the odds of giving birth to a baby with abnormal birth outcome was found higher than those mothers who attended antenatal care (AOR = 2.2, 95% CI: 1.1–4.2). In Ethiopia, non-attendance to antenatal care is one of the most important public health problems which preconception care intervention can solve. There is an evidence that the odd of uptake of antenatal care is higher among mothers who get preconception care than those who are not getting the service [21]. In Ethiopia, for the past two decades, the antenatal care service uptake remained very low. This is evident

Table 4 Predictors of child related adverse pregnancy outcome from backward stepwise (Wald) logistic regression, in Governmental health institutions, Hawassa Ethiopia, 2017

Predictors		Adverse pregnancy outcome (APO)		COR[95%CI]	AOR[95%CI]
		No APO	Yes APO		
Previous History of child related APO	Yes	87	48	2.3(1.3–4.1) *	4.2(2.5–6.9)***
	No	387	58	1§	1
Previous History of maternal APO	Yes	42	19	3.7(2.4–5.8) ***	1.7(0.8–3.6)
	No	432	87	1	1
Age of the Mother	20–34 Years	411	81	1	1
	18–19 Years	27	16	1.3(0.6–2.7)	1.5(0.6–3.7)
	35–45 Years	36	9	3.0(1.6–5.8) **	2.3(1.1–4.8) *
Attend at list one ANC visit	Not attended	40	19	2.4(1.3–4.3) *	2.2(1.1–4.3)*
	Attended	434	87	1	1
Duration b/n the current & previous pregnancies in months	1st pregnancy	229	38	1	1
	< 12 Months	21	14	4.0(1.9–8.6) ***	2.3 (0.9–5.4)
	12–17 Months	29	8	1.7(0.7–3.9)	1.3(0.5–3.3)
	18–23 Months	66	17	1.6(0.8–2.9)	1.6(0.8–3.3)
	> 24 Months	129	29	1.4(0.8–2.3)	0.7(0.4–1.3)
Anemia in current pregnancy	Yes	60	21	1.7(0.9–3.0)	1.5(0.8–2.8)
	No	414	85	1	1
Own cat in the house?	Yes	162	55	1.8(1.2–2.7) *	2.2(1.3–3.7) **
	No	312	51	1	1
Had any chronic disease/s	Yes	34	16	2.3(1.2–4.4)*	2.2(1.1–4.8)*
	No	440	90	1	1
Mothers' PCC knowledge	Good Knowledge	105	10	1	1
	Fair Knowledge	139	25	1.9(0.9–4.1)	2.2(0.9–5.5)
	Poor Knowledge	230	71	3.2(1.6–6.5) **	3.0(1.4–6.6) *
Monthly income	≤1000.0birr	133	41	1.8(1.1–3.3)*	1.4(0.7–2.7)
	1001.0-2000.0birr	99	20	1.2(0.6–2.3)	1.1(0.5–2.4)
	2001.0 -3675.0 birr	118	24	1.2(0.6–2.3)	1.2(0.6–2.4)
	≥ 3676 birr	124	21	1	1

Key 1 = references group, * = PV < 0.05, ** = PV < 0.001, *** = PV < 0.0001, *CI* confidence interval, *COR* crude odds ratio, *AOR* adjusted odds ratio, *ANC* antenatal care, *PCC* preconception care, *ETB* Ethiopian birr(1$ = 27ETB)

from those national demographic health survey reported an increase from 27% in 2000 to 62% in 2016 [2]. This sluggish increment in antenatal care attendance may be accelerated by the introduction of preconception service in the countries health care system. As one study denoted, despite the world health organization's recommendation, preconception care is not yet formally and officially introduced in the Ethiopian health care system [22].

The chance of developing an abnormal birth outcome among mothers with a previous history of child-related abnormal birth outcome was by four times higher than those mothers who had not had the history (AOR = 4.1, 95% CI:2.5–6.8). Having had a child with abnormal birth outcome, in the previous pregnancy/ies, is one of the most important predictors of all the five predictors identified in this study. A similar study conducted in Shire town of North Ethiopia showed the fact those mothers with the previous history of child related abnormal birth outcome are at greater risk of giving birth to a baby with [19]. There is well-established evidence that previous history of abnormal birth outcome is a risk factor to the occurrence of abnormal birth outcome in subsequent pregnancies. Significant proportion 135(23.3%) of the study participants, in the current study, had a history of child-related adverse pregnancy outcomes. Through preconception care the healthcare, the provider can screen out such risk factors prior to pregnancy. This preventive preconception care intervention is one of the recommended evidence-based practice to solve the occurrence of similar abnormal birth outcome in

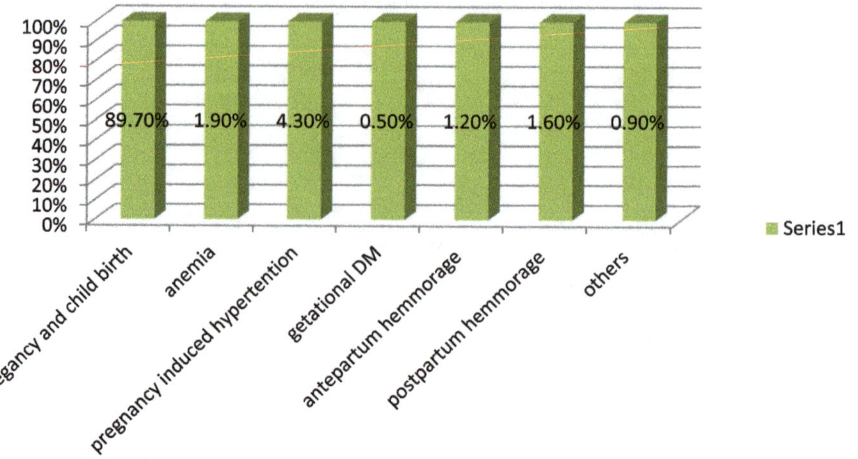

Fig. 1 Maternal related adverse obstetrics complications of women in Governmental health institutions in Hawassa town, southern Ethiopia, 2017. (*n*=580)

subsequent pregnancies. One study showed the need and uptake of preconception care are higher among women with previous history abnormal birth outcome [23].

Similarly, the odd of giving birth to a baby with abnormal birth outcome was by 2 times higher among women with chronic diseases than those who didn't have(AOR = 2.3, 95% CI: 1.1–4.9). This finding is consistent with a study conducted at Dessie [20]. Chronic diseases such as diabetes, hypertension, asthma, epilepsy, depression are well-known risk factors to abnormal birth outcome [24, 25]. Early identification and management of chronic diseases including mental health, prior to conception, is proven to bring a normal pregnancy outcome [4]. Delaying pregnancy until the control of the underlying chronic diseases is one of the objectives of preconception care. This is managed by using preconception family planning service and effective medical care. Nevertheless, there is high the unmet need for family planning among this group of people. Those women with chronic medical conditions are at risk of abnormal birth outcome demanding preconception care [26].There is evidence that advanced maternal age is a risk factor for the occurrences of both maternal and child related abnormal birth outcome s [27]. In line with these evidence, this study revealed a twofold higher odds of abnormal birth outcome among women in the age group 35–45 Years than those in the age group 20-34 years (AOR = 2.395% CI: 1.1–4.8). The co-occurrence of chronic diseases with pregnancy is common. This is one of the cases that complicate the outcome of pregnancies. Though, an advanced maternal age is one of the non-modifiable risk factors for pregnancy, early enrolment of women in preconception care may help couples to make a wise reproductive plan [26]. Those women with a poor knowledge of preconception health/care were 3 times (AOR = .3.0,95%, CI: 1.4–6.6) more likely to have an abnormal birth outcome than those who had good knowledge. A community-based study conducted at Adet, North Ethiopia, showed poor knowledge among the vast majority of the women [28]). If the woman has appropriate knowledge of preconception health and care, she can seek or easily attend to the preconception care service. This can help her to easily identify and effectively control the underlying risk condition that leads to abnormal birth outcome. Health care providers participated in one research reported that poor awareness or knowledge of preconception health and care as a barrier to the uptake and delivery of preconception care [28]. Another systematic study that investigated the reasons why women are not using preconception care reported poor PCC knowledge and awareness as a barrier to preconception care uptake [29].

The last predictor identified by the current study showed that those women who have cat in their house had two times higher odds of abnormal birth outcome than those who didn't have (AOR = 2.3, 95% CI: 1.4–3.8). The possible explanation for this result may be toxoplasmosis infection that uses cats as a reservoir can lead leads adverse birth outcome like premature birth and low birth weight. Studies conducted at different areas of Ethiopia showed high prevalence of Sero-prevalence of Toxoplasma gondii (T.gondii) antibodies for IgM among pregnant women [30–32]. This studies reported that contact with cat or cat ownership as factors that increased the odds of women's to T.gondii infection and recommended avoidance of contact with cats and avoidance of raw and under cooked foods [31–33]).

In general this study identified five preconception risk factors or that increased the mothers odds of giving birth to a baby with abnormal birth outcome. Nevertheless, his study is not without limitation. Some of participants of the study may not remember some of the questions. This may lead to underreporting of the findings reported in this study. For some of the variables, such as previous history of abnormal birth outcomes, this study relied on the study participants verbal response. This study never included abnormal birth outcomes s happening at an and post pregnancy period. This include abnormal birth outcome such as miscourage, pregnancy loss, neonatal and infant death. As a cross sectional study this study do didn't determined causal relationship and also temporal relationship. Despite this study, might tried to focus on preconception risk factors contributing to abnormal birth outcomes. To the best of authors best systematic search, there are not published articles reported preconception risk factors contributing to abnormal birth outcomes in Ethiopia.

Conclusion and recommendation

The prevalence of the overall adverse birth outcome is significant. Previous History of child related abnormal birth outcomes, women's poor knowledge of preconception health/care, having any chronic diseases, advanced maternal age (35–45 years), and having a cat in the house were all preconception risk factors that increased the likelihood of developing child related abnormal birth outcomes. Non attendance to antenatal care was the other factor that increased the odds of the occurrence of abnormal birth outcomes. Provision of preconception and inter-conception care is the best approach to the identification and early management of risk factors to abnormal birth outcomes. The continuums of the maternal and child health care services are incomplete without the inclusion of PCC. Adverse pregnancy outcome reduction strategies should consider early identification and management of the preconception risk factors. The preconception care should include educating all eligible or reproductive-aged couples about preconception care/health. Creating awareness about family planning methods type and efficacy for women of reproductive health is mandatory.

Abbreviations

ABO: Adverse birth outcome; AOR: Adjusted odds ratios; CI: Confidence interval; COR: Crudes odds ratios; CSA: Central Statistical Agency; EDHS: Ethiopian Demographic and Health survey; PCC: Preconception care

Acknowledgements

Our heartfelt gratitude is to supervisors, data collectors, and all study participants. Our particular appreciation goes to Mr. Arega Donka who supervised the overall data collection process. Finally, we would like to thank Hawassa University for funding the research project.

Funding

There was no any funding or sponsoring organization for this paper.

Authors' contributions

AK conceived the study and wrote the proposal, facilitated data collection, analysis, data interpretation, drafted the final report write up and prepared manuscript. BT, participated in developing the tools and data collection process, data analysis and involved in report write up. Both the authors revised the subsequent drafts of the paper and read and approved the final manuscript.

Consent for publication

Not applicable

Competing interests

The authors declare that they have no competing interests.

References

1. Howson CP, Kinney MV, McDougall L, Lawn JE. Born too soon: preterm birth matters. Reprod Health. 2013;10(1):S1.
2. Ehiopia: Ethiopian demographic health survey 2016.
3. WH. O. Success factors for women's and children's health. Ethiopia; 2015.
4. Lassi ZS, Haider BA, Bhutta ZA. Community-based intervention packages for reducing maternal and neonatal morbidity and mortality and improving neonatal outcomes. Cochrane Database Syst Rev. 2010;11(11):CD007754.
5. Kuganab-Lem RB, Dogudugu R, Kanton L. Birth preparedness and complication readiness: a study of postpartum women in a rural district of Ghana. Public Health Res. 2014;4(6):225–33.
6. Mengesha HG, Sahle BW. Cause of neonatal deaths in northern Ethiopia: a prospective cohort study. BMC Public Health. 2017;17(1):62.
7. EA AK, Kuku J, Lateef I, Ogundipe J, Mogbeyteren T, Banjo M. Birth preparedness and complication readiness of pregnant women attending the three levels of health facilities in Ife Cenral local government Nigeria. J Commun Med Primary Health Care. 2011;23(1–2):61–8.
8. Karkee R, Lee AH, Binns CW. Birth preparedness and skilled attendance at birth in Nepal: implications for achieving millennium development goal 5. Midwifery. 2013;29(10):1206–10.
9. Bloom T, Bullock LF, Sharps P, Laughon K, Parker BJ. Intimate partner violence during pregnancy. In: Family violence and nursing practice. New York: Edn.: Springer Publishing Co; 2010. p. 155–80.
10. Gudura TT, Debiso AT, Gudura TT. Factors associated with institutional delivery in Boricha district of Sidama zone, southern Ethiopia. Int J Public Health Sci (IJPHS). 2014;3(4):224–30.
11. Goel N, Gupta B. Maternal risk factors affecting perinatal mortality. Indian Pediatr. 2012;49:188–9.
12. Hurt KJ, Guile MW, Bienstock JL, Fox HE, Wallach EE. The Johns Hopkins manual of gynecology and obstetrics: Lippincott Williams & Wilkins; 2012.
13. Organization WH. International statistical classification of diseases and related health problems. 2010 [cited 2017 Mar 03]. http://www.who.int/lassifications/icd.ICD10volume2-en-2010pdf.
14. Gupta PCSS. Smokeless tobacco use, birth weight, and gestational age: population based, prospective cohort study of 1217 women in Mumbai, India. Bmj. 2004;328(7455):1538.
15. Mohammadbeigi A, Farhadifar F, Soufi Zadeh N, Mohammadsalehi N, Rezaiee M, Aghaei M. Fetal macrosomia: risk factors, maternal, and perinatal outcome. Ann Med Health Sci Res. 2013;3(4):546–50.
16. Fretts RC: Effect of advanced age on fertility and pregnancy in women. Up to date online http://www.uptodate.com 2007.
17. Ali A, Zahad S, Masoumeh A, Azar A. Congenital malformations among live births at Arvand hospital, Ahwaz, Iran-a prospective study. Pakistan J Med Sci. 2008;24(1):33.
18. Adane AA, Ayele TA, Ararsa LG, Bitew BD, Zeleke BM. Adverse birth outcomes among deliveries at Gondar University hospital, Northwest Ethiopia. BMC Pregnancy Childbirth. 2014;14(1):90.
19. Haftu A. Assessment of magnitude and associated factors of adverse birth outcomes among deliveries at Suhul hospital Shire, Tigray, Ethiopia from September, 2015 to February, 2016. Biomed J Sci Tech Res. 2017;1(7).
20. Niguss Cherie AM. Adverse birth out comes and associated factors amongDelivered mothers in Dessie referral hospital, north East Ethiopia. Nurs Health Care. 2018;1.
21. Dean SV, Lassi ZS, Imam AM, Bhutta ZA. Preconception care: promoting reproductive planning. Reprod Health. 2014;11(3):S2.
22. Biratu AK. Addressing the high adverse pregnancy outcomes through the incorporation of preconception care (PCC) in the health system of Ethiopia; 2017.

23. Batra P, Higgins C, Chao SM. Previous adverse infant outcomes as predictors of preconception care use: an analysis of the 2010 and 2012 Los Angeles mommy and baby (LAMB) surveys. Matern Child Health J. 2016;20(6):1170–7.
24. Farahi N, Zolotor A. Recommendations for preconception counseling and care. Am Fam Physician. 2013;88(8).
25. Lassi ZS, Imam AM, Dean SV, Bhutta ZA. Preconception care: screening and management of chronic disease and promoting psychological health. Reprod Health. 2014;11(3):S5.
26. Manaf RA, Ismail IZ, Latiff LA. Contraceptive use among women with chronic medical conditions and factors associated with its non-use in Malaysia. Global J Health Sci. 2012;4(5):91.
27. JA. S: Effect of advanced age on fertility and pregnancy in women: Literaturereview [\English]. USA2013 [updated Mar 29, 2013.; cited 2018 June 30]. Available from: http://www.uptodate.com.
28. Ayalew Y, Mulat A, Dile M, Simegn A. Women's knowledge and associated factors in preconception care in adet, west gojjam, Northwest Ethiopia: a community based cross sectional study. Reprod Health. 2017;14(1):15.
29. Poels M, Koster MP, Boeije HR, Franx A, van Stel HF. Why do women not use preconception care? A systematic review on barriers and facilitators. Obstet Gynecol Survey. 2016;71(10):603–12.
30. Abamecha F, Awel H. Seroprevalence and risk factors of toxoplasma gondii infection in pregnant women following antenatal care at Mizan Aman general hospital, bench Maji zone (BMZ), Ethiopia. BMC Infect Dis. 2016; 16(1):460.
31. Agmas B, Tesfaye R, Koye DN. Seroprevalence of toxoplasma gondii infection and associated risk factors among pregnant women in Debre Tabor, Northwest Ethiopia. BMC Res Notes. 2015;8(1):107.
32. Gebremedhin EZ, Tadesse G. A meta-analysis of the prevalence of toxoplasma gondii in animals and humans in Ethiopia. Parasit Vectors. 2015; 8(1):291.
33. M'hamdi HI, van Voorst SF, Pinxten W, Hilhorst MT, Steegers EA. Barriers in the uptake and delivery of preconception care: exploring the views of care providers. Matern Child Health J. 2017;21(1):21–8.

14

Exploring mistreatment of women during childbirth in a peri-urban setting in Kenya: experiences and perceptions of women and healthcare providers

Jackline Oluoch-Aridi[1*], Vania Smith-Oka[2], Ellyn Milan[3] and Robert Dowd[4]

Abstract

Background: In Kenya, indirectly caused maternal deaths form a significant portion of all maternal deaths within the health system. Many of these deaths are avoidable and occur during delivery and labor. Poor quality health service has been a recurring concern among women in Kenya, with women reporting interactions with healthcare workers that are often demeaning and abusive. This paper explores the experiences and perceptions of both female patients and healthcare workers regarding mistreatment during childbirth. This study aims to provide recommendations on how dignified care can be made the norm, specifically focusing on a peri-urban setting in Kenya.

Methods: The research was accomplished using qualitative research methods with focus group discussions and in depth interviews with women and healthcare workers. The aim was to gain a deeper understanding of the manifestations of mistreatment within the context of a peri-urban setting in Kenya.

Results: Female patients reported different forms of mistreatment, such as verbal abuse, physical abuse, neglect, discrimination, abandonment, poor rapport and failure of the health system to uphold professional standards. The healthcare workers described a health system that was weak and fragmented with poor policy support particularly for the new free maternity services policy leading to the mistreatment of women.

Conclusion: Newly formed County Governments need to provide resources for a functioning health system to ensure an enabling environment for the provision of high quality maternal health services. This process can include feedback loops with maternity clients to ensure woman-centered services. Policy makers need to strengthen oversight for the implementation of the free maternity services Community health volunteers can be trained to provide this information. Professional associations that govern the standards of quality care for healthcare workers need to address the mistreatment through retraining and norms transformation.

Keywords: Maternal health, Women, Mistreatment, Healthcare workers experiences, Peri-urban, Qualitative study, Kenya

* Correspondence: Jackline.A.Oluoch-Aridi.1@nd.edu
[1]Regional Research Programs Manager, The Ford Program in Human Development Studies and Solidarity, University of Notre Dame, Regional Office, East Africa, P.O. Box 49675-00100, Nairobi, Kenya
Full list of author information is available at the end of the article

Plain English summary

As many developing countries, Kenya has made little progress on reducing the number of maternal-related deaths within its population. Most of these deaths occur during labor and childbirth. Evidence is clear that access to facility-based deliveries and skilled birth attendance directly impacts the number of maternal deaths. However, many women are reluctant to access health facilities for childbirth services because of the type of treatment they encounter at many health facilities. Previous research in Kenya suggests that women are subject to mistreatment at health facilities, including physical abuse such as slapping and pinching, verbal abuse such as yelling, as well as other acts of abuse and negligence. In this study, qualitative research methods were used to explore both women and healthcare providers' experiences and perceptions of mistreatment of women during childbirth in the peri-urban setting of Dandora in Nairobi. The study found that mistreatment during facility-based delivery is widespread and is largely driven by weak maternal healthcare policies and poor rapport between different actors within the system, such as mothers, nurses, midwives, doctors, hospital administrators, and the larger healthcare system. It is necessary for the newly formed county governments in Kenya along with policy workers to seek solutions to mistreatment through provision of resources for maternity wards such as retraining as well as health systems improvements such as increasing the numbers of staff and providing adequate resources.

Background

Maternal mortality remains a global health challenge that promises little progress of subsiding under current conditions. Many countries have failed in efforts to reduce the rates of maternal deaths, with over 300,000 maternal deaths having occurred in developing countries in 2015 [2, 23]. Evidence suggests that a reduction of these deaths can be achieved through the use of a skilled birth attendant during delivery, facility-based delivery and ensuring access to good quality maternal health care [19, 35]. Any examination of maternal mortality must take into account whether deaths were due to direct (e.g. obstetric complications, interventions, use of incorrect treatment, etc.) or indirect causes (e.g. the presence of pre-existing conditions that developed during pregnancy and increased the risk during pregnancy) [36]. Though recent research by van den Akker et al. [33] suggests that this distinction needs to be re-examined, as it places too much emphasis on direct causes while ignoring the indirect causes that might, in fact, be more significant factors in maternal mortality (see also [20]).

Kenya has experienced little progress on maternal mortality indicators as per the MDG targets of 2015. The country's current maternal mortality rate is 362 per 100,000 deaths [18]. Most of these deaths occur during labor and childbirth. The proportion of women delivering in a health facility in Kenya had increased from 44 to 60%; despite this increase many women in Kenya continue to shun health facilities, choosing to deliver their babies elsewhere [18]. Poor quality of care as well as fear of abuse and disrespect perpetuated by healthcare workers may be some of the reasons shaping women's decisions [1]. The provision of high quality healthcare is central to improving maternal health services and female patients' satisfaction. Quality of care, specifically for maternity care, needs to include several components, including being safe (minimizing risk), effective (care based on existing evidence-based guidelines), timely (making sure to reduce delays care), efficient (maximizing resource use), equitable (where everyone receives good care regardless of background), and people-centered (taking into account local needs). QoC for pregnant women and newborns in facilities requires competent and motivated human resources and the availability of essential physical resources [32].

There has been an increased scholarly attention to the context within which mistreatment arises [3, 5, 13, 24]. Some of these studies have been conducted with an aim of identifying typologies for mistreatment. Bohren et al. [6] identified seven forms of mistreatment of women during facility-based delivery in sub-Saharan African settings. These forms included, physical abuse, sexual abuse, verbal abuse, stigma and discrimination, failure to meet professional standards of care, poor rapport between female patients and providers and health systems conditions and constraints. Bradley et al. [9] elaborated on the context for mistreatment as well as the drivers of mistreatment at the meso-, micro-, and macro-level. Qualitative studies exploring perceptions and experiences of both female patients and healthcare workers in diverse sub-Saharan African countries, such as Nigeria, Guinea, and Tanzania, demonstrate that mistreatment during facility-based childbirth is not only prevalent but is a growing concern [4, 8, 22].

Research in Kenya shows that mistreatment during childbirth is also prevalent. One study using exit interviews in a small rural public hospital in Western Kenya described women's experiences with the health system as being unsatisfactory [27]. Another study comparing thirteen health facilities estimated that disrespect occurred in at least 20% of cases [1]. An additional study by Warren et al. [34], which compared care in seven counties describe the manifestations of mistreatment of women and shows that female patients expressed frustration with a lack of confidentiality during delivery, a lack of autonomy, an abandonment by providers, and unsanitary maternity settings.

A critical policy change that was relatively new during the time of this research was a free maternity health policy initiated by a presidential decree in 2013. This policy allowed all women in Kenya to access free delivery services in all public health facilities. This policy led to a considerable shift in service delivery and expectations. The subsequent high workload also brought about by the free delivery services decree led to increases in the number of women accessing delivery services particularly in the public sector (Calhoun et al., 2018). This subsequently led to high workload with women who previously used private health facilities making trade-offs and attending already busy maternity health facilities hence frustrating already overworked healthcare workers.

Research conducted in peri-urban settings have often focused on the poor quality of services, wherein they experience higher maternal mortality rates [14, 40]. Despite the fact that Kenya has many peri-urban areas, where a large proportion of its impoverished populations live, there have been no studies of the manifestations of maternal mistreatment among its population. This is an important gap, which we aim to fill. We thus describe the manifestations of the different forms of disrespect and abuse and its connection to human dignity. Dignity is defined as health care that has understanding, compassion and empathy at its core [11]. Our ultimate goal is to explore solutions on how to improve the delivery experiences of women living in peri-urban settings and incorporate dignified healthcare practices among healthcare workers.

Methods

Study setting

The main objective of this study was to explore female patients' and health care providers' experiences and perceptions of mistreatment of female patients during childbirth. The location was the peri-urban setting of Dandora in Nairobi, Kenya. Dandora has a population of approximately 300,000 people and is situated in Embakasi-North sub-county, Nairobi. The City of Nairobi's garbage fill is located in Dandora; there is significant criminal activity in the area, which is raising insecurity levels. Dandora lacks basic amenities such as clean water and garbage disposal, which leads to many health and development issues for its population. The setting was selected as a study site because it is a peri-urban setting, and thus serves to help answer questions of maternal health in these areas. Studies conducted in peri-urban settings close to Dandora have estimated maternal mortality at 700 per 100,000 [40]. Additionally because of the location's insecurity, the area is largely understudied and the maternal health situation is not well understood.

Within Dandora there are two secondary care public health centres, four private health centres (of varying size). The two other major maternities that participants mentioned are outside of Dandora. These are referral maternities, however some of the women do go there to deliver. There is a major referral hospital, which is also outside of Dandora, near Nairobi's city centre.

Prior to choosing the site, the research team engaged in many months of continuous community engagement sessions with the local population. These sessions were facilitated by the Dandora Human Development project (established in 2011), which is a community based organization that has worked to address the development challenges by empowering the community through facilitating community engagement and enhancing people's dignity and sense of agency. One of the community engagement sessions identified the issue of lack of quality of maternal health services for women residing in Dandora as a key developmental challenge.

Study participants and recruitment

The study participants included nurse-midwives, doctors, and administrators from six different health facilities within the Dandora area. Using random sampling, the women were recruited during their antenatal care services at the Holy Cross parish's Brother Andre Medical Centre. The same system of random sampling was used to recruit healthcare workers from their workstations at the different health facilities within the Embakasi-North sub-county health office, which has contacts for healthcare workers. The healthcare workers were included to triangulate the information obtained from the female patients and to ensure a balanced view about the women's perceived experiences. Healthcare workers who had not served in a maternity ward setting were ineligible to participate in the study.

Data collection and management

The first phase of the study was conducted between October and December 2016. The data were collected through 46 in-depth individual (IDI) semi-structured interviews and 15 focus group discussions (FGDs) with women who had given birth during the previous five years. The second phase was conducted between January and March 2017 and was done through observations and 20 in-depth interviews with healthcare workers.

Data collection was a joint effort between the principal investigators, two research assistants, a medical officer, a graduate student, and a community mobilizer attached to the Dandora Human Development Project. The FGDs were coordinated by the first author, who is a health policy specialist and also fluent in Swahili (the local language). The interviews with the healthcare workers were conducted by the third author, a graduate student who was accompanied by a Kenyan medical doctor who helped facilitate the conversations with the healthcare workers and ensured that they did not view the interviews as an audit on their work. One of the unforeseen situations was a medical workers strike in early 2017, which created a difficulty in accessing healthcare workers at their workstations. All study participants provided informed consent through a written consent form, which they read and signed. The interviews lasted between one to one and a half hours and were audio recorded for verbatim accounts. Selected healthcare workers who were interviewed outside their work areas were reimbursed for their transport and lunch costs at a rate of 1000Ksh (10 USD). Interviews were done in English were transcribed, while the interviews that took place in Swahili were transcribed, translated, and back translated by the research assistants. The transcripts were de-identified and stored in a password-protected computer.

Study instruments

The study employed a semi-structured discussion guide for the interviews (Additional files 1 and 2).

Ethical considerations

Written informed consent was obtained from all study participants prior to participation. The Focus group discussions (FGDs) with the women were conducted in a safe setting away from the facility (on the grounds of the parish) where they could speak in confidence about their experiences. This location offered the requisite privacy that the women needed. To enhance additional confidentiality, all FGD participants were encouraged not to discuss each other's opinions outside the FGD setting. The names of the respondents or any personal information were not recorded in the manuscript, so as to make it unlikely for their opinions to be linked to their identities. Research approval for the study was provided by the National Council for Research and Technology Institute (NACOSTI) in Kenya. Local ethical approval was provided by Strathmore University Institutional Review Board. Additional Ethical approval was provided by the University of Notre Dame Institutional Review Board.

Data analysis

The data analysis was conducted by the first and third author. The approach used was thematic analysis as described by Braun and Clarke [10]. Line by line coding was done on a sub-section of the transcripts independently to obtain emerging codes inductively. The software used to organize the data prior to analysis was *Nvivo 11* [28]. The data was classified and organized according to emergent key themes and categories, such as different forms of abuse or neglect. A codebook was designed using these inductively emergent codes and an existing literature typology on mistreatment of women (specifically [7] work), which was adapted to the Kenyan context (see Additional file 1). This codebook expressed high-level themes and code families. The similarities and differences within the themes were highlighted and analyzed. To establish inter-coder reliability, some of the coded transcripts were reviewed by an independent author.

Results

Two data collection methods were used during this research: (1) 15 FGDs with participating women, which included between five to seven participants, and (2) 46 individual in-depth interviews. Because of the sensitive nature of the information, some women preferred to speak about mistreatment individually and in confidence, which is why there are more than three times as many interviews as FGDs. The average age reported by the women was 30 years; the majority (74%) were married, and most of the women (91%) were Christian. In terms of tribal representation, the Luo and Kikuyu tribes were most heavily represented, with 61% claiming at least one of these. Almost 50% of participants had attained at least a secondary education, and described their job as housewife. Sixty one percent of participants had previously delivered between 2 and 3 children (see Table 1). A total of 20 healthcare workers were interviewed (6 doctors, 2 clinical officers, 8 nurses/midwives and 4 hospital administrators). Details for the demographics characteristics of the healthcare workers are presented in Table 2.

Mistreatment experiences of women

The following presents the emergent themes from the data collected on the female patients' and healthcare worker's perceptions of mistreatment. As was mentioned in the introduction, Bohren et al. [7] identified the following typology of mistreatment: Physical abuse, sexual abuse, verbal abuse, stigma and discrimination, poor rapport between healthcare workers and women, failure to meet professional standards and health systems constraints Our data fell within all the six major themes aforementioned with the exception of sexual abuse. Because of the prevalent stigma around the issue of sexual abuse among most populations in Kenya, participants did not mention its manifestations to us. Additionally, because of the prevailing power imbalance between healthcare workers (who are often of higher socioeconomic status than the women) it is unlikely that the women would report any instances of sexual abuse.

Physical abuse

The women reported physical abuse occurring during their delivery. The physical abuse was often described in terms of beatings and slaps. One woman described her experience as below;

Table 1 Sociodemographic characteristics of the women of reproductive health interviewed through In-depth individual Interviews

Characteristic	n (%)
Age in years	
20–24	4 (9%)
25–29	10 (22%)
30–34	13(28%)
35–39	11(24%)
40+	8(17%)
Marital status	
Single	12(26%)
Married	34(74%)
Religion	
Christian	42 (91%)
Muslim	2 (4%)
Other/Missing	2 (4%)
Ethnicity	
Luo	16 (35%)
Kikuyu	15 (33%)
Kamba	3 (7%)
Kisii	2 (4%)
Luhya	8 (17%)
Other	2 (4%)
Education	
Primary	18(39%)
Secondary	32(50%)
Tertiary	7(4%)
None	2
Employment	
Private Sector	5 (11%)
Civil servant	1(2%)
Housewife	23(50%)
Tailor	3(7%)
Trader	7(15%)
Other	7(15%)
Number of living children	
0–1	5(11%)
2–3	28(61%)
4–5	10(22%)
5 and above	3 (7%)

"...At this public hospital the doctors are usually nice, they walk around the wards and when they find you seated, they encourage you to walk. The only problem there is when you disturb them during the delivery process they beat you up, a slap will just land on you or they could beat you up with a plank of wood..." (Woman, age public hospital).

Table 2 Sociodemographic characteristics of healthcare workers interviewed through In-depth individual Interviews

Characteristics of healthcare workers	Doctors (n = 6)	Nurses (n = 8)	Clinical Officers (n = 2)	Hospital Administrators (n = 4)
Age in years				
20–29	4	1	1	0
30–39	2	4	1	3
40–49	0	2	0	0
50+	0	1	0	1
Marital Status				
Single	6	2	1	0
Married	0	6	1	4
Gender				
Female	3	6	0	4
Male	3	2	2	0
Years of Experience				
0–4	6	3	2	0
5–9	0	0	0	2
10–15	0	3	0	1
15+	0	2	0	1
Type of health facility				
Private	0	5	1	4
Public	6	3	1	0

The women we spoke with experienced fear, panic, a sense of helplessness, bitterness, and psychological pain as a result of the beatings meted out by the healthcare workers. Another woman interviewed described some of the harsh treatments she was subject to;

"...I could see how people were giving birth and the doctors were harsh, beating people seriously and you were next and you don't even know what you were are going to do..." (Woman, aged 23, FGD, delivered in public hospital).

The female participants explained that they knew that the nurses were slapping them in order to assist them in their delivery of their babies, but also noted that they were never given explicit reasons for why the beating was necessary, leaving them confused and perplexed. This abuse was especially shocking for first time mothers who admitted having bitter feelings towards the nurses after these experiences, and thus considered never returning to the health facilities for any future delivery.

Our data show that there were conflicting views from healthcare workers regarding the physical abuse. When asked, the nurses particularly justified the slaps as a tool of obtaining compliance and cooperation from the women during the pushing phase of birth, citing the urgency required to save the lives of a mother and baby during the active phase of childbirth. A few of the midwives justified the physical abuse by citing their training, saying they were taught to be 'firm' with the women. They thus learned to obtain compliance through physical means, with the end goal of ensuring good health outcomes for the women and their babies. Nurses and midwives described their patients' lack of cooperation and compliance, especially during labor put the women at risk of losing their lives and harming their child during a critical time as illustrated below:

> *"...You know some mothers are uncooperative because of the pain you find a woman if you are so gentle with them they become unruly but if you are so gentle and so you can find some of them even injuring the baby so you have to be 'firm'..." (IDI, Nurse-Midwife at private health facility)*

The nurse-midwives interviewed used terms such as "uncooperative", "unruly", "wild" and "rude" to describe some of the women. They also described a special class of women that they labeled "difficult women." These women tended to be either underage women with no children, older women who were multiparous, or women who had not attended antenatal care services. They described these women as woefully unprepared for the eventualities surrounding childbirth. One doctor interviewed mentioned that he had encountered some very young women who were likely victims of sexual assault. He said they were extremely hostile and were hence at risk of verbal or physical abuse because of the perceived lack of compliance to medical instructions during labor and childbirth.

Almost all the different kinds of healthcare workers attempted to justify physical abuse. They stated that because female patients in labor were undergoing intense pain, their emotional state was questionable. They went on to add that these patients were unable to comply with the rigorous instructions issued, and hence the healthcare workers were forced to become physical with them. This kind of justification of physical abuse represents a clear illustration of the normalization of physical abuse during childbirth.

Verbal abuse

Female participants described how healthcare workers attempted to silence them from asking about their own care during labor and delivery. They mentioned that the nurse-midwives predominantly asserted their power over them by using sarcastic words when they asked questions related to their care. The women also complained that the nurses castigated them for their sexuality and told them they were not present when the women were conceiving and so the women should not expect help from them. The nurses were reported to have regularly used abusive language, especially during the process of labor to suppress the noises women made during pushing. Interestingly, women were also castigated during seemingly mundane tasks, such as when they made their beds, as illustrated by the quotes below;

> *"...In the wards nurses and workers were shouting at mothers, if they notice that you have soiled the bed sheets you are in trouble; that is the time you are told to wake up quickly and bathe with cold water; and at that time you are weak and can only move slowly..." (Woman, aged 26, FGD, delivered in public hospital).*

> *"...I was in labor pains for three days and the nurses were saying that my cervix had not opened and eventually an artificial rupture of membranes was conducted by the nurses who were assisting me... They looked at me with contempt and used abusive language when I was pushing the baby... They could tell me to push or don't push that really confused me. After a long struggle I told them to take me for an operation because I thought I could not manage [and] the head of the baby was already out. I was terrified to see the nurses hold my legs and forcing me to push the baby, because they had sensed danger. Eventually my baby was safe but I didn't like how I was handled..." (Woman, aged 24, FGD, delivered in major public maternity hospital).*

Almost half of all women in the focus group discussions used terms such as "they are very harsh", "they insult you", "they were rude", "they can't handle someone in a good way", "they look down upon you" and "they abuse you". They claimed that the nurses abused them verbally for the most menial transgressions, for instance, the clothes they wore. They also said that they used insinuations surrounding their sexuality. These verbal abuses illustrated a power imbalance between the nurses and the women, which seemed to normalize the unwarranted verbal abuse.

> *"...Sometimes maybe a mother has not been attending clinic, she has come with nothing because you have to conduct an ANC profile and know her HIV status. Some are just like they have not gotten any health education outside there. And also primiparous women do not attend clinic.so we have to shout at them..." (IDI, Clinical officer at private facility).*

Stigma and discrimination

Stigma and discrimination appear in the following ways: (1) Discrimination based on age; (2) As ethnic-based discrimination; (3) Structural discrimination based on continuity of care from prenatal to post-natal period; 4) Discrimination based on parity; 5) Discrimination based on disease status; and 6) Discrimination based on socioeconomic status. Some women stated that if they were young, the healthcare workers would mistreat them for being involved in sexual relations and having babies prematurely. Healthcare workers would thus neglect them during labor or deny them care altogether. Other women described discrimination due to their ethnic background. They reported that they perceived that women of "higher" ethnicities were given preferential treatment over those of "lower" ethnic groups, as described by one woman,

> *".... One looks at a card and sees this is Jane and this is Mary, they would call Jane first (because her name indicates her ethnicity) and she gets attended to with priority and Mary will stay there until at night someone complains (about the queue jumping) and only then do they use the order (in which the patients arrived). This is not right as we are one tribe, just one tribe..." (Woman, aged 30, FGD, delivered at Major Referral Hospital A).*

Another unexpected dimension of discrimination was based on continuity of care from antenatal care services to delivery care. That is, women who received their antenatal services at the hospital where they were intended to deliver were given preferential treatment in comparison to those who had not.

> *"...They shouldn't dwell on where one has gone to the antenatal clinic; they get to attend to those who went to private hospitals first and leave those who have been going to the city council hospital. For example at [major maternity Hospital A], those that used to attend city council's clinic were attend to first while those who were attending private clinics were put aside and they could actually die from there..." (Woman, aged 20, FGD, delivered at a private hospital)*

As with both verbal and physical abuse, multiparous women were also discriminated against. That is, they experienced neglect because healthcare workers assumed that their multiple experiences giving birth gave them the ability to know what to do with their current birth. As has been noted by other scholars, women with a certain disease status (specifically HIV+) experienced discrimination. They reported in confidence that healthcare workers did not want to handle them or would embarrass them by loudly calling out their disease status in the presence of other women.

Poor rapport between women and healthcare workers

As can be imagined based on the narratives described thus far, for many women, rapport between them and their providers was a major challenge. The women described a lack of supportive care as well as inattentiveness and insensitivity regarding their experiences of pain. They stated that they felt that healthcare workers deliberately ignored their plight. When women attempted to call the doctors they were rebuked and left to deliver on their own.

> *"...I tried calling the doctor who said I had just arrived [and] it wasn't still time. ... I actually forgot, [and] so I took myself to the ward and climbed into bed. In the process my water broke; they then came started making noise at me asking why I had made the place dirty. When [the nurse] left, the child came out and she just heard the child crying; the child almost slid and fell because of that water. I delivered on my own; they came and assisted me with the cutting [of the cord] but I just delivered on my own..." (Woman, aged 28, FGD, delivered in a public maternity).*

The healthcare workers reported that the women always expected to receive high quality health care services, privacy, and personalized attention, such as counseling, despite the acute shortages of healthcare workers. Participating nurses reported that female patients seemed to expect better quality service from private facilities than public health facilities. Healthcare workers also described how an increasing number of women delivering their babies expected to receive all their services for free, including miscellaneous items such as free clothes. The reason behind this was the Kenyan Government's newly introduced policy of free maternity services at all public health facilities. Detailed instructions on implementation of this policy to healthcare workers were lacking and this lack resulted in great confusion and frustration for most healthcare workers. This underlying frustration led them to justify their many forms of mistreatment to the women.

> *"...Because it's free maternity they think they'll walk in and walk out with everything for the baby. So most of the times when they come, they come without children's clothes. So when they come, they find out it's only the service that is free, everything else they're supposed to bring for themselves. So this is usually the biggest problem most times ..." (IDI, Doctor in Major Maternity Hospital A).*

The healthcare workers we interviewed felt that the women did not understand how the health system worked and were therefore imposing their expectations for a high quality care. Despite the fact that this was a heavily constrained health system (which, as was stated earlier, was undergoing a strike) patients continued to demand good quality services and personalized care. The health workers in response to their female patients' expectations deliberately failed to build a rapport with them and would be rude towards them. The healthcare workers would mistreat them as a way of expressing discontent with the women's attitude towards the free delivery services.

Failure to meet professional standards

Women described feeling neglected and that their care was abandoned at critical moments during the delivery due to healthcare workers claiming that they had other competing demands. One woman in a focus group stated that:

> *"...I called the doctor when I began feeling the baby coming down, but the doctor refused to come and so I delivered on my own. And that is when the doctor was called by the other people. When the doctor came he cut the umbilical cord and before the doctor could attend to me there was another woman nearby also giving birth. The doctor left my child uncovered and unattended and went to the other woman and came back after she had delivered and took my child to the nursery..." (Woman, aged 23, FGD, delivered in a private health facility).*

What is interesting about this above description is that the doctor does, indeed, have other competing claims. While we hear the concern from the patient herself, who felt abandoned, we can also identify how the doctor was trying to attend to two patients at once, given the shortage of workers and time constraints. The women emphasized a dearth of supervision of deliveries because of the shortage of staff and the work demands of the busy maternity sections. They described women being left with trainee clinicians who were often inexperienced and would make mistakes. The women construed these mistakes as deliberate mistreatment, even though it could be argued that the doctors were trying to manage an almost impossible situation as best they could.

The women described that a few healthcare workers were clearly inebriated and were responsible for enacting physical violence on their patients, as described below.

> *"...At this point there were only two trainees in the ward, one doctor was drunk and was sleeping, when the trainee gets stranded with anything. He comes and when you try to argue with him he beats you up. When I was about to start pushing the baby, the trainee came and was unable to help me. When the doctor came he painfully pressed my stomach and I told him he was hurting me and he said that this was not his work ....His work was to deliver the baby and asked if I hadn't called for him; but I gave birth well..." (Woman, aged 27, FGD, delivered in Major Referral hospital).*

In the above narrative there are two healthcare workers, one drunk and unable to manage the work, and another who enacted what was likely the Kristeller maneuver (or fundal pressure), consisting of pushing down on the fundus to move the baby out. This procedure is considered to be a standard, but unnecessary and very aggressive, practice within obstetrics, with many medico-legal implications [21].

Women described other unnecessary procedures, such as episiotomies, or other procedures done repeatedly by students and different healthcare workers without their consent as illustrated below.

> *"...I have three kids my firstborn was born at [Maternity hospital A] but I used to go to [small clinic B] where I had high blood pressure so it forced me to attend clinic weekly. On my last weeks of pregnancy I was referred to [Maternity hospital A] where I was examined by students and the real doctors were nowhere to be found. It took me around two hours before I gave birth to a baby was weighing 2.5kg. It made me wonder why they did [an] episiotomy and they also took a lot of time to stitch me. The reasons I was given was that they were waiting for the higher ranked doctors who supervise them to guide them on what or how they should do it. After waiting for a long time they decided to stitch [me]. Unfortunately after 15 mintues, when the doctors came, it was redone. I felt a lot of pain..." (Woman, aged 30, FGD, delivered in Maternity hospital).*

Health systems conditions and constraints

The women mentioned that some of the mistreatment was as a direct result of poor quality of service exhibited by the overcrowding at public hospitals and acute shortages of healthcare workers. They suggested that the number of healthcare workers needed to be increased to improve the quality of care offered during delivery services. One participant stated,

> *"...They should add more nurses. The existing nurses are few in and the patients are many. That's why they were going from this side to that side and they are*

tired because they are also looking for a salary increment. If they have good salary they will handle people with care and if they attend to two people they don't get tired. They should employ more nurses to avoid one nurse attending to 10 patients and to improve their services..." (Woman, aged 22, IDI, delivered at public health facility).

Some women suggested that the lack of bed spaces available at the major hospitals for delivery services was due to the increased number of female patients accessing medical services. They added that the government could add the required space needed for the delivery beds. This deficiency in infrastructure generally led to women receiving poor quality services. For instance, women sometimes shared beds with other patients, gave birth on the floor, or were ignored and neglected by healthcare workers. Women defined these lacks as forms of mistreatment. Two women describe their experience below;

"...The women were seated outside on the bench when one delivers. That is when the other one then gets a bed. The room was small. They could add another room because I don't know if people are still giving birth as much. The doctors there wanted to assist but the beds were occupied. They would ask if people didn't want to go elsewhere even though the delivery process there was free. Therefore, women had to wait by the bench; when a woman would report that they were in pain, they would be told to go home and come back the following day; they were unable [to do that] and some would sit by the bench for days. The delivery beds were few..." (Woman, aged 28, IDI, delivered in Maternity Hospital B).

"...I don't know about [Major Maternity Hospital A]. I don't know what they could add because there were a lot of people during that time. Probably they could add a room as I think they added doctors at [Major Maternity Hospital B]. The room was small; the delivery room was small at that time; it had two beds on one side and two on the opposite side. There were 4 beds in total..." (Woman, aged 34, IDI, delivered in Maternity Hospital A).

Healthcare workers concurred with the women's descriptions of the health facilities. They similarly described the state of the public health facilities as deplorable, citing that the capacity of the health system was lacking. They claimed that the main government maternity hospitals serving women in peri-urban settings such as Dandora lacked basic physical facilities, such as sufficient number of delivery wards, beds, and waiting rooms. They described the facilities as few and lacking in quality to meet the needs of the women accessing services. They added that there were acute shortages of basic supplies, such as gloves and surgical equipment, as well as general utilities such as electrical power and water. These latter two were frequently unavailable, which not only inconvenienced the healthcare workers, but also compromised the quality of services they could offer. This situation thus resulted in poor patient outcomes. The quote by the medical officer illustrates the issue;

"...Sometimes you use ergometrine (medication used to cause contractions of the uterus to treat heavy vaginal bleeding after childbirth) and we don't have sterile gloves. Sometimes you want to remove a retained placenta, you don't have the gynecology gloves and you have to improvise. You cut up the other gloves and patch it up. Sometimes in the [operating] theatre you don't have suturing material... are you serious? It's something that is quite sad. Sometimes in the middle things can be running smoothly then all of a sudden there is no suture material, there is no water, just like that. There is no water, there is no electricity..." (IDI, Doctor in Major Public Maternity Hospital B).

Healthcare workers described the maternity and labor ward settings especially in the larger referral hospitals as chaotic scenes that were routinely understaffed. Midwives described situations where they were simultaneously helping patients in labor and triaging the ones ready for delivery. They went on to say that the female patients who were perceived to be difficult were often left on their own, an action which the patients later construed as abandonment. The midwives claimed that their working environment where there was a lack of assistance made them easily prone to stress. This situation led them to lose their tempers with 'difficult' women more frequently. Additionally, the healthcare workers expressed frustration at their workload, with one midwife vividly describing having to regularly attend to multiple women during critical phases of labor simultaneously, leading her to prioritize only the cases that seemed most urgent in her perspective.

"...So like I once took a patient to [Public Maternity B]... You see someone [attending to] almost 10 mothers... One mother is calling the other is also calling... In fact they even look as if they are confused. So (they try to hurry), they try to sew one while another patient in the second stage of labor is calling them and its only one nurse. So you find that this time factor makes the stress of work too much. The patient nurse ratio is, I don't know, it is very, very low. A whole room is just attended by one person. So you just

empathize [with their predicament]..." (IDI, Nurse-midwife currently at private facility).

Another main frustration with the health system was the ineffective referral systems in most health facilities that subsequently lead to the delays in care. Women constantly interpreted this phenomenon as mistreatment in the form lack of support and attention to their needs. The healthcare workers, especially those stationed at maternity hospitals, mentioned that they frequently received women who had been referred from far-off smaller facilities who were brought in after botched deliveries. The healthcare workers said that the patients often arrived with heavy bleeding, and they were expected to attend to them despite the obvious adverse clinical consequences of late referrals.

> *"...They always refer when it's too late... There are situations where they stay with a mother who has been bleeding for quite a while, so when they see they are not going to help the mother they bring [her] here to our facility... The number one cause for most of the mothers [losing] their lives is postpartum hemorrhage... despite making the necessary interventions on time..." (IDI, Medical officer in public maternity hospital B).*

Culture of blame

There was a prevailing culture of blame in these medical settings. Healthcare workers, particularly those at lower end of the hierarchy, strongly felt that they took the 'direct hit' for any adverse outcomes on the women or children. They also expressed fears at being blamed for outcomes that they largely thought were a result of non-compliance by the women. They said they were blamed by those higher up in the medical hierarchy (such as doctors). Additionally, they stated that blame was meted out at different levels and by different people. Sometimes it was doctors blaming midwives and sometimes it was the patient's family blaming both doctors and midwives. Workers mentioned that this fear of blame is what drove them towards harsh treatment.

> *"...You know generally as human beings, it's something natural that when someone is grieving, the first person you see is the one you want to blame. [...]. And as human beings we always blame the person, then ask questions later. These relatives don't want to know and most of them don't understand how the system works..." (IDI, Doctor at Major public Maternity B).*

> *"...Makes them less cooperative (laughs) and then complicates the delivery most of the time. Psychologically they get traumatized, you can see them withdrawn and if they have a problem they won't be free enough to ask you for help because they are not sure how you'd react to them..." (Medical officer in Public Maternity Hospital A).*

When asked why the women thought they were mistreated by healthcare workers, many didn't seem to know the answer to the question, adding that they pleaded with healthcare workers to be patient with them during labor. They expressed fear around resuming care seeking activities at facilities where they had been mistreated and considering other options for childbirth, including home births.

Occasionally, patients and their families reported the mistreatment to medical regulatory agencies or sued healthcare workers in cases that resulted in maternal mortality. Despite this, many women expressed frustrations that there were no formal avenues set up in public and private sectors to discuss mistreatment or redress poor quality services. They added there were no feedback mechanisms at the hospitals to lodge complaints about poor quality services. Many said they were afraid of the consequences and future retaliation that they would face from the healthcare workers during subsequent visits to the health facilities if they ever took action. These fears were compounded by the distinct power and class dynamics inherent in the patient-caregiver relationship.

Additional findings

The primary focus of this article has been to understand the ways that mistreatment in Kenyan hospitals occurs. It is important to add that there were also a few female participants who experienced positive birth experiences. They mentioned that the nurses who assisted them during the delivery process were extremely helpful. They described being accompanied throughout the entire delivery process. Several women referred to one mission hospital that consistently had high quality care. At this particular hospital, the women described the doctors and nurses as "being with you all the way" and provided detailed examples of what their positive experiences were. One woman described the experience as "relaxing" and confirmed that she gave birth to all her children at this particular hospital. She said,

> *"...I had to now go to [Mission Hospital A] every other week. They kept examining me to know what the problem was. Everything was relaxing; the doctors are with you all the way; if you begin having pains they ask you what you would want; if you turn this way they apologize; they rub your back. When the baby begins to come out, they come and assist you and if you have to be stitched they do it there. They wash the baby and you also get to shower; they treat people*

well. I gave birth to all my children there..." (Woman, aged 25, FGD, delivered at Mission Hospital A).

Discussion

This qualitative study explored female patients' and healthcare workers' perceptions and experiences of mistreatment during labor/delivery. As other studies on mistreatment during childbirth have noted [7, 17, 23], our data shows that not only was abuse prevalent, it tended to match maternal abuse found elsewhere. Participants mentioned that the most frequent was a failure to meet professional standards, followed by verbal abuse, physical abuse, health systems constraints, and a poor rapport between healthcare workers and women; the least frequent were stigma and discrimination.

In our study lack of professional standards during delivery was identified as a major problem. We discovered that younger women, multiparous women and women who failed to attend ANC were most frequently mistreated. This pattern has been identified in similar studies assessing prevalence of disrespect and abuse that found that women under the age of 19 were more likely to be mistreated by healthcare workers (Second Author 2013; [1]). The healthcare workers participated and reinforced the culture of blame, by not only blaming the women for getting pregnant, but by also increasing the level and form of abuse (through reducing their privacy or shouting at them for their lack of knowledge of their bodies).

Verbal abuse was very prevalent in this setting; indeed, contempt and use of derogatory terms was commonplace. Verbal abuse and comments about a woman's sexuality was mentioned by almost every female participant interviewed. The most popular rebuke mentioned was the scolding about how the women had enjoyed sexual intercourse but were now expressing pain during birth; this abuse has been identified in several different contexts, especially amongst women of lower socioeconomic status ([7, 16, 26, 39]; Second Author 2013) It is likely that, because the women in this study were from a lower socioeconomic status, the healthcare workers abused their position of power. This form of abuse was intertwined with discriminatory practices based on age, parity, socioeconomic status, antenatal care attendance, and ethnicity [31]. Our female participants felt that because of their income status, healthcare workers who were from higher socioeconomic status would mistreat them and offer them little or no guidance or explanations when providing care. This abuse arose either because of healthcare provider frustrations with their patients and the system, or was a deliberate way to exert power on populations that would not fight back. There were a few incidences of women resisting but most of them said they were afraid of being denied future services and would instead just take the verbal abuse.

As with other studies across the world, physical abuse was prevalent. What was surprising, however, was how much the women did not question the physical abuse. Several women seemed to be accepting of some forms of physical abuse, such as the slaps and pinches, stating that they were for the sake of their health and their babies during pushing. Such forms of abuse have been observed in studies within the African context [12, 22, 25]. Social norms and attitudes around such violence allow the normalization of these forms of physical abuse in this context. As Bohren [5] state in their work in Nigeria, the abuse is seen as a way of 'rescuing' the lives of mother/infant. The nurses in our study, at the end of a delivery, would often convince the patients that without the beatings their children would have been harmed and had adverse outcomes. Conversely to the concerns expressed by the women, the healthcare workers prided themselves on having been taught to be "firm" with their patients. We argue that it is thus important to understand and investigate the social norms of acceptability of mistreatment not only to understand how and why they occur, but also to examine them as facets arising within a gender-based violence frame [38].

Health systems constraints were mentioned by almost all the healthcare workers citing the mistreatment as unintentional and largely due to staff shortages and lack of resources. Such health constraints (including a lack of resources and facility culture) in Kenya have been identified as drivers for mistreatment [34]. Some women seemed to understand these health system constraints, and thus perceived the mistreatment as unintentional, while others claimed that the mistreatment was deliberate and intentional. However studies by Freedman and Kruk argue that despite disrespect and abuse being perceived differently by women and healthcare workers in the context of health system constraints, there are certain practices that are "unambiguously disrespectful" ([15]:e42). These practices should be identified in each context, while the social norms surrounding their acceptability needs to be challenged. We would argue that behavioral anomalies amongst healthcare workers that drive cultures of mistreatment within health institutions need to be not only addressed, but also challenged.

The poor rapport between women and healthcare workers primarily manifested as abandonment and neglect during labor and delivery. The women described several instances where the neglect led to fatal consequences. This practice has been witnessed in settings where nurse-midwives want to create social distance between themselves and the people they are serving. This situation was described by Jewkes et al. [16] in their study of nurses in a South African context. In this study there were several instances where healthcare workers, particularly nurse midwives, wanted to exert control over their patients and the childbirth process, which led to patients feeling mistreated. Avenues for redress for this situation need to be particularly created with women have access to accountability mechanisms especially to professional associations whose role is to regulate their membership.

The drivers of mistreatment in our study seemed to stem from a general perception of the women that healthcare workers and the institutions they work in fail to provide professional care. According to a framework put forward by Freedman and Kruk [15] mistreatment can manifest itself and be driven at the individual, structural, and policy level. In our study all three levels interacted to promote mistreatment. At the individual level between the healthcare workers and the women evidence pointed to a need for healthcare workers to promote abusive behavior as a way of asserting control of the women ((see, for instance, [9, 16]).. At the structural level, institutions such as health facilities, either promoted cultures that condoned mistreatment or were largely unaware of it and its manifestations. Lack of supervision of medical staff and shortages of medical staff increased this unintentional mistreatment. Other institutions such as medical schools were also implicated in this situation, as they were the places where healthcare workers learned how to interact with patients. Professional bodies governing the conduct of healthcare workers were also largely uninvolved in the regulation of their members in the mistreatment. At the policy level the new free maternity policy was a factor increasing the mistreatment due to the elevated expectations for quality maternity care simply because of its free status. Interventions that increase the understanding of the entitlements, such as deploying community health volunteers at the health facilities to inform women of the coverage package under the free maternity services, can help assist women to reduce the friction between themselves and healthcare workers regarding expectations and greatly reduce mistreatment driven by mismatched expectations.

Limitations of the study

One main limitation of the study is the self-reporting of abuse. This method makes it difficult to detect underreporting or exaggeration, especially around a sensitive and highly subjective topic like mistreatment [29]. Additionally, because of the sensitivity of the topic, access to health facilities for observations is limited (see [30]). An important limitation was the location for the interviews (within the compound of the church within range of the health facility), which might have prevented participating women from speaking openly. Finally, the focus on only the negative experiences might be an additional limitation, as only in conversations did positive experiences of delivery emerge ((see also [34]).

Recommendations on interventions for reducing mistreatment

We want to end this article with a discussion of some of the recommendations for reducing mistreatment. Female participants suggested that healthcare workers needed to show more compassion and patience to women in labor. They emphasized the need for a system to provide feedback on poor quality of care at public facilities. Professional societies that govern healthcare workers such as the Nursing Councils and the Kenya Medical Practitioners and Dentists Boards need to be consulted about health facilities whereby reports have been lodged regarding mistreatment of women, these institutions should strengthen accountability mechanisms and support processes for legal redress. Additionally these professional associations should seek to re-train their healthcare workers especially cadres such as nurse midwives who were predominantly involved the management of labor and childbirth. This training should include elements that address soft skills such as interpersonal relationships such as treating patients with dignity and avoidance of discrimination based on background. Previous studies in Kenya such as [34] described strategies for healthcare workers such as value clarification and attitude transformation workshops as well as stress management [34].

There is a need for greater support from the County Government that manages the public maternity hospitals in peri-urban settings where a lot of the mistreatment was described as happening. The County Government needs to provide adequate resources in terms of adequate numbers of supervised staff and supplies as well as strengthen education on the package of interventions available for free maternity service. The need The County Government needs to have a feedback mechanism for redress for complaints of mistreatment. The need for greater support is in line with guidelines that have been provided by WHO [37]. This statement also calls for Governments to be involved particularly in research as well as implementation of interventions to improve disrespect and abuse in maternity settings. The healthcare workers suggest that the county government needed to investment in health education for women particularly during antenatal care on what to expect particularly for the young first time mothers and identification of victims of sexual abuse and provision of counselling services for them.

Implementation of the relatively new government policy on maternal health services needs to be improved with supplementary health education to the women on what the included minimum package of interventions that is covered including excluded services. The implementation of the policy needs to be clarified at all levels of the health system and women need to be educated by trained community health volunteers so as to curb the unrealistic expectations described particularly by low educational status women in peri-urban settings such as the ones in this study. This will in turn help reduce common forms of mistreatment verbal abuse that results from the misunderstanding about entitlements of the policy.

Conclusion

This study has shown that mistreatment of women during facility based delivery is rife in peri-urban settings as appreciated by the vivid descriptive accounts by both women and healthcare workers. This mistreatment is largely driven by an unbalanced relationship between healthcare workers and the women they serve due to socioeconomic status and institutional norms that normalize mistreatment. Despite the fact that there is free delivery service as a policy oversight for its implementation needs to be strengthened to clarify expectations through providing adequate information to women accessing delivery services on the coverage of services as well as exclusions to reduce misunderstandings. Medical Professional associations need to be involved in addressing the mistreatment issue amongst their members through research and creating accountability procedures. County Governments need to address mistreatment through providing resources for a functioning health system that can provide an enabling environment for the provision of high quality maternal health services and ensuring women give birth in a dignified manner.

Acknowledgements

This research was funded by the Kellogg Institute of International Studies, Keough School of Global Affairs. The authors would like to thank the women of Dandora community who participated in this study by providing information on their mistreatment experiences as well as the healthcare workers at the different health facilities we visited in Nairobi, without you this study would not have been possible. We would also like to thank Bro Andre Medical Centre staff and the Parish priest of Dandora Holy Cross Parish Fr Alex Okidi (CSC) for allowing us to interview women within your premises and healthcare workers stationed at your health facility. Great thanks to Dr. Anne Ndungu, Sandra Masira and Christine Achieng who all facilitated the contacts and participated in data collection within Dandora. The researchers would also like to thank Fr. Bob Dowd (CSC) Director of the Ford Family Program in Human Development Studies and Solidarity who graciously provided the time and opportunity to engage in this important study.

Funding

The funding for the research was provided by the Kellogg Institute of International Affairs through a Faculty grant. The funding body had no role in influencing design of the study and collection, analysis, and interpretation of data as well as in writing the manuscript.

Individual data

The manuscript submitted does not contain any individual data for any of the respondents interviewed. To enhance confidentiality any names provided in transcripts were redacted for the protection of the individual identities.

Authors' contributions

JOA, VSO, and RD conceptualized and designed the study and its data collection tools. EM supported the design of the data collection tools. JOA and EM administered and transcribed the interviews with healthcare workers, and supervised the data collection. EM supervised the transcription of the FGDs. All authors participated in the data analysis. JOA wrote the first draft of the manuscript, with revisions provided by the other authors. VSO and JOA worked on the revisions and resubmission for the journal. All authors read and approved the final manuscript.

Consent for publication

Not applicable.

Competing interests

The authors declare that they have no competing interests.

Author details

[1]Regional Research Programs Manager, The Ford Program in Human Development Studies and Solidarity, University of Notre Dame, Regional Office, East Africa, P.O. Box 49675-00100, Nairobi, Kenya. [2]Department of Anthropology, University of Notre Dame, 248 Corbett Family Hall, Notre Dame, IN 46556, USA. [3]Eck Institute for Global Health, University of Notre Dame, 120 Brownson Hall, Notre Dame, IN 46556, USA. [4]The Ford Program in Human Development Studies and Solidarity, Kellogg Institute of International Affairs, University of Notre Dame, 2167 Nanovic-Jenkins Hall, Notre Dame, IN 46556, USA.

References

1. Abuya T, Warren CE, Miller N, Njuki R, Ndwiga C, Maranga A, Mbehero F, Njeru A, Bellows B. Exploring the prevalence of disrespect and abuse during childbirth in Kenya. PLoS One. 2015;10(4):e0123606. https://doi.org/10.1371/journal.pone.0123606.
2. Alkema L, Chou D, Hogan D, Zhang S, Moller AB, Gemmill A, Fat DM, Boerma T, Temmerman M, Mathers C, Say L. Global, regional, and national levels and trends in maternal mortality between 1990 and 2015, with scenario-based projections to 2030: a systematic analysis by the UN maternal mortality estimation inter-agency group. Lancet. 2016;387(10017):462–74. https://doi.org/10.1016/S0140-6736(15)00838-7.
3. Balde MD, Diallo BA, Bangoura A, Sall O, Soumah AM, Vogel JP, Bohren MA. Perceptions and experiences of the mistreatment of women during childbirth in health facilities in Guinea: a qualitative study with women and service providers. Reprod Health. 2017;14(1):3. https://doi.org/10.1186/s12978-016-0266-1
4. Balde MD, Bangoura A, Sall O, Balde H, Niakate AS, Vogel JP, Bohren MA. A qualitative study of women's and health providers' attitudes and acceptability of mistreatment during childbirth in health facilities in Guinea. Reprod Health. 2017;14(1):4. https://doi.org/10.1186/s12978-016-0262-5.
5. Bohren MA, Vogel JP, Tunçalp Ö, Fawole B, Titiloye MA, Olutayo AO, . . . Hindin MJ. By slapping their laps, the patient will know that you truly care for her: A qualitative study on social norms and acceptability of the mistreatment of women during childbirth in Abuja, Nigeria. SSM - population health. 2016;2:640–55. https://doi.org/10.1016/j.ssmph.2016.07.003
6. Bohren MA, Hunter EC, Munthe-Kaas HM, Souza JP, Vogel JP, Gulmezoglu AM. Facilitators and barriers to facility-based delivery in low- and middle-income countries: a qualitative evidence synthesis. Reprod Health. 2014;11(1):71. https://doi.org/10.1186/1742-4755-11-71.
7. Bohren MA, Vogel JP, Hunter EC, Lutsiv O, Makh SK, Souza JP. The mistreatment of women during childbirth in health facilities globally: a mixed-methods systematic review. PLoS Med. 2015;12. https://doi.org/10.1371/journal.pmed.1001847

8. Bohren MA, Vogel JP, Tunçalp Ö, Fawole B, Titiloye MA, Olutayo AO, Ogunlade M, Oyeniran AA, Osunsan OR, Metiboba L, Idris HA. Mistreatment of women during childbirth in Abuja, Nigeria: a qualitative study on perceptions and experiences of women and healthcare providers. Reprod Health. 2017;14(1):9. https://doi.org/10.1186/s12978-016-0265-2.
9. Bradley S, McCourt C, Rayment J, Parmar D. Disrespectful intrapartum care during facility-based delivery in sub-Saharan Africa: a qualitative systematic review and thematic synthesis of women's perceptions and experiences. Soc Sci Med. 2016;169:157–70. https://doi.org/10.1016/j.socscimed.2016.09.039.
10. Braun V, Clarke V. Using thematic analysis in psychology. Qual Res Psychol. 2006;3(2):77–101. https://doi.org/10.1191/1478088706qp063oa.
11. Clark J. Defining the concept of dignity and developing a model to promote its use in practice. Nurs Times. 2010;106(20):16–9.
12. D'Ambruoso L, Abbey M, Hussein J. Please understand when I cry out in pain: women's accounts of maternity services during labour and delivery in Ghana. BMC Public Health. 2005;5:140. https://doi.org/10.1186/1471-2458-5-140
13. Diamond-Smith N, Sudhinaraset M, Melo J, Murthy N. The relationship between women's experiences of mistreatment at facilities during childbirth, types of support received and person providing the support in Lucknow. India Midwifery. 2016;40. https://doi.org/10.1016/j.midw.2016.06.014
14. Fotso JC, Mukiira C. Perceived quality of and access to care among poor urban women in Kenya and their utilization of delivery care: harnessing the potential of private clinics? Health Policy Plan. 2012;27(6):505–15. https://doi.org/10.1093/heapol/czr074.
15. Freedman LP, Kruk ME. Disrespect and abuse of women in childbirth: challenging the global quality and accountability agendas. Lancet. 2014;384. https://doi.org/10.1016/s0140-6736(14)60859-x
16. Jewkes R, Abrahams N, Mvo Z. Why do nurses abuse patients? Reflections from South African Obstetric Services. Soc Sci Med. 1999;47:1781–95.
17. Jewkes R, Penn-Kekana L. Mistreatment of women in childbirth: time for action on this important dimension of violence against women. PLoS Med. 2015;12(6):e1001849.
18. Kenya National Bureau of Statistics, Ministry of Health/Kenya, National AIDS Control Council/Kenya, Kenya Medical Research Institute, Population, N. C. f., & Development/Kenya. (2015). Kenya Demographic and Health Survey 2014. Retrieved from Rockville, MD, USA: http://dhsprogram.com/pubs/pdf/FR308/FR308.pdf
19. Kuruvilla S, Schweitzer J, Bishai D, Chowdhury S, Caramani D, Frost L, Cortez R, Daelmans B, Francisco AD, Adam T, Cohen R. Success factors for reducing maternal and child mortality. Bull World Health Organ. 2014;92(7):533–544b. https://doi.org/10.2471/blt.14.138131.
20. MacCormack C. In: Sargent CF, Brettell CB, editors. Risk, prevention, and international health policy. Gender and Health: An International Perspective; 1996. p. 326–37.
21. Malvasi A, Zaami S, Tinelli A, Trojano G, Montanari Vergallo G, Marinelli E. Kristeller maneuvers or fundal pressure and maternal/neonatal morbidity: obstetric and judicial literature review. J Matern Fetal Neonatal Med. 2018; 1–10. https://doi.org/10.1080/14767058.2018.1441278
22. McMahon SA, George AS, Chebet JJ, Mosha IH, Mpembeni RN, Winch PJ. Experiences of and responses to disrespectful maternity care and abuse during childbirth; a qualitative study with women and men in Morogoro Region, Tanzania. BMC Pregnancy Childbirth. 2014;14:268. https://doi.org/10.1186/1471-2393-14-268
23. Miller S, Abalos E, Chamillard M, Ciapponi A, Colaci D, Comandé D, Diaz V, Geller S, Hanson C, Langer A, Manuelli V. Beyond too little, too late and too much, too soon: a pathway towards evidence-based, respectful maternity care worldwide. Lancet. 2016;388(10056):2176–92.
24. Moyer CA, Rominski S, Nakua EK, Dzomeku VM, Agyei-Baffour P, Lori JR. Exposure to disrespectful patient care during training: Data from midwifery students at 15 midwifery schools in Ghana. Midwifery. 2016;41:39–44. https://doi.org/10.1016/j.midw.2016.07.009
25. Moyer CA, Adongo PB, Aborigo RA, Hodgson A, Engmann CM, Devries R. "It's up to the woman's people": how social factors influence facility-based delivery in rural northern Ghana. Matern Child Health J. 2014;18(1):109–19. https://doi.org/10.1007/s10995-013-1240-y.
26. Okafor II, Ugwu EO, Obi SN. Disrespect and abuse during facility-based childbirth in a low-income country. Int J Gynaecol Obstet. 2015;128(2):110–3. https://doi.org/10.1016/j.ijgo.2014.08.015.
27. Okwako JM, Symon AG. Women's expectations and experiences of childbirth in a Kenyan public hospital. Afr J Midwifery Womens Health. 2014;8(3):115–21. https://doi.org/10.12968/ajmw.2014.8.3.115.
28. NVivo qualitative data analysis Software; QSR International Pty Ltd. Version 10, 2012. http://www.qsrinternational.com/nvivo/support-overview/faqs/how-do-i-cite-nvivo-for-mac,-nvivo-11-for-windows
29. Savage V, Castro A. Measuring mistreatment of women during childbirth: a review of terminology and methodological approaches. Reprod Health. 2017;14(1):138.
30. Sen G, Reddy B, Iyer A. Beyond measurement: the drivers of disrespect and abuse in obstetric care. Reprod Health Matters. 2018;1–13. https://doi.org/10.1080/09688080.2018.1508173
31. Spangler, S. (2011). "To Open Oneself Is a Poor Woman's Trouble": Embodied Inequality and Childbirth in South-Central Tanzania (Vol. 25).
32. Tunçalp Ö, Were WM, MacLennan C, Oladapo OT, Gülmezoglu AM, Bahl R, Daelmans B, Mathai M, Say L, Kristensen F, Temmerman M. Quality of care for pregnant women and newborns—the WHO vision. BJOG Int J Obstet Gynaecol. 2015;122(8):1045–9.
33. van den Akker T, Nair M, Goedhart M, Schutte J, Schaap T, Knight M. Maternal mortality: direct or indirect has become irrelevant. Lancet Glob Health. 2017;5(12):e1181–2.
34. Warren CE, Njue R, Ndwiga C, Abuya T. Manifestations and drivers of mistreatment of women during childbirth in Kenya: implications for measurement and developing interventions. BMC Pregnancy Childbirth. 2017;17(1):102. https://doi.org/10.1186/s12884-017-1288-6.
35. WHO. Making pregnancy safer the critical role of the skilled attendant. 2004. http://www.who.int/maternal_child_adolescent/documents/9241591692/en/
36. WHO. The WHO Application of ICD-10 to deaths during pregnancy, childbirth and the puerperium: ICD-MM. 2012. http://apps.who.int/iris/bitstream/handle/10665/70929/9789241548458_eng.pdf
37. WHO. (2014). The prevention and elimination of disrespect and abuse during facility-based birth [Press release].
38. Williams CR, Jerez C, Klein K, Correa M, Belizan JM, Cormick G. Obstetric violence: a Latin American legal response to mistreatment during childbirth. BJOG. 2018;125(10):1208–11. https://doi.org/10.1111/1471-0528.15270
39. Zacher Dixon L. Obstetrics in a time of violence: Mexican midwives critique routine hospital practices. Med Anthropol Q. 2015;29(4):437–54.
40. Ziraba AK, Madise N, Mills S, Kyobutungi C, Ezeh A. Maternal mortality in the informal settlements of Nairobi city: what do we know? Reprod Health. 2009;6:6. https://doi.org/10.1186/1742-4755-6-6.

15

Early initiations of first antenatal care visit and associated factor among mothers who gave birth in the last six months preceding birth in Bahir Dar Zuria Woreda North West Ethiopia

Yibeltal Alemu* and Amanu Aragaw

Abstract

Background: Timing of Antenatal care booking is one of the basic components of antenatal care services; that helps to early detection, managing, and prevention of problems during the pregnancy and helps the mother to receive full packages of antenatal care services. However, in the world including Ethiopia, significant numbers of pregnant mothers were not booking the follow up on the recommended time. The main aim of this study was to assess the prevalence and factors that associated with the early timing of antenatal care visit in Bahir Dar Zuria District, North West Ethiopia.

Methods: A community-based cross-sectional study was conducted. A total of 410 mothers have participated. Data were collected through the interview from March 1 to 30/2018 using a structured and pre-tested questionnaire. Data were clear, code, and enter into Epi-info version 7.1 and export to SPSS for farther analysis. Both bivariate and multivariate analyses were used. On bivariate analysis *p*-value, less than 0.2 were used to select the candidate variable for multivariate analysis. *P*-value and confidence interval were used to measure the level of significance on multivariate analysis and those variables whose *P*-value < 0.05 were considered as statically significant.

Results: The prevalence of early timing of ANC in the study area was 46.8%; with [95% CI 40.5, 51.8]. Distances [AOR 2.47, 95% CI; 1.4, 4.2], Knowledge on the timing of ANC [AOR 2.1; 95% CI; 1.2, 3.7], No under-five children [AOR 2.7; 95% CI; 1.3, 5.8], having one under-five children [AOR 2.2; 95% CI; 1.1, 4.5], and wanted pregnancy [AOR 2.4, 95% CI, 1.3, 4.7] were affects the early timing of ANC.

Conclusions: The prevalence of early timing of ANC was high when compared to the national figure and the Sub-Saharan country. Accessibility of health services, knowledge on the timing of ANC, under-five children, and desire for pregnancy were factors that affect the early timing of ANC.

Keywords: ANC, Maternal health, Pregnancy, Utilization, Ethiopia

* Correspondence: yibeltalalemu6@gmail.com
Department of Reproductive Health, College of Medicine and Health Science, Bahir Dar University, P.O.Box 79, Bahir Dar, Ethiopia

Plain English summary

Antenatal care is the care which provided for the mother during pregnancy to improve the health of the mother and unborn baby. World health organization is recommended for booking the services before the first trimester or 12 weeks of gestation. However, according to our country Ethiopia ministry health, it's acceptable until 16 weeks of gestation. This study was trying to answer the level and associated factors through structured interview questionnaires.

The participants were asked their socio-demographic characteristics, reproductive characteristics, about antenatal care service utilization, and the challenges they face during antenatal care service utilization.

Of 400 participants 187 of the participants were initiated the follow-up before 16 weeks of gestation. This study reveals that the average month mothers were starting antenatal care visit at 16 weeks and 5 days. Short distances from the facilities, knowledge on the timing of ANC, not having under-five children, having one under-five child, and wanted or planned pregnancy was the main factor that affects the early timing of antenatal care visit.

In conclusion, the prevalence of early timing of ANC visit in the study area was high in comparison to the national figure. Factors that responsible for early initiation of ANC services were the accessibility of the services, knowledge about the timing of ANC, a desire of pregnancy, and under-five children. Policy action will be required to farther improve the timely booking of ANC.

Background

Pregnancy is one of the most important periods in the life of a woman, a family, and a society [1]. While, because of these physiological changes that occur during pregnancy, mother and her baby were facing life treating problems. To avert the problem, there are different maternal health care services were provided for minimizing the problem. One of the services is Antenatal care (ANC) [2]. The aim of ANC service is to prevent health problems that affect both the fetus and mother and to ensure that each newborn child has a good start [3].

Nevertheless, true progress has been made globally in terms of increasing access and use, there are high numbers of maternal deaths and stillbirths were occurred [4]. Globally around 2.6 million stillbirths annually and 830 maternal deaths every day occur due to the pregnancy-related cause. Among all deaths, 99% occurred in the developing countries as compared as 1% in developed countries [5]. Many maternal and prenatal deaths occur in women who have not received timely, inadequate and no utilization of ANC [6]. Early antenatal care attendance during the first three months of gestation plays a major role in detecting and treating complications that occur during pregnancy [2].

The timing of Antenatal care booking is one of the basic components of ANC services. It helps to early detection, managing, and prevent problems that occur during the pregnancy time. According to WHO Focus antenatal care model recommendation, all pregnant mothers are better to start ANC booking within the first trimester of pregnancy (within 12 weeks) [3]. In addition, now a time World Health Organization adopt a new ANC model that recommend to increase the numbers of contact from four visits to eight contacts for the aim of reducing prenatal mortality and to improve women experiences of care [3, 7]. Actually, this new Antenatal care model still is not practicable in Ethiopia. However, according to the Federal Democratic Republic of Ethiopia Ministry of Health recommendation, the timing of ANC booking is acceptable until 16 weeks of gestation [8].

Existing evidence in the global shows that the prevalence of early timing of antenatal care visits were around 43%. According to the report, there is a high discrepancy between developed and developing regions [9]. The report showed that 85% of mothers in the developed region start their ANC follow up earlier but it was below 45% and less than 25% in the developing countries and sub-Sahara region respectively [10]. According to different demographic health survey report in sub-Sahara countries shows that the prevalence of early timing of ANC visit ranges from 17.6 to 20% [8, 11, 12].

According to Ethiopian demographic health survey, 2016 report indicates that 20% of pregnant mothers started their Antenatal care visit at the first trimester of pregnancy from that 44% of the mothers live in the urban, start ANC visit at the first trimester of pregnancy compared to 17% in the rural community [8]. Different literature conducted in Ethiopia also shows that the prevalence of early timing of ANC visit ranges from 17 to 41% [13–15].

Studies conducted in developing countries showed that residence, educational status of the mother, husband occupation, parity and planned or wanted pregnancy was factors for late ANC booking [16, 17]. Studies conducted in the urban Ethiopia shows that age of the mother, educational status of the mother, previous history of ANC, perceive adequacy of ANC, low monthly income, receiving advice on when to start ANC visits, household food insecurity, parity, urine test as a means of pregnancy recognition, and unplanned pregnancy was a determinant of the early timing of ANC visits [13, 14, 18–22].

Studies conducted in rural Ethiopia showed that age of the mother, parity, planned pregnancy, media access, knowledge about the time of ANC booking, and advised to book within 12 weeks was affected the timing of antenatal care visit [23, 24]. There are limited finding on the prevalence and factors associated with the early timing of ANC booking in the study area as well as in the country. For this situation, a cross-sectional study is important to address the gap. Therefore assessing the prevalence and factors that associated with early timings of antenatal care visit are important for setting intervention that helps to improve the utilization of ANC services.

Methods and materials

Study area

The study was conducted at Bahir Dar Zuria District; it is founded around Bahir Dar city administration 564 km far from the capital Addis. The District consists of 9 rural clusters. The total population of the District was estimated 220,410 from those, around 48.6% were female. Two thousand five hundred ninety-nine mothers in the district gave birth from August first to January last 2018; of that 86.4%, mothers have a history of ANC. In the District, there are 9 health centers, and 224 health professionals and 32 health extension workers were enrolled [25].

Study design and period

A Community-based cross-sectional study was conducted from March 1 to 30, 2018.

Source populations

All mothers who have a history of ANC and gave birth in the last six months in Bahir Dar Zuria district.

Study population

Those selected mothers who have a history of ANC and gave birth in the study in the last six months during data collection period in Bahir Dar Zuria district.

Inclusion criteria

All mothers who have a history of ANC and gave live birth.

Exclusion criteria

Women excluded from the study were those who are not hearing and seriously ill during the data collection period.

Sample size determination

The sample size for the study was calculated using a single population proportion formula with the following assumptions. Based on findings from a previous study conducted in the central zone of Tigray (Ethiopia) [26]. The proportion of women who start ANC before the fourth month was found to be 41% By assuming a margin of error of 5%, $Z_{\alpha/2}$ = value for 95% CI (1.96), proportion = 41%, and the non-response rate of 10%, a sample size of 410 women obtained.

Sampling procedures and technique

All 9 clusters in the study area were included. The health extension workers immunization registration book was used to easily identify mothers who gave birth for the last six months in the District and whether they have a history of ANC from August 1 to January 30, 2018, G.C. Subsequently, the lists of the entire mother who have history ANC were found from the health extension worker registration books. Then the simple random sampling technique was used to select the study participants from those who have a history of ANC.

Data collection tools and procedures

Data were collected using a structured questionnaire which adopted and modified from Ethiopian DHS and other previous studies. The questionnaire was prepared in English and it translated into Amharic then translated back to English to check for consistency.

Data were collected via interview. Seven diploma holder nurses were recruited for data collection, 3 supervisor degree holder nurses were assigned for supervisory activities along with the principal investigator.

Data quality controls

The prepare questionnaire and tools were translated into Amharic and then translated back to English for consistency. The Amharic version of the questionnaire was pre-test among 41(10%) of the sample population in the Cluster not include in the study. Training was provided for the data collectors and supervisors on the objectives, relevance of the study, how to keep the confidentiality of the information and techniques of interviews for two consecutive days. The supervisors have supervised the data collection process every day and the principal investigator also cheeks the collected questionnaire for completeness every other day.

Data processing and analysis

Data were cleaned, code and entered into Epi-info version 7.1 then exported to SPSS version 23 for analysis. Descriptive analysis was carried out to see the distribution of independent variables. Binary logistic regression was used to examine associations between the dependent variable and each independent variable. Based on the bivariate analysis those factors whose crude associations to the timing of antenatal care booking at $p < 0.2$ was entered into the multivariate analysis to get adjusted odds ratio.

The strength of association was determined by using a crude odds ratio in the bivariate analysis and adjusted odds ratio in multivariate analysis. *P*-values and 95% confidence interval was used to determine the level of significance of the association. $P < 0.05$ considered as statistically significant. Hosmer and Lemeshow Test were used for checking the model fitness of logistic regressions.

Results

Out of 410 mothers who have a history of Antenatal care follow up in Bahir Dar Zuria District, 400 complete the interview administer questionnaires. Therefore the data analysis was made based on 400 respondents that have been completed the interview. The response rate was 97.56%.

Socio-cultural characteristics

Among the total participants, one hundred twenty-eight (32%) of the respondents were in the age group of 25-29 years. The mean ages of the respondents were 28.47 (SD ± 5.47). Three hundred ninety-four (98.5%) of the respondents were followers of Orthodox religion the rest were Muslim. Three hundred ninety-eight (99.5%) of the respondents were Amhara ethnicity. Three hundred-ninety (97.6%) of the respondents were married. Fifty (12.5%) of the respondents were attended formal education.

Eighty-four (21%) and 85 (21.5%) of the household were rich and richest wealth index respectively. Two hundred sixty-two (65.5%) of the respondents were poor household decision making power. One hundred fourteen (28.5%) of the respondent traveling more than one hour to reach the ANC services. The median time travel to reach the ANC services was 60 min. Three hundred sixty-seven (91.8%) of the respondents were traveling on foot. (Table 1).

Reproductive history

Three hundred twenty-two (80.2%) of the respondent were knowledgeable about the timing of antenatal care. Two hundred-thirteen (53.3%) of the respondents were multi-gravid. Two hundred twenty-five (56.3%) of the respondents were multi-Para. Fifty-six (14%) of the participants has had an unwanted pregnancy. (Table 2.

Prevalence of early timing of antenatal care booking

Among the participants one hundred eight-seven (46.7%) with 95% CI [40.5, 51.8] of the respondents, were booking there first ANC visit before four months of pregnancy. The average months of starting the follow up were 16 weeks and 5 days. One hundred fifty-seven (39.3%) of the respondents were started the follow up at four to five months. (Fig. 1).

Table 1 The socio- cultural characteristics of the mother in Bahir Dar Zuria district North West Ethiopia 2018($n = 400$)

Variables	Frequency	Percent (%)
Age		
< 20 years	9	2.3
20–24 years	89	22.2
25–29 years	128	32
30–34 years	113	28.3
≥35 years	61	15.2
Educational status of the mother		
Not attained formal education	350	87.5
Primary level (Grade 1to 8)	41	10.3
Secondary (Grade 9 to 12)	9	2.2
Marital status		
Single	6	1.5
Married	390	97.6
Divorced	3	0.8
Widowed	1	0.3
Occupation of the mother		
Farmer	384	96
Trader	12	3
Student	3	0.75
Governmental employer	1	0.25
Wealth index		
Poorest	67	16.75
Poor	74	18.5
Middle	90	22.5
Rich	84	21
Richest	85	21.25
Accompanion during ANC visit		
Yes	267	66.8
No	133	33.3
Family size		
1–3	89	22.2
4–5	142	35.5
Above 5	169	42.3
Numbers of under five children		
No under five	108	27
One under five	234	58.5
Two under five	58	14.5
Distance		
Less than 30 min	146	36.5
30 min to one hour	140	35
More than one hour	114	28.5

Table 2 reproductive characteristics of the mother in Bahir Dar Zuria district North West Ethiopia 2018(n = 400)

Variable	Frequency	Percent
Numbers of pregnancy		
One	80	20
2 to 5	213	53.2
≥ 5	107	26.8
Parity		
Primipara	91	22.7
Multi-para	225	56.3
Grand multi-para	84	21
Knowledge of the mother on the timing of ANC		
Knowledgeable	322	80.5
Not knowledgeable	88	19.5

Factors that associated with early initiations first antenatal care visit

In the bivariate analysis, family size, decision-making power, distance, wealth index, knowledge, under five, age, accompanying person, urine test, a desire of pregnancy were candidate variable for multivariate analysis. And on multivariate analysis, distances, knowledge, under-five children, and desire for pregnancy were true determinants of early time antenatal care visit at the p-value less than 0.05.

The factors that directly affect the early timings of Antenatal care visit were short distances from the facility, knowledge on the timing of ANC, not having under-five children, having one under-five child, and wanted or planned pregnancy were factors that affect the early timing of antenatal care visit.

The odds of early timing of ANC visit among mothers who travel less than 30 min to reach ANC services were 2.47 times higher than those who travel more than one hour [AOR 2.47, 95% CI; 1.4,4.2]. The odds of early timing of antenatal care visit among mothers who were knowledgeable on the timing of ANC visit were 2.1 times higher than the counterparts [AOR 2.1; 95% CI; 1.2, 3.7]. The odds of early timing of ANC visit among mothers who have no under five children 2.7 and one under five children 2.2 times higher than those who had two under-five children [AOR 2.7; 95% CI; 1.3,5.8], [AOR 2.2; 95% CI; 1.1,4.5] respectively. In addition to this, the odds of early timing of ANC visit among mothers with wanted pregnancy were 2.4 times higher than the counterparts [AOR 2.4, 95% CI, 1.3, 4.7]. (Table 3).

Discussion

The prevalence of early timing of ANC visits was 46.8%. The factors that directly affect the early timing of ANC visits were distances, knowledge of the mother on the timing of ANC, numbers of under-five children, and desire of pregnancy.

This finding shows that the prevalence of early first time antenatal care visits was 46.8 with 95% CI [40.5, 51.8] which is in line with the prior study conduct in Gonder Ethiopia 47.4% [18], and central Tigray Ethiopia 41% [14]. However the finding of this study was lower than study conduct in Addis Ababa Ethiopia 58% [27], and Nepal 70% [17]. The difference might be due to the study area in Addis Ababa there are accessible and available services and more aware of the existing services than the study area.

The finding of this study was higher than study conduct in Gedeo Zone Ethiopia 35.4% [20], Ethiopian DHS 20% [8], and in the Global estimate 24% [10]. This inconsistency could be attributed to the scope of the study, the fact that EDHS covered more remote. It is also significant to note down the time gap between the EDHS and this study.

This study also shows that mothers who live within short distances from the health facility were more likely early initiate ANC visit than those who travel more than one hour. This finding was in line with the finding of previous study conduct in Cameron [28]. This might be due to women live

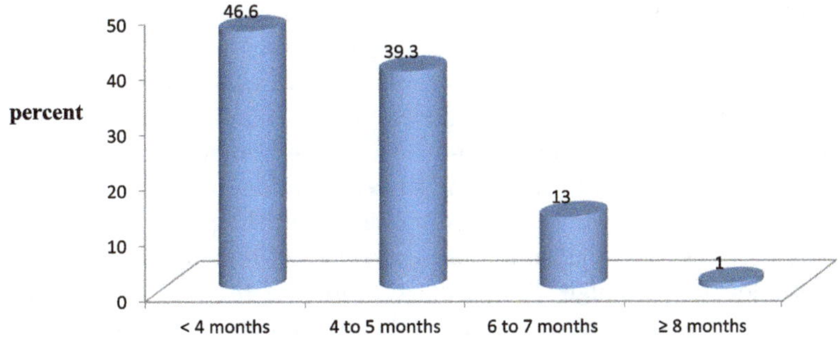

Fig. 1 Timing of first ANC booking among ANC utilized mothers in Bahir Dar Zuria District North West Ethiopia 2018. The figure showed that among all participants, 46.7% of the respondents, were booking there first ANC visit before four months of pregnancy and 39.3% of the respondents were started the follow up at four to five months. In addition, 13 and 1% of the respondents were booking there first ANC at six to seven; and eight and after months respectively

Table 3 Bivariate and multivariable association of factors, with the timing of ANC initiation in Bahir Dar Zuria District, North West Ethiopia 2018. (n = 400)

Variable	Early ANC initiation		COR (95% CI)	AOR (95% CI)	p-value
	Yes	No			
Distance					
Less than 30 min	70	44	3(1.9,5.3)	2.47(1.4,4.2)*	0.002
30 min to 1 h	70	76	1.8(1,2.9)	1.6(0.98,2.6)	0.71
More than 1 h	47	93	1	1	
Accompanying person					
Yes	135	132	1.59(1,2.4)	1.3(0.86,2.2)	
No	52	81	1	1	
Family size					
< 5	92	71	1.94(1.3,2.9)	1.4(0.62, 2.1)	
≥ 5	95	142	1	1	
Knowledge on ANC					
Knowledgeable	165	157	2.67(1.5,4.5)	2.1(1.2,3.7)*	0.016
Not knowledgeable	22	56	1	1	
Numbers of under five children					
No under five	58	50	4 (1.9,8.3)	2.7(1.3,5.8)*	0.014
One under five	116	118	3.4 (1.6, 6.6)	2.2(1.1,4.5)*	0.030
Two under five	13	45	1	1	
Age of the mother					
≤ 24 years	58	40	2.39(1.2,4.6)	1.7(0.85,3.5	
25 to 34	106	135	1.29(0.7,2.3)	1.2(0.66, 2.25)	
≥ 35	23	38	1	1	
Wanted or planned pregnancy					
Yes	173	171	3(1.6,5.7)	2.4(1.3,4.7)*	0.008
No	14	42	1	1	

in a developing country spent more times for activities like drawing water, household chores, rearing children and for agricultural activities rather than their health. As a result, they didn't think to attain the health facility for receiving ANC services because they have no time to go there. In addition to this, it may impose them for extra costs for transportation as well as loss from agricultural production.

This study also explains that mothers who have had knowledgeable on the timing of ANC were more likely to early initiate the ANC services than those not knowledgeable. This finding was consistent in meta-analysis study conduct in Ethiopia [29], and Southern Ethiopia [30, 31] this might be due to knowledge is important to realize the existing services and the timing of initiating ANC visits. In addition to this, high illiteracy level in the community may cause poor knowledge in the community.

Mothers who want her pregnancy were more likely to start the follow up early than the counterpart. This finding was in line with previous study conduct in Debre Markos Ethiopia [32], Sothern Ethiopia [33], Ethiopia [29], Tigray Ethiopia [34], South Africa [35], and Nepal [17]. This might be due to when the mother prefers the pregnancy she is eager to keep the health of the baby. Due to that, they are excited to attain the follow up earlier.

In addition in this study the odds of early initiations of ANC visit among women who have no under-five children 2.7 and one under-five children 2.2 times higher than those who had two under-five children [AOR 2.7; 95% CI; 1.3,5.8], [AOR 2.2; 95% CI; 1.1,4.5] respectively. There are limited finding with regard to the relation between timing of initiation and numbers of under-five children in the previous study but in this study numbers of under-five children was one of the determinant factors for the timing of initiation of ANC. This might be due to women may responsible for caring for their baby.

Conclusion

The prevalence of early initiation of ANC in the study area was high in comparison to the national prevalence of the country. The factor that responsible for early initiation of ANC services were distance, knowledge on the timing of ANC, a desire of pregnancy, and less and family size.

Recommendation

For federal and regional health bureau to increase the awareness of timings of antenatal care utilization and increase access and availability of family planning method for preventing unintended pregnancy.

Limitation

The finding of this study was not triangulated on qualitative finding.

Abbreviations

ANC: Antenatal Care; DHS: Demographic Health Survey; E.C: Ethiopian Calendar; EDHS: Ethiopian Demographic Health Survey; FANC: Focus Antenatal Care; Km: Kilometer; SDG: Sustainable Development Goals; SPSS: Statistical Package for Social Sciences Software; UN: United Nation; UNICEF: United Nations International Children's Emergency Fund; USAID: United State Aid for International Development; WHO: World Health Organization

Acknowledgements

First of all, I would like to thank Bahir Dar University College of Medicine and Health Sciences, School of Public Health.

I would like to also thank the Bahir Dar Zuria District health office staff, health professional they work in the health centers and health extension workers in the Cluster for their invaluable support through the whole process.

Finally, I am also grateful to the supervisors and data collectors who have committed themselves throughout the study period and to all participants who were a volunteer to participate in the study.

Funding

Bahir Dar University has funded this research.

Authors' contributions

Y.A. performs the development of manuscript, develop the survey questioners, supervised the data collection and analysis of the data. A.A. supports the methodology of the study. All authors read and approved the final manuscript.

Ethics approval and consent to participate

The ethical clearance was received from Bahir Dar University College of Medicine and Health Science ethical and clearance review committee with the ethical protocol number of 014/18–01. The permission letter was received from Amhara regional state health bureau, West Gojjam Health office, and Bahir Dar Zuria District health office.

Informed verbal consent was taken in every questionnaire for every mother and based on her agreement the data collections took place. Information was provided for all participants about the objective, the purpose or the contents of the study as well as their rights to refusal and discontinuation of the study and reassuring the confidentiality how to handle and use the data.

Competing interests

The authors declare that they have no competing interests.

References

1. World Health Organization (WHO), Pregnancy 2018.
2. Abou-Zahr CL, Wardlaw TM. Antenatal care in developing countries: promises, achievements, and missed opportunities: an analysis of trends, levels, and differentials, 1990-2001. In: World Health Organization; 2003.
3. World Health Organization (WHO). Antenatal care randemization trial. Geneva; 2002.
4. World Health Organization (WHO). Provision of effective antenatal care: integrated management of pregnancy and childbirth (IMPAC). Geneva: Standards for maternal and neonatal care (1.6), Department of making pregnancy safer; 2006.
5. World Health Organization (WHO). In: M.a.R. Health, editor. Maternal Mortality, global health observation data; 2016.
6. Oyerinde K. Can antenatal care result in significant maternal mortality reduction in developing countries. J Community Med Health Educ. 2013;3(2):2–3.
7. World Health Organization (WHO), New ANC recommendation for positive pregnancy experience 2016.
8. Ethiopian Central Statistics Agency (ECSA), Ethiopian demographic health survey (EDHS). 2016.
9. World Health Organization (WHO). In: S.a.r. health, editor. More women worldwide receive early antenatal care, but great inequalities remain; 2018.
10. Moller A-B, et al. Early antenatal care visit: a systematic analysis of regional and global levels and trends of coverage from 1990 to 2013. Lancet Glob Health. 2017;5(10):e977–83.
11. Kenya National Bureau of Statistics, Kenyan Demographic, And health survey 2014.
12. The National Population Commission Federal Republic of Nigeria, Nigeria demographic and health survey 2013. 2014.
13. Gebremeskel F, Dibaba Y, Admassu B. Timing of first antenatal care attendance and associated factors among pregnant women in Arba Minch town and Arba Minch district, Gamo Gofa zone, South Ethiopia. J Environ Public Health. 2015;2015.
14. Gebreamlak G, et al. Timing of first focused antenatal care booking and associated factors among pregnant mothers who attend antenatal care in central zone, Tigray, Ethiopia. BMC research notes. 2017;10(1):608.
15. Sanni Y, et al. Timing and adequate attendance of antenatal care visits among women in Ethiopia. PLoS One. 2017;12(9):e0184934.
16. Thin A, et al. Late initiation of antenatal care and its determinants: a hospital-based cross-sectional study. International Journal Of Community Medicine And Public Health. 2017;3(4):900–5.
17. Paudel YR, Jha T, Mehata S. Timing of first antenatal care (ANC) and inequalities in early initiation of ANC in Nepal. Front Public Health. 2017;5:242.
18. Belayneh T, Adefris M, Andargie G. Previous early antenatal service utilization improves timely booking: a cross-sectional study at the University of Gondar Hospital, north West Ethiopia. J Pregnancy. 2014;2014.
19. Gebrekidan K, Worku A. Factors associated with late ANC initiation among pregnant women in select public health centers of Addis Ababa, Ethiopia: unmatched case-control study design. Pragmatic and observational research. 2017;8:223.
20. Abuka T, Alemu A, Birhanu B. Assessment of timing of first antenatal care booking and associated factors among pregnant women who attend antenatal Care at Health Facilities in Dilla town, Gedeo zone, southern nations, nationalities and peoples region, Ethiopia, 2014. J Preg Child Health. 2016;3(258):2.
21. Kondale M, et al. Timing of first antenatal care visit and associated factors among pregnant women attending antenatal clinics in Halaba Kulito governmental health institutions, 2015. J Women's Health Care. 2016;5(308): 2167–0420.1000308.
22. Zegeye AM, Bitew BD, Koye DN. Prevalence and determinants of early antenatal care visit among pregnant women attending antenatal care in Debre Berhan Health Institutions, Central Ethiopia. Afr J Reprod Health. 2013;17(4).
23. Getasew, M., K. Teketo, and A. Mekonnen, Antenatal care service utilization and its associated factors among mothers who gave live birth in the past one year in Womberma Woreda, north West Ethiopia. Epidemiology: Open Access, 2015. 5(Special Issue 2).
24. Geta MB, Yallew WW. Early initiation of antenatal care and factors associated with early antenatal care initiation at health facilities in southern Ethiopia. Advances in Public Health. 2017;2017.

25. Bahir Dar Zuria district, Quarterly and Yearly report 2017.
26. Gidey G, et al. Timing of first focused antenatal care booking and associated factors among pregnant mothers who attend antenatal care in central zone, Tigray, Ethiopia. BMC research notes. 2017;10(1):608.
27. Gulema H, Berhane Y. Timing of first antenatal care visit and its associated factors among pregnant women attending public health facilities in Addis Ababa, Ethiopia. Ethiopian journal of health sciences. 2017;27(2):139–46.
28. Tolefac PN, et al. Why do pregnant women present late for their first antenatal care consultation in Cameroon? Maternal health, neonatology and perinatology. 2017;3(1):29.
29. Tesfaye G, et al. Delayed initiation of antenatal care and associated factors in Ethiopia: a systematic review and meta-analysis. Reprod Health. 2017; 14(1):150.
30. Dembelu M, et al. Assessment of timely initiation of first ANC visit and associated factors among pregnant mothers in Wolayita Soddo public health facilities. Soddo Town: Wollayita Zone, SNNPR, Ethiopia; 2016.
31. Geta MB, Yallew WW. Early Initiation of Antenatal Care and Factors Associated with Early Antenatal Care Initiation at Health Facilities in Southern Ethiopia. Advances in Public Health. 2017;2017(Article ID: 1624245:6.
32. Ewunetie AA, et al. DELAY on first antenatal care visit and its associated factors among pregnant women in public health facilities of Debre Markos town, north West Ethiopia. BMC Pregnancy and Childbirth. 2018;18:173.
33. Gebremeskel F, Dibaba Y, Admassu B. Timing of First Antenatal Care Attendance and Associated Factors among Pregnant Women in Arba Minch Town and Arba Minch District, Gamo Gofa Zone, South Ethiopia. J Environ Public Health. 2015;2015(ID 971506):7.
34. Lerebo W, Kidanu A, Tsadik M. Magnitude and Associated Factors of Late Booking for Antenatal Care in Public Health Centers of Adigrat Town, Tigray, Ethiopia. Clinics Mother Child Health. 2015;12:171. https://doi.org/10.4172/2090-7214.1000171.
35. Ebonwu J, et al. Determinants of late antenatal care presentation in rural and peri-urban communities in South Africa: a cross-sectional study. PLoS One. 2018;13(3):e0191903.

Preference of specimen collection methods for human papillomavirus detection for cervical cancer screening: a cross-sectional study of high-risk women in Mombasa, Kenya

Griffins O. Manguro[1*], Linnet N. Masese[2], Kishor Mandaliya[3], Susan M. Graham[4,5], R. Scott McClelland[4,5] and Jennifer S. Smith[6,7]

Abstract

Objectives: Self-collection of genital specimens for high-risk types of human papillomavirus (hrHPV) detection may increase cervical cancer screening uptake. We hypothesized that women would prefer self-collection to clinician-collection of genital specimens. To test this hypothesis, and women's preference between two different self-collection approaches, a total of 199 women were enrolled in a cross-sectional study in Mombasa, Kenya.

Materials and methods: Participants provided self-collected specimens using the Evalyn cytobrush (Rovers) stored in a dry tube and the Viba cytobrush (Rovers) stored in wet Aptima media (Hologic). A clinician also collected cervical specimens for hrHPV testing and for cytology, and performed visual inspection using acetic acid. A post-examination questionnaire assessed preferences for the different methods of specimen collection. To test the difference in proportions for each collection method, we performed an exact binomial probability test, under the null hypothesis that women would prefer each specimen-collection method equally.

Results: Most women preferred clinician-collection over self-collection (68% versus 32%, $p < 0.01$). For self-collection, dry-self collection with the Evalyn brush was preferred over the wet-selection with the Viba brush (53% versus 27%, p < 0.01). There was no association between preference for self-collection and preference for a particular self-collection cytobrush.

Conclusion: Further research to understand and address obstacles to self-collection of genital specimens may be needed to improve the uptake of self-collection for cervical cancer screening, especially in settings with poor access to trained healthcare providers.

Keywords: HrHPV, Self-collection, Clinician-collection, Cervical cancer, Screening, Kenya

* Correspondence: gmanguro@uw.edu
[1]Kenyatta National Hospital, P.O. Box 91109, Mombasa 80103, Kenya
Full list of author information is available at the end of the article

Plain English summary

Testing for high-risk sub-types of human papillomavirus (hrHPV) is an effective way of screening for cervical cancer. Unlike Pap smears which have to be performed by a clinician, women can self-collect genital samples for HPV testing. Such samples often produce results that are as accurate as those obtained from clinician-collected samples.

Between August 2013 and April 2015, we conducted a study among 199 women at high risk of sexually transmitted infections (STIs) and HIV in Mombasa, Kenya. Our aim was to find out if the women preferred to collect their own genital samples or have samples collected by a clinician, and between two self-collection brushes, which one they would like most. Study participants performed self-collection in a private room, followed by clinician-collection and a pap smear.

More than two thirds (68%) of the women preferred to have a clinician collect the genital samples. For self-collection, majority of women (53%) preferred the Evalyn brush, which was stored and transported without any preservative (dry) compared to the Viba brush, which was stored and transported in a liquid preservative.

Further research is needed to find out reasons why women in this setting prefer to have genital samples collected by a clinician rather than to collect samples themselves, considering that self-collected vaginal samples is likely to be easier, more comfortable, less embarrassing and just as accurate as those collected by a clinician. Understanding such factors may help to scale-up self-testing, which may increase the number of women who screen for cervical cancer.

Background

Detection of high-risk human papillomavirus (hrHPV) in genital specimens is current being used in conjunction with (co-testing) or as an alternative to Papanicolau (Pap) smears for primary cervical cancer screening [1–6]. Testing for hrHPV in genital specimens has demonstrated significantly greater sensitivity as compared to conventional Pap smear for detecting high-grade cervical intra-epithelial neoplasia (CIN 2+) [2, 6, 7]. Additionally, women can self-collect cervico-vaginal specimens for hrHPV testing. These self-collected specimens demonstrate similar sensitivity and specificity to clinician-collected specimens for detecting high-grade cervical lesions (CIN 2+), and may improve access to screening [8]. Studies conducted in Europe, North and South America looking at the acceptability of self-collection of genital specimens for hrHPV testing indicate that self-collected HPV genital specimens were preferred compared to the conventional Pap smears for HPV screening. In the latter one study from South America, age and level of education were strongly correlated with increased preference for self-collection [4, 9]. Few studies [10, 11] have explored the acceptability of self-collection of genital specimens in Africa, where cultural and religious beliefs concerning both clinician and self-collection of genital specimens may be an important consideration. Understanding women's preference for self-collection versus clinician-collection of specimens will help to guide future interventions for cervical cancer screening.

Our study, conducted in a cohort of high-risk women in Mombasa, Kenya, assessed women's preference for self-collection versus clinician-collection of genital specimens for detection of hrHPV for primary cervical cancer screening. We also explored women's preference between two different self-collection devices, the Viba cytobrush (Rovers®, Netherlands), which required a liquid transport media, and the Evalyn cytobrush (Rovers®, Netherlands), which did not. Based on existing data, we hypothesized that women would prefer self-collection over clinician collection [9]. Due to the presumed ease of collection, we also hypothesized that Evalyn cytobrush (dry) would be preferred over the Viba cytobrush (in liquid media) for self-collection of specimens.

Materials and methods

Study design

We conducted a clinic-based, cross-sectional study from August 2013 to April 2015. A total of 200 women participating in a cohort study of women at high risk of acquiring sexually transmitted infections (STIs) and HIV in Mombasa, Kenya were enrolled. Clinical procedures, including self-collection of hrHPV specimens, were performed at the Ganjoni Health Centre in Mombasa. Study procedures were integrated into the ongoing follow-up procedures for the Mombasa Cohort [12, 13]. Briefly, the Mombasa Cohort is an open cohort study of female sex workers (FSWs) established in 1993 as a HIV incidence cohort. FSW are recruited from major sex work venues in Mombasa. Those interested are referred to the research clinic, located in the Ganjoni Municipal Clinic. Women are invited into this parent cohort if they are 18–45 years old, reside in Mombasa area, are self-identifying as exchanging sex for payment in cash or in kind and are able to provide informed consent. Routine cohort visits are scheduled every month. Every 3 months, the scheduled visit procedures include collection of genital specimens for *Chlamydia trachomatis* and *Neisseria gonorrhea* nucleic acid amplification testing (NAAT). For this ancillary study, we invited women whose study visits coincided with the NAAT specimen collection visit. We used convenience sampling to enroll those who agreed to participate from among those who were eligible.

Study visit procedures

A study nurse briefly introduced the study to eligible women and invited them to participate. Women who agreed to participate were referred to the study counselor, who provided further information and responded to questions. Following this discussion with the counselor, interested participants were required to provide written informed consent.

Self-collection of genital specimens was conducted in a private room at the health facility. A study nurse provided verbal instructions on self-collection procedures, after which participants performed the procedure on their own. Pictorial diagrams with detailed instructions on self-collection were also available in the room. Each woman performed self-collection using the two different specimen brushes, the Evalyn cytobrush (Rovers®, Netherlands), and the Viba cytobrush (Rovers®, Netherlands). To minimize potential bias from the order of specimen collection, women had study numbers assigned to them based on their enrollment into the study, and those with odd study numbers self-collected using the Evalyn brush first, while those with even study numbers self-collected using the Viba cytobrush first. The physical characteristics and specimen handling slightly differ between these two devices (Fig. 1). For both cytobrushes, self-collected specimens were obtained by inserting the collection brush and following the manufacturer's instructions to sample cells from the cervico-vaginal wall.

The Evalyn cytobrush is pink in color, and consists of a plunger containing white bristles made of polyethylene at the tip, a transparent casing, and a transparent cap. For self-collection, women were instructed to squat, pull the plunger down into the clear casing to protect the bristles, and gently insert the brush into the vagina. Next, they pushed the plunger back up to expose the bristles, and rotated the brush through five complete turns in the same direction for specimen collection. Each complete rotation was accompanied by an audible click on the device. Self-collection using the Evalyn brush was "dry," in that there was no need to place the specimens in a preservative for transportation to the laboratory.

The Viba brush consists of a blue handle and an easily removable white tip. The tip contains bristles made of similar material as the Evalyn brush. The Viba brush was provided with a cryovial containing 1 ml of Aptima media (Hologic®, USA). After self-collection, participants broke off the brush head at the tip of the cytobrush and deposited it into the cryovial containing Aptima media.

After self-collection, a study clinician performed a speculum-assisted pelvic examination, which included collection of cervical specimen for hrHPV testing. Clinician-collection of specimens was performed using a cervical specimen collection brush (Hologic®, USA). Unlike self-collected specimens, clinician specimens were collected from the endocervix. Similar to the Viba brush, clinician-collected specimens were stored in Aptima media (Hologic®, USA). After hrHPV specimen collection, the clinician performed visual inspection under acetic acid and a conventional Pap smear. All clinicians in this study had extensive training and experience in

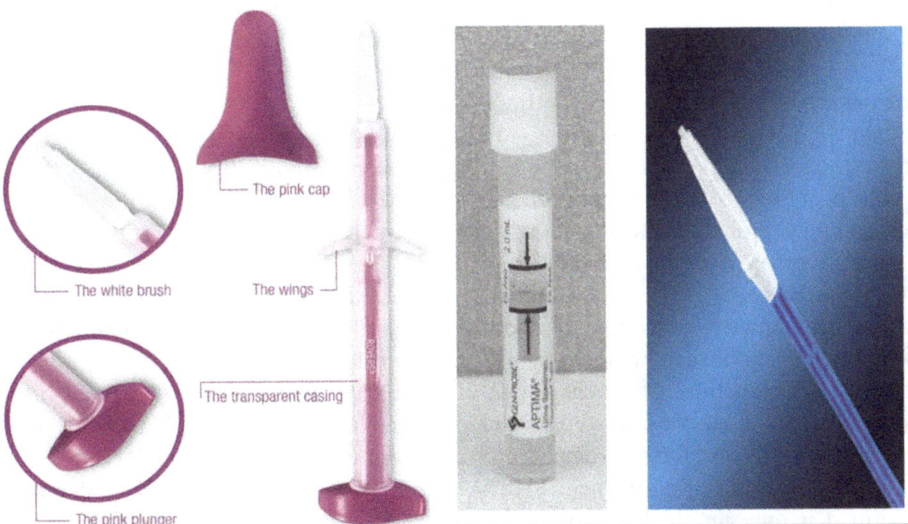

Evalyn cytobrush (Rovers®, Netherlands)

The Viba cytobrush (Rovers®, Netherlands) with cryovial containing Aptima media (Hologic)

Fig. 1 The Evalyn cytobrush (left side) and the Viba cytobrush with cryovial containing Aptima media (right side)

genital examination and specimen collection as part of the procedures in the Mombasa Cohort.

Post-examination questionnaire to assess women's preference

Following the clinical examinations, women participated in a structured interview using a standardized questionnaire to assess their preferences for different methods of specimen collection. For the question on self-collection versus clinician-collection, women were asked, "If you were to be tested for hrHPV infection again, how would you like the specimen to be collected?" They gave their answers as either self-collection or clinician-collection.

To assess women's preferences between the Evalyn and Viba cytobrushes, they were asked, "Which of the two brushes you collected yourself did you like best?" They were then asked to select one of three possible responses; "I liked the blue brush (Viba brush)," "I liked the pink brush (Evalyn brush)," and "I liked them both equally". To explore women's perceptions of specific characteristics of the two brushes, they were asked four questions. Their responses to these questions were graded on a 5-point Likert scale, with a range of one for "strongly agree", two for "agree somewhat"; three for "neutral"; four for "disagrees somewhat"; and five for "strongly disagree." The four questions were: "Was the brush comfortable to insert?" "Were you concerned about hurting yourself with the brush?", "Were you concerned about using the brush properly?", and, "Were the instructions for self-collection using the brush easy to understand?"

Statistical analysis

The primary aim of the study was to test the hypothesis that women would prefer self-collection to clinician-collection of genital specimens. To test the difference in proportions for each collection method, we performed an exact binomial probability test, under the null hypothesis that women would prefer each specimen-collection method equally (i.e., $p = 0.50$ for selecting self-collection or clinician-collection). To determine which self-collection cytobrush was most preferred, we compared the proportion of women who preferred the Evalyn brush to those who preferred the Viba brush and to those who preferred them both equally. To determine the statistical significance of this difference, we performed a one-sample t-test, with responses distributed between 0 for the Viba brush, 1 for no preference, and 2 for the Evalyn brush, testing the null hypothesis of no difference in preference (i.e., mean preference = 1.0).

Log-binomial regression analyses were performed to explore the predictors of preference for clinician collection versus self-collection. The variables tested were identified a priori through a review of the literature. We included factors associated with self-testing for other conditions (HIV) and those associated with screening for cervical cancer. These included women's age at first sexual intercourse [14], current age [15], level of education [16, 17], marital status [16], parity [15], and religion [18].

To explore predictors of preference for the dry self-collection brush, wet self-collection brush, and preference for both equally, we performed a multinomial logistic regression analysis, with no preference as the referent category. The predictors included in the models were similar to those included in our analysis of predictors of preference for self-collection versus clinician-collection. Relative risk ratios greater than 1 in this analysis indicated a higher probability of preferring the brush specified, relative to having no preference. Conversely, relative risk ratios less than 1 indicated a lower probability of preferring the brush specified, relative to having no preference. We performed chi-squared tests to explore whether there was an association between preference for self-collection and preference for a particular collection device. Finally, to better understand women's preferences for specific collection devices, we explored their perceptions about characteristics of the two brushes. Median and interquartile ranges were used to summarize the responses to each question that was graded on a Likert scale. Wilcoxon signed-ranks tests were performed to analyze differences in paired responses to each of these questions for the Evalyn brush compared to the Viba brush. All analyses were performed using STATA version 13.

Results

Between August 2013 and April 2014, a total of 200 women were enrolled into the cervical cancer screening study. Of these, 199 (99%) participated in the post-examination interview and were included in analyses. Mean age of study participants was 37.6 years, range (30–44) and approximately half were HIV-positive (Table 1).

Of 199 women, 63 (32%) reported preference for self-collection compared to 136 (68%) who reported preference for clinician-collection (exact binomial probability test, $p < 0.001$). Baseline demographic and clinical characteristics were broadly similar between women who preferred clinician-collection and those who preferred self-collection. Univariate log-binomial regression analyses of predictors of preference for self-collection found that older age at sexual debut was significantly associated higher with preference for clinician-collection versus self-collection (odds ratio [OR] 1.10, 95% confidence interval [CI] 1.02–1.10, $p = 0.02$) (Table 2).

Table 1 Baseline characteristics of 199 female sex workers from Mombasa, Kenya

Characteristic	Mean (SD) or Number (percent)
Age (years)	37.6 (9.5)
Age at first sex (years)	16.9 (2.3)
> 8 years of education (At least some high-school)	91 (46%)
Ever pregnant	183 (92%)
Ever married	120 (60%)
Religion	
Christian	176 (89%)
Muslim	18 (9%)
Other[a]	5 (3%)
Using modern contraception other than condoms alone	
No contraceptive method	63 (32%)
Hormonal contraceptive use	53 (27%)
Non-hormonal contraceptive use	83 (41%)
HIVseropositive	101 (51%)

[a]Includes traditional African religions and no religious affiliation

For self-collection, the Evalyn brush was generally preferred ($n = 105$; 53%), compared to the Viba brush ($n = 50$; 25%), and equal preference for both brushes ($n = 44$; 22%) (One-sample t test $p < 0.001$). We found no association between preference for specimen collection method self-versus clinician) and preference for self-collection cytobrush (Chi-square test, $p = 0.69$). In univariate multinomial logistic regression analyses, age, parity, comfort when using the brush and concerns of getting hurt while using the brush were significantly associated with preference for a particular self-collection method (Table 3). In multivariable analyses, increased comfort with the Evalyn brush was associated with lower probability of selecting the Viba brush (OR 0.48, 95% CI 0.32–0.71), and increased concerns about hurting themselves with the Viba brush were associated with an increased probability of selecting the Evalyn brush (OR 1.33, 95% CI 1.05–1.71).

Table 4 presents responses to questions comparing women's experience with the Evalyn and Viba cytobrushes, together with p-values from the test for differences in paired responses to each of these questions. Participants strongly agreed that instructions for both

Table 2 Univariate log-binomial regression analyses exploring predictors of women's preference for clinician-collection versus self-collection of genital specimens

Variable	Overall Number (Percent) of women who prefer self-collection $N = 199$	Women who prefer clinician-collection $n = 136$ Mean (SD) or Number (Percent)	Women who prefer self-collection $n = 63$ Median (IQR) or Number (Percent)	Relative Risk (95% CI) for preference of clinician versus self-collection	p-value
Age (years)		38.2 (9.7)	36.4 (9.1)	0.99 (0.97–1.0)	0.25
Age at first sex (years)		16.6 (2.2)	17.4 (2.4)	1.10 (1.02–1.19)	0.02
Parity					
Nulliparous	44%	9 (7%)	7 (11%)	Reference	
Ever pregnant	31%	127 (93%)	56 (89%)	0.71 (0.39–1.28)	0.26
Education					
8 years and less	27%	79 (58%)	29 (46%)	Reference	
v > 8 years	37%	57 (42%)	34 (54%)	1.39 (0.92–2.10)	0.11
Marital status					
Never married	30%	55 (40%)	24 (38%)	Reference	
Ever married	33%	81 (60%)	39 (62%)	1.07 (0.70–1.63)	0.75
HIV status					
HIV-negative	35%	64 (47%)	35 (56%)	Reference	
HIV-positive	28%	72 (53%)	28 (44%)	0.79 (0.52–1.20)	0.27
Religion					
Christian		122 (90%)	54 (86%)	Reference	
Muslim		18 (9)	8 (13%)	1.45 (0.83–2.54)	0.20
Other[a]		5 (3)	1 (2%)	0.65 (0.11–3.82)	0.64

[a]Traditional African religions and no religious affiliation

Table 3 Multinomial regression analysis exploring predictors of women's preference for the Viba or the Evalyn cytobrush

Variable	Prefers Viba cytobrush		Prefers Evalyn cytobrush	
	Relative risk ratio (95% CI)	*p*-value	Relative risk ratio (95% CI)	*p*-value
Age (years)	0.92 (0.88–0.97)	0.001	0.94 (0.91–0.98)	0.004
Age at first sex (years)	1.07 (0.89–1.28)	0.47	1.05 (0.90–1.23)	0.55
Parity				
Nulliparous	Reference		Reference	
Ever pregnant	0.68 (0.52–0.90)	0.008	0.82 (0.65–1.02)	0.07
Education				
No high school education	Reference		Reference	
At least high school-level	1.22 (0.54–2.78)	0.63	1.42 (0.70–2.88)	0.34
Marital status				
Never married	Reference		Reference	
Ever married	0.81 (0.35–1.85)	0.62	0.95 (0.46–1.95)	0.88
HIV status				
HIV-negative	Reference		Reference	
HIV-positive	1.16 (0.51–2.63)	0.72	0.62 (0.31–1.26)	0.19
Religion				
Christian	Reference		Reference	
Muslim	0.35 (0.07–1.93)	0.23	0.92 (0.30–2.83)	0.89
Other[a]	2.66 (0.27–26.62)	0.41	0.42 (0.03–6.87)	0.54
Evalyn brush more comfortable to insert[b]	0.64 (0.46–0.89)	0.009	1.38 (0.92–2.06)	0.12
Viba brush more comfortable to insert [b]	1.48 (1.01–2.16)	0.04	0.69 (0.55–0.87)	0.002
Concerned about hurting themselves with Evalyn brush [b]	1.25 (0.98–1.58)	0.07	0.89 (0.72–1.09)	0.25
Concerned about hurting themselves with Viba brush [b]	0.93 (0.74–1.18)	0.56	1.38 (1.12–1.69)	0.002

[a]Traditional African religions and no religious affiliation

[b]For this analysis, the rating scale for these questions was reverse coded (5 strongly agree, 4 agree somewhat, 3 neutral, 2 disagree somewhat, 1 strongly disagree) so that increasing ratings indicated agreement with each item and higher relative risk ratios indicated a higher probability of preferring the brush specified

self-collection brushes were easy to understand. In terms of analyses comparing women's experience with the Evalyn and the Viba cytobrushes, for the questions, "Were the instructions for self-collection using the brush easy to understand?" and, "Were you concerned about using the cytobrush properly?" women rated both self-collection cytobrushes equally and favorably. For the question "Were you concerned about hurting yourself with the brush?" responses were more favorable for the Evalyn brush as compared to the Viba brush. For the question "Was the brush comfortable to insert?" a significantly greater proportion of women reported comfort with the Evalyn brush compared to the Viba brush.

Discussion

In this study of 199 high-risk Kenyan women participating in an HIV incidence cohort, significantly more participants preferred to have specimens for hrHPV testing collected by a clinician rather than self-collected sampling. When directly comparing the two self-collection

Table 4 Median scores and interquartile range for responses to questions on experience when using the cytobrushes and *p*-values from the Wilcoxon signed ranks test for differences in each paired response

Question	Evalyn	Viba	*p* value
	Median (IQR)	Median (IQR)	
Were the instructions on using brushes easy to understand?	1 (1–1)	1 (1–1)	0.08
Were you concerned about using the brush properly?	2 (1–4)	2 (1–4)	0.15
Were you concerned about hurting yourself?	4 (1–5)	2 (1–5)	0.0004
Was the brush comfortable to insert?	1 (1–1)	1 (1–4)	< 0.001

(1 strongly agree, 2 agree somewhat, 3 neutral, 4 disagree somewhat, 5 strongly disagree)

devices, most women preferred the self-collection Evalyn brush stored "dry" to the Viba brush stored in liquid media. Women strongly agreed that both self-collection brushes were comfortable during use, and the instructions easy to follow. For both self-collection approaches, most women somewhat agreed that they were concerned about performing self-collection properly.

Women in several studies from the US and Europe reported a preference for self-collection compared to clinician-collection for hrHPV specimen collection [4, 19, 20]. A meta-analysis including eight studies from Europe and two from North America also reported that, among women who did not routinely screen for cervical cancer, compliance was better when using self-collected genital specimens as initial screening as opposed to pap smears [4]. In contrast, one study from Cameroon reported that while women found self-collection more comfortable and less embarrassing, a greater proportion of women still preferred to have genital specimens collected by a clinician (62% vs. 29%, $p < 0.001$) [21]. In this African population, women reported greater concerns about the reliability of results from self-collected specimens as compared to clinician-collected specimens (59% vs. 1%). Our results suggest that Kenyan women may have similar concerns about the reliability of self-collected specimens. When asked, "Were you concerned about using the cytobrushes properly?" most of the women's response was "agreed somewhat" (Table 4). This is in contrast to their responses on questions pertaining to the specific characteristics of the brushes, which were consistently very favorable. Most women, for example, felt that the self-collection brushes were comfortable to use, and instructions for self-collection easy to follow.

While the overall rating for both cytobrushes was positive, the Evalyn cytobrush was generally more preferred. Importantly, the majority of women in this study who reported greater preference for the Evalyn brush also found the cytobrush more comfortable to insert, and reported greater fears of hurting themselves with the Viba cytobrush. These two may be explained by the difference in physical characteristics of the Evalyn cytobrush. The cytobrush has a plunger, which allowed the women to pull down the bristles into the transparent casing at the point of insertion. The Evalyn brush also has wings which marks the furthest point the cytobrush can be inserted into the vagina. It is possible that these two characteristics may contribute to the greater comfort and less fears of hurting themselves when using the Evalyn brush. Additionally, women did not have to detach the tip of the Evalyn brush and insert into the liquid transport media and merely replaced the plastic cap after self-collection as the cytobrush was stored and transported dry. The finding that women reported a preference for one cytobrush over the other for self-collection is important for the potential scale-up of self-collection programs in this region. However, it is important to note that it is unknown whether women's preference for the Evalyn brush would have a meaningful impact on self-collection program coverage if only an alternative like the Viba brush were offered.

It is interesting to note that while findings from our study and the Cameroonian study [21] agree, the study populations are distinctly different. Our study was conducted in female sexual workers at a notably high risk of infection with HIV and STIs, who regularly attended clinic and had frequent pelvic examinations. In contrast, the study from Cameroon was conducted in general population with limited exposure to pelvic examinations. The parallel findings from these two distinct populations of African women may point towards a general preference for clinician-collected genital specimens among women from this region, although more research is warranted to confirm these findings.

Our study has several strengths. Few other studies in sub-Saharan Africa have evaluated women's preference between different methods of genital specimen-collection for hrHPV testing. East Africa contributes a significant burden of invasive cervical cancer globally, and reports one of the lowest proportion of reproductive-aged women having been screened for cervical cancer [22]. In addition, our study was conducted in a cohort of women at a particularly high risk for hrHPV and high-grade cervical lesions. Interventions aimed at improving hrHPV testing in this population are, therefore, likely to be of great benefit in terms of reducing preventable cervical cancer and associated mortality.

One important limitation of our study was that self-collection of genital specimens was conducted in a clinic setting. Women had to present to a health facility to conduct the self-test. Part of the challenge of cervical cancer screening in East Africa is poor access to health facilities. It is plausible that women would appreciate self-collection more if they were offered the additional convenience of self-collection at home or in another non-clinical setting. Another limitation was that this study was conducted in a group of women who were part of an ongoing cohort study in which pelvic examinations with collection of genital specimens for STI screening is routine. It is possible that the women in this population have grown more comfortable with clinical examinations compared to women in the general population.

Conclusion

In conclusion, our findings suggest that high-risk women in sub-Saharan Africa may prefer clinician-collection, rather than self-collection, for hrHPV testing. Areas with inadequate healthcare infrastructure, especially those with few trained clinicians to conduct pelvic examinations, would benefit greatly from scale-up of self-collection for cervical cancer screening. In this regard, education about the validity, safety and ease of self-collected specimens for hrHPV detection will be important to enhance uptake of self-collection of genital specimens for cervical cancer screening.

Abbreviations

CI: Confidence interval; CIN: Cervical intraepithelial neoplasia; HIV: Human immunodeficiency virus; HrHPV: High-risk human papillomavirus; Pap : Papanicolau smear; STI: Sexually transmitted infections

Acknowledgements

We acknowledge the support received from all clinical staff at the Ganjoni Municipal clinic, Mombasa, Kenya.

Funding

Specimen collection and processing was supported by a grant from Hologic (Boston, MA, USA), and the UNC Gillings Innovation Laboratory through JSS. HPV self-collection kits were donated by Rovers Medical Devices (Amsterdam, The Netherlands). GM was a scholar in the International AIDS Research and Training Program, supported by the Fogarty International Center; NIH Research Grant D43 TW009580. RSM receives support for mentoring through NIH K24 HD88229. Infrastructure and logistical support for the Mombasa research site was received from the University of Washington & Fred Hutchinson Cancer Research Center's Center for AIDS Research (NIH grant P30-AI27757). The content is solely the responsibility of the authors and does not necessarily represent the official views of the National Institutes of Health.

Authors' contributions

GOM, RSM, JSS and SMG conceptualized the study. GOM and LNM carried out the research procedures, including clinical examination and post-examination interviews. KM analyzed specimens and was a major contributor in writing the manuscript. GOM, LNM and SMG analyzed the data. RSM and JSS reviewed the manuscript. All authors read and approved the final manuscript.

Competing interests

The authors declare that they have no competing interests.

Author details

[1]Kenyatta National Hospital, P.O. Box 91109, Mombasa 80103, Kenya. [2]Department of Epidemiology, University of Washington, P.O Box 357236, Seattle, WA, 98195, USA. [3]Pathcare Laboratories, Mombasa, Kenya. [4]Departments of Epidemiology, Global Health, and Medicine, University of Washington, P.O Box 359909, Seattle, WA, USA. [5]Institute of Tropical and Infectious Diseases, University of Nairobi, Nairobi, Kenya. [6]University of North Carolina at Chapel Hill, Chapel Hill, NC, USA. [7]Lineberger Cancer Center, Chapel Hill, NC, USA.

References

1. Arbyn M, Anttila A, Jordan J, et al. European guidelines for quality assurance in cervical Cancer screening. Second Edition—Summary Document. Ann Oncol. 2010;21(3):448–58.
2. Arbyn M, Ronco G, Anttila A, et al. Evidence Regarding Human Papillomavirus Testing in Secondary Prevention of Cervical Cancer. Vaccine. 2012;30(Supplement 5):88–99.
3. McGraw SL, Ferrante JM. Update on prevention and screening of cervical cancer. World J Clin Oncol. 2014;5:744–52.
4. Racey CS, Withrow DR, Gesink D. Self-collected HPV testing improves participation in cervical cancer screening: a systematic review and meta-analysis. Can J Public Health. 2013;104:159–66.
5. Snijders PJ, Verhoef VM, Arbyn M, et al. High-risk HPV testing on self-sampled versus clinician-collected specimens: a review on the clinical accuracy and impact on population attendance in cervical cancer screening. Int J Cancer. 2013;132:2223–36.
6. Wright TC, Stoler MH, Behrens CM, et al. Primary cervical cancer screening with human papillomavirus: end of study results from the ATHENA study using HPV as the first-line screening test. Gynecol Oncol. 2015;136:189–97.
7. Whitlock EP, Vesco KK, Eder M, et al. Liquid-based cytology and human papillomavirus testing to screen for cervical Cancer: a systematic review for the U.S. preventive services task force. Ann Intern Med. 2011;155:687–97.
8. Jentschke M, Chen K, Arbyn M, et al. Direct comparison of two vaginal self-sampling devices for the detection of human papillomavirus infections. J Clin Virol. 2016;82:46–50.
9. Arrossi S, Ramos S, Straw C, et al. HPV testing: a mixed-method approach to understand why women prefer self-collection in a middle-income country. BMC Public Health. 2016;16:832.
10. Mahomed K, Evans D, Sauls C, et al. Human papillomavirus (HPV) testing on self-collected specimens: perceptions among HIV positive women attending rural and urban clinics in South Africa. Pan Afr Med J. 2014;17:189.
11. Adamson PC, Huchko MJ, Moss AM, et al. Acceptability and accuracy of cervical Cancer screening using a self-collected tampon for HPV messenger-RNA testing among HIV-infected women in South Africa. Liu X, ed. PLoS One. 2015;10:9.
12. Martin HL, Jr., Nyange PM, Richardson BA, et al. Hormonal contraception, sexually transmitted diseases, and risk of heterosexual transmission of human immunodeficiency virus type 1. J Infect Dis 1998;178:1053–1059.
13. Graham SM, Holte SE, Peshu NM, et al. Initiation of antiretroviral therapy leads to a rapid decline in cervical and vaginal HIV-1 shedding. AIDS. 2007;21:501–7.
14. Lee CH, Peng CY, Li RN, et al. Risk evaluation for the development of cervical intraepithelial neoplasia: development and validation of risk-scoring schemes. Int J Cancer. 2015;136:340–9.
15. Cerigo H, Coutlee F, Franco EL, et al. Factors associated with cervical cancer screening uptake among Inuit women in Nunavik, Quebec, Canada. BMC Public Health. 2013;13:438.
16. De Vito C, Angeloni C, De Feo E, et al. A large cross-sectional survey investigating the knowledge of cervical cancer risk aetiology and the predictors of the adherence to cervical cancer screening related to mass media campaign. Biomed Res Int. 2014;2014:304602.
17. Ezechi OC, Petterson KO, Gbajabiamila TA, et al. Predictors of default from follow-up care in a cervical cancer screening program using direct visual inspection in South-Western Nigeria. BMC Health Serv Res. 2014;14:143.
18. Padela AI, Peek M, Johnson-Agbakwu CE, et al. Associations between religion-related factors and cervical cancer screening among Muslims in greater Chicago. J Low Genit Tract Dis. 2014;18:326–32.
19. Rosenbaum AJ, Gage JC, Alfaro KM, et al. Acceptability of self-collected versus provider-collected sampling for HPV DNA testing among women in rural El Salvador. Int J Gynaecol Obstet. 2014;126:156–60.
20. Dzuba IG, Diaz EY, Allen B, et al. The acceptability of self-collected samples for HPV testing vs. the pap test as alternatives in cervical cancer screening. J Womens Health Gend Based Med. 2002;11:265–75.
21. Berner A, Hassel SB, Tebeu PM, et al. Human papillomavirus self-sampling in Cameroon: women's uncertainties over the reliability of the method are barriers to acceptance. J Low Genit Tract Dis. 2013;17:235–41.
22. Global Burden of Disease Cancer Collaboration. The global burden of Cancer 2013. JAMA Oncol. 2015;1:505–27.

17

An awareness-raising framework for global health networks: lessons learned from a qualitative case study in respectful maternity care

Meaghan O'Connor*, Kayla McGowan and R. Rima Jolivet

Abstract

Background: The increase in global health networks as mechanisms for improving health and affecting social change has been recognized as a key component of the global health landscape today. To successfully raise awareness of shared causes, global health networks need tools to help them plan successful campaigns and evaluate the impact of their work, as well as to coordinate and reinforce each other's efforts. One global health network, the Respectful Maternity Care (RMC) Global Council, can be credited with raising the profile of the issues of disrespect and abuse (D&A) in childbirth and the need for RMC within global maternal health. We set out to learn from the work of the RMC Global Council and the RMC movement at large to develop a tool—a framework for planning and evaluating awareness-raising efforts—useful for networks focused on global health and human rights.

Methods: We reviewed the literature for theoretical models on awareness raising and, finding a lack of appropriate tools, developed a new, draft framework using components of the Framework for Effective Campaigns, the SpitFire SmartChart 3.0, and Network Theory. We conducted semi-structured interviews with members of the RMC Global Council to validate the draft framework and identify any additional strategies or tactics that were used during their efforts to raise awareness of D&A and RMC. We also interviewed "influenced" individuals to validate inputs from the influencers and determine the key documents, events, individuals, and organizations that made the greatest contribution to the increased awareness of D&A/RMC. Data were analyzed using deductive and inductive qualitative research methods.

Results: The validated awareness-raising framework includes five strategies that characterize a successful awareness-raising effort. Each strategy has a set of tactics that can operationalize those strategies. Each tactic is classified as essential, helpful, or variable based on the number of key informants who utilized it.

Conclusion: This case study offers an example of how global health networks can create a movement that effects change at global and local levels by providing an empirically-grounded framework to help plan, coordinate, and evaluate future campaigns designed to raise awareness and create momentum in global health, human rights, and quality of care.

Keywords: Respectful maternity care, Disrespect and abuse, Global health networks, Awareness raising, Case study

* Correspondence: meaghancoconnor@gmail.com
Maternal Health Task Force, Women and Health Initiative, Harvard T.H. Chan School of Public Health, 651 Huntington Avenue, Boston, MA 02115, USA

Plain English summary

Today, networks of organizations and individuals are working together to meet global goals and improve health worldwide. These networks need tools to plan, coordinate, and evaluate their efforts in the most effective way. The global Respectful Maternity Care (RMC) movement, launched by the RMC Global Council, is an example of a network that worked together and effectively raised awareness of the mistreatment of women in childbirth facilities and women's right to high quality, respectful care before, during, and after childbirth. To learn from this success, we used a case study approach to develop and validate a framework for awareness raising. We reviewed the literature on awareness raising and developed a new, draft framework drawing from the Framework for Effective Campaigns, the SpitFire SmartChart 3.0 tool, and Network Theory. We interviewed members of the RMC Global Council to compare their efforts to the items in our draft awareness-raising framework and note any additional strategies or tactics that they used. We also interviewed individuals who were influenced by the RMC movement to identify the key documents, events, individuals, and organizations that contributed to their increase in awareness. Data were analyzed using qualitative methods. The result of the research is an awareness-raising framework with five strategies for a successful awareness-raising effort. Each strategy has a set of tactics, labeled integral, helpful, or variable for awareness-raising efforts. Global health networks in many fields can use this tool when planning and assessing awareness-raising efforts.

Introduction

Over the last seven years, the issues of disrespect and abuse in childbirth (D&A) and the need for respectful maternity care (RMC) have become key components of the global maternal health agenda. Much of the work that brought these issues to light was guided by the RMC Global Council, a network of individuals and organizations working collaboratively to raise awareness of D&A and RMC through research, programming, and advocacy. Today, global health networks like the RMC Global Council are more common than ever, bound together by "a common purpose oriented towards social change" and "durable relationships among the actors who constitute them" [1]. Indeed, Shiffman et al. write that "the proliferation of global health networks represents one of the most dramatic shifts in global health governance over the past three decades" [1]. To successfully raise awareness of shared causes—in particular those related to norms, such as respectful care—however, networks need tools to help them plan and coordinate their work, ultimately allowing them to reinforce rather than duplicate each other's efforts [2]. Furthermore, monitoring and evaluating awareness raising has historically been a challenge for researchers and program implementers, and work is needed to provide tools to track progress and impact in this area.

Health messages that reach the entire spectrum of stakeholders at once—from patients, caregivers, and health facility managers, to local, state, national, and global policymakers—versus those that just reach a single group of stakeholders are more likely to raise awareness of an issue [3], but few organizations have the resources to implement such a comprehensive undertaking. A network of organizations and/or individuals can pool its resources and tap into its individual connections to facilitate efforts that can reach beyond the capacity of a single actor [4, 5]. However, unlike individual organizations or formal alliances guided by a specific contract, network members nearly always participate on a voluntary basis and leadership is often spread out among the members [1]. Thus, guiding frameworks and tools are especially important when many groups are working together, bringing different resources and perspectives to the table.

The RMC movement, catalyzed by the RMC Global Council, provides a particularly interesting case for examining and learning from the work of a global health network. The council, formed in 2011, now includes more than 300 individuals from around the globe, all of whom have a keen interest in advancing and protecting the rights of childbearing women. The council meets regularly and engages in advocacy and information-sharing globally and locally. We set out to learn from the success of the RMC Global Council and the RMC movement it helped engender to develop a tool—a framework for awareness raising—useful for networks focused on global health and human rights.

Raising awareness

Networks can play a key role in raising awareness of an issue, which is often the first step in catalyzing change. Awareness messages "provide general background ... and can be used to reinforce the importance of informed action and behavioral change" [6]. Many issues in global health—including maternal health—have gained traction through the efforts of networks [3, 4, 7]. A historic document, a landmark event, an engaging or powerful champion, and the persistence of many dedicated advocates can direct attention to an issue, raising both awareness and resources. A recent systematic review of efforts to raise awareness of maternal health rights found that "efforts that pursued multi-level, stakeholder and sectoral pathways were likely to build synergies that sustain the promotion of rights over the long term" [5].

Nevertheless, evaluating the effectiveness of awareness-raising activities is challenging, particularly in the case of policy and advocacy and when traditional media (e.g. television, radio) with existing standards for measurement are not employed. A 2014 high-level convening of the Global Policy & Advocacy and Measurement & Evaluation teams at the Bill & Melinda Gates Foundation (BMGF) emphasized that when evaluating awareness related to policy and advocacy, "the field ... is still evolving" and "the focus should be on contribution, not attribution" [8]. Interestingly, Shiffman identifies a similar challenge when describing the difficulty of attributing change to the work of a network: "Detecting network influence is more difficult as one moves from outputs to policy consequences to impact" [1]. The consensus that emerged from the high-level convening was that monitoring and evaluation (M&E) practices, such as the application of behavior change theories and the development of indicators, can provide structure to awareness-raising efforts that can aid in tracking progress [2, 8].

Focusing on contribution rather than attribution, we can use at least two "tracer" indicators to track the success of the RMC Global Council and its members' work to raise awareness of RMC: research papers and news articles published and national dialogues conducted. These tracers can signal the contributions of the council and its members' work. A PubMed search for "respectful maternity care," "disrespect and abuse," or "obstetric violence" published between 2000 and 2009 results in zero papers, while the same search terms yield 82 papers on the topic published in 2010 or later. Indeed, more than half of those papers were published within the last two years. In popular culture, a Google News search for "respectful maternity care" articles published between 2000 and 2009 again finds zero articles, while the same search results in 42 news articles published since 2010. The specific search strategy can be found in Table 1.

Furthermore, since 2010, RMC has been a topic of national dialogue among law- and decision-makers in Nigeria, Afghanistan, Nepal, and Malawi, resulting in the specific inclusion of RMC in laws or professional standards [9–13]. Taking this as evidence of an increased

Table 1 "Respectful maternity care" 1 publications search strategy

PubMed
("respectful maternity care"[All Fields] OR "disrespect and abuse"[All Fields]) OR "obstetric violence"[All Fields] AND ("2000/01/01"[PDAT] : "2009/12/31"[PDAT])
("respectful maternity care"[All Fields] OR "disrespect and abuse"[All Fields]) OR "obstetric violence"[All Fields] AND ("2010/01/01"[PDAT] : "2018/3/29"[PDAT])
Google News
"respectful maternity care"[All Fields] AND ("2000/01/01":"2009/12/31")
"respectful maternity care"[All Fields] AND ("2010/01/01":"2018/3/29")

awareness of D&A and RMC within the period in which the RMC Global Council was active, we looked for explanatory frameworks that could help explain *how* RMC awareness-raising efforts led to the observed impact. Our search for tools and frameworks for raising awareness yielded topic-specific tools and toolkits with indicators and social or behavioral change theories [14–17] that are not necessarily applicable to other health issues or audiences. For example, toolkits for raising awareness on managing household mercury waste [18], literacy in Europe [19], and gender roles and political participation in the Middle East and North Africa [20] do not share common measures of success or even social or behavioral change theories. Thus, a gap remains, leaving a need for a broader tool that can help networks to effectively raise awareness of any topic across many stakeholder groups.

Disrespect & Abuse/Respectful Maternity Care

D&A—also known as "mistreatment" or "obstetric violence"—includes physical, verbal, and sexual abuse, violations of privacy, confidentiality, and/or consent, and detainment of the woman or her baby for failure to pay for the services provided at a facility [21–23]. Childbirth is a uniquely vulnerable time, and what happens during this period can have lasting effects on the health and wellbeing of both mother and baby. RMC applies human rights principles to maternity care to ensure that all women and their newborns receive high-quality interpersonal care throughout the childbearing process. As the White Ribbon Alliance (WRA) describes, RMC is a "universal human right due to every childbearing woman in every health system" [24].

In the 1970s, women's rights advocates first exposed cases of women being disrespected or abused in health facilities during labor and delivery [22]. In the 1990s, work by Rachel Jewkes [25] in South Africa and the primarily-Latin American movement to combat *violencia obstetrica* (obstetric violence) [26–28] continued to underscore the need for increased attention to women's rights during childbirth. Later, as more women around the world were encouraged to seek facility-based care during pregnancy and childbirth [29], research thrust provider behaviors and facility and health system failures into the spotlight [30]. Despite this important work, the global magnitude and significance of D&A remained a silent, veiled issue. Anecdotally, many providers and pregnant or postpartum women expressed familiarity with such injustice, but the lack of public awareness about D&A and its effect on utilization of facilities led to continued silence and mistreatment [30–32].

In 2010, the United States Agency for International Development (USAID) allocated funding towards research and advocacy on the subject, convening members of the global community to initiate a concerted effort against D&A. USAID initially commissioned the seminal paper, "Exploring Evidence for Disrespect and Abuse in Facility-based Childbirth: Report of a Landscape Analysis," by Diana Bowser and Kathleen Hill [30], which was followed by funding for projects in Kenya and Tanzania to study the prevalence and drivers of D&A and design tailored interventions to address it, led by the Population Council and the Averting Maternal Death and Disability (AMDD) program at Columbia University, respectively [33–35]. USAID-funded advocacy activities, led by the WRA, centered on convening stakeholders, developing strategies, and undertaking activities that would raise awareness of D&A and the need to provide RMC for all women. To do so, WRA formed the RMC Global Council, whose first joint action was the development of "Respectful Maternity Care: Universal Rights of Childbearing Women," more commonly referred to as the "RMC Charter," which was released in 2011 [36]. Since then, the council has encouraged research into and dialogue around RMC by conducting a global survey on RMC, creating a publicly-available wiki page online to act as a repository for RMC resources, and releasing briefs on RMC in different contexts, among other activities [37].

In concert with the formation of the RMC Global Council and the momentum created by the studies in Kenya and Tanzania, several other programs and activists began to adopt RMC-related work. USAID continued to fund research as well as implementation programs through the Maternal and Child Health Integrated Program (MCHIP) and, later, the Maternal Child Survival Program (MCSP). But what was it about these activities—and subsequent events—and the individuals and organizations driving the movement that helped land RMC on the global and national maternal health agenda?

The RMC Global Council's work from 2010 to 2016 provides an illustrative example of how a global health network can successfully raise awareness of an issue across multiple groups of stakeholders, from individual women seeking maternal health care to the global organizations that set the agenda for millions. The purpose of this case study is to learn from the experiences and successes of the RMC Global Council to inform the development of a validated, empirically-grounded strategic framework that outlines the critical success factors for effectively raising awareness of a policy- and human rights-related issue. Although the framework is likely most effective when employed by a network, many of its components also apply to individual activists.

Methods

Case study approach

To identify the critical success factors that raised the visibility of and concern for RMC within the global maternal health agenda, we selected a qualitative case study approach. Case studies are well suited to examine a real-life phenomenon in depth and in context [38]. Given that the work of the RMC Global Council was executed by numerous organizations and individuals and was intended to reach a broad audience, the case study approach is an appropriate method for capturing and compiling the various strategies and tactics used by the different council members and organizations into a coherent framework. Furthermore, to our knowledge there are no other close examinations of awareness raising in the context of maternal health and human rights. The case of RMC is thus unique, as is our approach of examining the phenomenon of RMC from the perspective of both those implementing the awareness-raising efforts—the "influencers"—and those affected by the efforts—the "influenced."

Framework development

We reviewed the literature on theories and frameworks for raising awareness in public health, human rights, and communication to guide the development of study tools. Given the absence of one theoretical model or tool that provided a suitable explanatory framework for the case of D&A/RMC movement, we combined three relevant resources into a new draft framework for raising awareness: the Framework for Effective Campaigns (FfEC) [39], the Spitfire SmartChart 3.0 tool (Smart Chart) [40], and Network Theory [41]. The FfEC is not a formal theory but provides recommendations for developing public information campaigns meant to influence decision-makers at the policy level. Given that addressing D&A and normalizing RMC requires changes at the interpersonal as well as policy level, this framework's recommendations—encompassing multiple perspectives—are particularly relevant to the case at hand. The SmartChart is a tool to help nonprofit organizations create effective, strategic communication campaigns. WRA used the SmartChart to guide its advocacy strategy development during the period under study, thus making it a pertinent tool against which to evaluate the case of RMC. (Note that for the purposes of this paper, we defined "campaign" as organized efforts intended to achieve a common goal with a focus on awareness raising, including but not limited to advocacy, public information, or communications.) Finally, Network Theory examines the way associated individuals and groups interact, partner, and share resources with one another in order to achieve individual and shared goals. This mix of resources was chosen strategically: because of the multi-disciplinary, multi-stakeholder nature of the RMC Global Council—and the varied approaches the council members took to awareness raising (e.g. research, communications, and policy advocacy)—it made sense to cast a wide net and consider scholarly frameworks, job aids and tools, and broader social theories, in order to capture the complexities of such a diverse network. Together, these three resources address the spectrum of characteristics underpinning the RMC awareness-raising effort: policy change, formal communication planning, and strategic partnerships and networks. Using the FfEC, the SmartChart, and Network Theory, we drafted a theoretical framework—using language from the three resources—for raising awareness across multiple audience levels to be validated with data gathered through qualitative research methods. Some of the elements can be found in more than one of the resources (e.g. "define and describe the target audience"), while others are unique to a particular source or are a modification of an existing element. Table 2 outlines the different elements and indicates the resource from which it was derived.

Study participants

Study participants were categorized into the following two groups: the "influencers"—or those who implemented the awareness-raising efforts—and the "influenced"—those who were affected by the efforts. An initial list of influencers was generated through purposive sampling using the list of names on the RMC Charter [42]. The influencers included researchers, program implementers, human rights specialists, legal advocates, educators, and individuals associated with donor agencies. The list of influenced individuals included those who have initiated and/or participated in RMC-related efforts at global, national, and local levels, such as researchers, program implementers, government officials, and community activists. This list was generated using snowball and purposive sampling. Theorizing that the council's global work would drive national changes, we

Table 2 Draft awareness-raising framework

A successful awareness-raising effort ...	FfEC	SmartChart	Network Theory	New
...is supported by a clearly-defined strategic plan.				
Define your position		X		
Define the ultimate goal		X		
Assess (continually) the current context and environment				X
...targets the right audience and aims to capture its attention.				
Define and describe the target audience, including their readiness and core concerns	X	X	X	X
Select appropriate communication channels and expose the audience sufficiently	X	X		
Stand out and be noticeable	X			
...delivers a credible, understandable message.				
Select a credible source and messenger	X	X	X	
Craft a clear message	X			
Fit the message with prior knowledge and the current context and environment	X			X
...delivers a message that influences the audience.				
Provide information	X		X	
Direct attention	X			
Trigger norms	X		X	
Change underlying values and/or preferences	X			
Select overall theme and tone of message		X		
Expose the audience sufficiently		X		
...shapes contexts and environments.				
Leverage the problems and pressures that govern behavior	X			
Involve the audience	X			
Use multiple channels	X			
Coordinate with like-minded partners/organizations/individuals			X	X
...is supported by sufficient resources.				
Identify and allocate human and financial resources		X		

FfEC: Framework for Effective Campaigns
SmartChart: Spitfire SmartChart 3.0
Network Theory: Network Theory

asked several members of the RMC Global Council to recommend individuals who have pushed RMC at a national level with whom we could speak (snowball sampling). We also used a Google search to identify professional organizations and researchers engaged in D&A/RMC-related work (purposive sampling). Interviews with the influenced individuals assessed the effectiveness of the activities and efforts undertaken by the influencers. Although many of the influenced individuals later became influencers themselves, the two groups were divided based on whether they participated in the development of the RMC Charter, given the charter's role as one of the first group efforts of the RMC Global Council. Ethics approval for this study was granted by the Harvard T.H. Chan School of Public Health Office of Human Research Administration.

Data collection

Data were collected using semi-structured key informant interviews that were conducted via online conferencing platform and directed by interview guides (see Additional files 1 and 2). During the interviews, influencers and the influenced individuals provided details of their individual activities and interest in D&A/RMC as well as the activities or approaches of the organizations with whom they were working during the study period. The interview guide for influencers organized questions around each of the components of the framework for raising awareness with the aim of validating those components (by identifying whether the component was utilized, or "present"), extracting any additional themes, and identifying the events, individuals, organizations, and documents that both participant groups considered most impactful over the study period. The questions included in the interview guide for influenced individuals aimed to identify:

a. the messages being sent by the influencers and their respective organizations;
b. the appealing aspects of the D&A/RMC-related messages; and
c. the messengers, events, and documents that were particularly influential in raising their awareness of D&A/RMC.

For consistency, one member of the study team (MO'C) conducted the interviews and took detailed notes; interviews were recorded for reference only. Prior to commencing the interviews, each study participant provided informed consent which was captured in the notes and on interview recordings. Two members of the study team (MO'C and KM) analyzed the interview notes using deductive and inductive thematic coding. First, the interview notes were coded to identify those components of the draft awareness-raising framework that were present, not present, or not mentioned in each transcript. Next, inductive thematic analysis was used to identify any themes not included in the framework. The emergent themes were discussed and refined. All data and themes were analyzed using Nvivo 11.4.1 software (QSR International, USA). Prior to commencing analysis as a whole, the study team selected three sets of interview notes, coded them each independently, and compared the results to test inter-rater reliability. Once the study team reached an inter-rater reliability greater than 80%, the remaining 25 sets of interview notes were compared to the framework and coded. The study team also noted the events, documents, and individuals that each informant identified as being most influential in raising awareness of D&A and advancing the RMC agenda.

Results

Twenty-eight individuals were interviewed, including 20 "influencers" and eight "influenced." The influencers came from research and academia, health professional organizations, non-governmental organizations, government and donor agencies, human rights law, program implementation, and advocacy. The influenced individuals represented six countries and worked in the fields of research and academia, health professional organizations, non-governmental organizations, and government organizations. Data from the interviews informed the refinement and validation of the framework for awareness raising.

Primary results: Validated framework for awareness raising

The final, validated framework for raising awareness includes five strategies that characterize a successful awareness-raising effort.

1. The effort utilizes elements of strategic planning
2. The effort aims to capture the attention of key stakeholders
3. The effort delivers a consistent persuasive message
4. The effort creates a receptive environment
5. The effort maximizes all existing and potential resources

Within each strategy is a set of tactics—framed as actions—that can operationalize the strategy. The resulting 20 tactics are organized into three groups based on the proportion of key informants who described using a component in their work: integral (reported by 80% or more influencers), helpful (reported by 50–79% of influencers), and variable (reported by fewer than 50% of influencers). See Table 3 below.

Overall, 14 of the 20 elements in the draft framework were used by 80% or more of the influencers and can thus be considered integral to create a successful

Table 3 Validated awareness-raising framework

A successful awareness-raising effort …	Score	Integral	Helpful	Variable
...utilizes elements of strategic planning.				
Clearly define your position on the topic	.90	X		
Clearly define your end goal or objectives	.75		X	
Constantly assess and adapt to the environment and context in which you are working	.95	X		
...aims to capture the attention of key stakeholders.				
Clearly define the target audience	.95	X		
Identify and pay attention to the different levels of influence (take a multi-level approach to identifying and approaching the target audience)*	.65		X	
Use communication channels that are appropriate given your target audience's preferences and behaviors	.90	X		
Find ways to stand out and be noticeable	.25			X
...delivers a consistent, persuasive message.				
Ensure that your message is delivered by a credible messenger and uses credible sources	.95	X		
Ensure that your message is clear	.90	X		
Ensure that your message aligns with the target audience's prior knowledge and the current context	.85	X		
Establish a shared, consistent language/lexicon, particularly when working with a loose coalition*	.70		X	
Ensure that the message is informative	.75		X	
Use your message and tactics to lead the target audience's attention to your topic	.50		X	
Leverage the norms that guide your target audience's behaviors	.80	X		
Leverage the target audience's values and preferences and find ways to change or shift those	.80	X		
Select a consistent and appealing theme or tone for your message	.85	X		
Ensure that the audience is exposed to the message sufficiently for it to sink in	.40			X
...creates a receptive environment.				
Leverage the problems and pressures that govern the audience's behavior(s)	.85	X		
Involve the audience in your efforts to develop or spread the message	.60		X	
Use multiple channels to reach the audience	.85	X		
...maximizes all existing and potential resources.				
Coordinate with like-minded partners (individuals and organizations)	1.0	X		
Identify your internal and external human and financial resources and allocate them wisely	1.0	X		
Leverage individuals' passion for the topic especially when the work is largely unfunded*	.70		X	

*Emergent theme

awareness-raising effort as they were constant across nearly all influencers regardless of setting, context, goal, or resource capacity. Of those 14 elements, eight were used by 90% or more of the influencers. For example, 90% ($n = 18$) of the influencers reported outlining a clearly defined position on RMC. Among those, the positions (of both individuals and organizations) fell into three categories: RMC as a human right, RMC as a quality of care issue, and RMC as a behavioral norm. A constant awareness of the current environment and willingness to adapt the effort and message accordingly was also integral (reported by 95% of influencers). Researchers and advocates took into account the existing legal, political, medical-cultural, and system factors/norms that might influence their audience's beliefs and behaviors around pregnancy or childbirth. For example, one influencer working in Latin America explained that, "It was a favorable context [for RMC] in Bolivia, Ecuador, and Mexico. There was a strong consolidation of women's groups and good media coverage of women's/indigenous rights, and constitutional frameworks. It was a context in which there was accountability and awareness of the duty bearer's responsibility." Context shaped the way the influencers approached their work, and often, changes to goals or positions were in response to changes in the environment. Several respondents used the term "evolved" or "evolving" to describe the environment and context as well as their approach to promoting RMC.

Nearly all of the influencers (95%, $n = 19$) stated that they had a clearly defined target audience. Although not all influencers were concerned with the same audiences, the influencers reported targeting pregnant women, indigenous women's groups, consumer groups, medical and midwifery students and practitioners, doulas, health care facility administrators, local parliamentarians, lawyers, academics, researchers, donors, and international development agencies. Some influencers focused on one audience while others found ways to reach multiple groups: one influencer explained, "[as an organization we] were trying to target maternity services worldwide. But as an obstetrician, I have been targeting medical education in personal work; with both medical students and qualified doctors as well as NHS midwives to make them aware of human rights in childbirth, respectful maternity care, and obstetric violence." Influencers also reported using appropriate (i.e., relevant to the target audience's information-consumption habits) communication channels (90%, $n = 18$) and employing credible messengers and sources (95%, $n = 19$) to share a clear message (90%, n = 18). "Using appropriate channels" meant attending and presenting at key maternal health technical meetings and human rights fora for some, or for others, creating posters on D&A/RMC and distributing them to health facilities. Credible messengers included leaders in maternal health from donor agencies (e.g. USAID), academia and research (e.g. AMDD), and professional organizations (e.g. IMBCO, DONA International).

For most of the influencers, the messages used were closely tied to each organization's or individual's position and centered on the basic concepts of human rights, respect for women (and providers), respect for culture and the variety of experience, and quality of care. The messages also differed slightly depending on the target audience in order to make the message as appealing as possible. As one influencer explained, "Because [our organization] works at so many levels (global, country-level and national and subnational levels) we strategically target our RMC messaging to specific audiences, using messages that we think will resonate with distinct stakeholders: [for example, we focus on] professional ethics for provider professional associations, human rights for women's groups, increasing institutional delivery for policymakers, quality of care for Ministry of Health stakeholders, providers and clients, etc." Another influencer working in research and implementation noted that her organization "had three levels of messages: policy level ... health facility, and the community."

Importantly, this research evaluated awareness-raising efforts that extended beyond traditional message dissemination. Because few of the influencers were engaged in formal communications campaigns, other actions such as funding programs or conducting research related to RMC conveyed the message that RMC was a priority. All influencers also reported identifying and strategically allocating human, financial, and material resources (100%, $n = 20$). Finally, all influencers reported partnering with other likeminded individuals and organizations (100%, n = 20), highlighting the importance of partnerships for successful awareness raising. As one influencer from an international development agency explained, "Coming from a health system perspective and structural perspective, when thinking about things that are non-health but that still affect health, you begin to put together a network [of organizations]. Nothing that's important to be done can be done by a single group. You can't change policy or be proactive alone, much less sustain those changes over time. We all need to be good colleagues and think about large ecological frameworks. Thinking about continuity is important, and partnerships are a part of that."

Four of the 20 elements from the draft framework were used by 50–79% of respondents and can be considered "helpful" when creating and executing an awareness-raising effort. Defining an end goal or objectives (75%, $n = 15$), creating an informative (70%, $n = 14$) and attention-getting (50%, $n = 10$) message, and involving the target audience in the effort to raise awareness (60%, $n = 12$) were all helpful tactics for influencers. Participants described various ways in which they involved the target audience. One influencer videotaped providers during a birth and played it back for them so that they could see their own behavior—both respectful and disrespectful—firsthand. Another influencer described creating opportunities for dialogues between women and health providers "so they can exchange ideas about good practices ... *best* practices" related to RMC.

Three additional elements—not included in the original draft framework—were identified through thematic analysis and fall into the "helpful" group: 1) identify and pay attention to the different levels of influence in maternity care (described further below); 2) use a shared, consistent lexicon around D&A/RMC; and 3) leverage individuals' passion for RMC and human rights to support work when funding is low or nonexistent.

Sixty-five percent ($n = 13$) of the influencers noted that they identified and took into consideration the different levels of influence affecting maternity care when planning their work. These levels of influence include individual care providers, pregnant women, facility administrators, national decision makers, and global influencers, such as the World Health Organization (WHO). For example, one influencer explained that, "a big part for us is articulating a comprehensive strategy with different elements and targets—at the policy systems level, point of care with providers, and rights and demand perspective from women themselves." On the other hand, an influencer whose work focused on research and facility-level solutions remarked that theirs was, "a very multipronged approach to look at whatever seemed to be a driver [of disrespect and abuse] in the facility."

Seventy percent ($n = 14$) of respondents expressed the importance of having a shared language or lexicon regarding D&A/RMC among all of the different organizations and individuals acting as influencers; by using the agreed-upon term "respectful maternity care," influencers felt they could support and complement, rather than distract from, the work being done by partners and other likeminded advocates. One influencer noted that, "as the debate [about D&A] has become more refined, there's been more clarity. 'Respectful maternity care' is a good way of framing it. And that became a catch phrase, or a good hook for what's fundamentally a moral and ethical orientation." Another influencer highlighted the importance of using the term consistently: "We developed our measurement [of D&A] based on Bowser and Hill's work, but since [the WHO] paper on different groupings of mistreatment, we're using that. And ... we won't stop calling it [respectful maternity care] now, because the movement is there."

A passionate commitment to RMC, high-quality care, and women's rights were identified as central to the effort to raise awareness of D&A/RMC. More than half of the influencers ($n = 14$) described themselves or their colleagues as "volunteers," all driven by the same commitment to RMC and women's health and rights in general. One influencer described herself and her network of colleagues working on RMC as "a coalition of the willing." Another influencer explained: "We're also part of what is a growing movement where we interact with many people with no expectation of money changing hands or formal engagement. We're just working toward a shared goal."

Finally, two of the 20 elements from the draft framework were used by fewer than half of the respondents and thus can be considered "variable." One quarter of influencers reported that they tried to find ways to stand out and be noticeable; for example, one influencer cited a promotional book tour that provided an opportunity to meet with women and speak about respectful maternity care. While only 40% ($n = 8$) of influencers reported that they made an effort to expose the audience sufficiently to their message, such efforts may have been captured in another component of the framework (see "use multiple channels").

Secondary results: Insights from influenced individuals

The influenced individuals reported hearing RMC-related messages that were well aligned with the messages being shared by the influencers: that RMC is a quality of care issue, a human right, and/or a behavioral norm. The messages were appealing to the influenced individuals primarily because of alignment with their existing work or interests. Participants reported that they could easily connect the need for RMC to their work at various levels of the health system, for example, in prevention of mother-to-child transmission (PMTCT) of HIV, the Sustainable Development Goals and the WHO Quality of Care Network, and gender-based violence. The influenced individuals also noted that the emergence of a single term ("respectful maternity care") from the global community was meaningful, but that it was important that influencers also allowed for tailoring the messages and materials to local languages and contexts. For example, one influenced individual explained that in the local context in which he works, "the direct translation of 'disrespect and abuse' [into the local language] isn't the same—it's much stronger—and [health care workers] don't think they're engaging in such harsh behaviors. So we say 'lack of respect.'"

Influenced individuals also noted the key role that the engagement and partnerships of influential, trusted players in global maternal health played in encouraging involvement in the RMC movement. One researcher described a technical meeting on RMC featuring a number of international and national development organizations: "Everyone was sharing their experiences and the complexities of trying to define RMC and conduct research. And from that ... is what launched [our organization's] work in the area."

Validating influential events, documents, and individuals

The research team also reviewed the interview transcripts to identify the individuals, organizations, documents, and events that both groups of respondents cited as instrumental in raising awareness of D&A and RMC. Using these data, we created two word clouds (see Fig. 1 below) that show the similarities and differences regarding what was considered most influential in raising awareness of D&A and RMC during the study period. For the influencers, the most influential documents, events, organizations, and individuals in the effort to raise awareness of D&A and the need for RMC tended to be at a higher global level. For example, many of the influencers cited the work of Bowser and Hill [30], as well as individual RMC champions at WHO and USAID. The events, documents, or individuals that the influenced participants felt were particularly influential in raising awareness of D&A/RMC, however, tended to be those that operated at a more local level, engaging the specific countries and communities in which they (the influenced participants) were working, such as the WRA, Population Council, and AMDD.

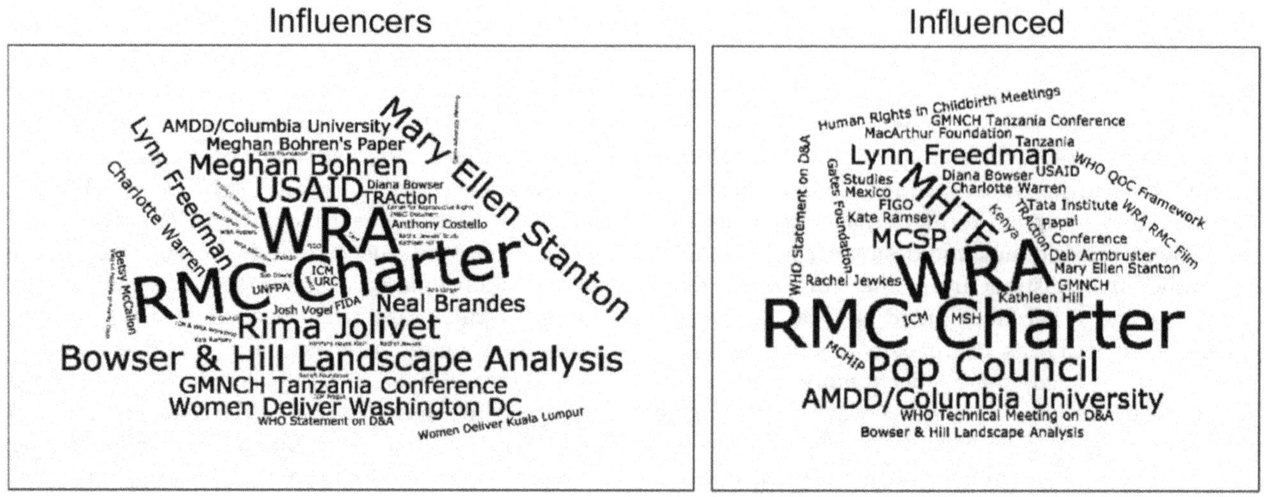

Fig. 1 Word clouds depicting key individuals, organizations, documents, and events in the in the D&A/RMC awareness-raising effort, by key informant type

Discussion

The results of this case study suggest that the increase in awareness of D&A/RMC can be attributed to the use of the five strategies and their accompanying tactics outlined in the validated framework described above. By utilizing these strategies and tactics, the RMC Global Council was able to plan wisely and use their resources effectively in order to share the right messages with the appropriate stakeholders and create an environment that was and is receptive to the concept of respectful maternity care.

Beyond identifying and validating specific, successful strategies and tactics for raising awareness, the results suggest that the respectful maternity care movement also benefited from the RMC Global Council taking an approach that valued consistency, flexibility, and collaboration.

Consistency in position, message, language, and target audience among the influencers helped to create a unified message despite the lack of a formal, overarching communications, public information, or advocacy campaign guiding the actors' work. The influencers who chose to align D&A/RMC within human rights and quality of care positions linked to two larger current issues in maternal health, giving them the ability to utilize existing networks of allies, resources, and language. It also allowed them to embed their message into those of their allies, as evidenced by the data indicating that RMC was appealing to individuals and organizations working in various fields, from global maternal health directives to gender-based violence to PMTCT. Those whose position framed RMC as a behavioral norm were able to tap into the target audiences' core values. Both positions also tied closely to what Smith and Shiffman describe as the existing global health community's understanding of maternal survival as an issue of social justice and women's rights [3]. The messages that influencers selected were closely tied to their chosen positions and centered on the concepts of human rights, respect for women (and care providers), respect for culture and the variety of experience, and quality of care. A relatively consistent use of the term "respectful maternity care" among multiple influencers likely helped create a stronger, more cohesive message. While RMC was not the only term used—others were selected based on local contexts—the use of this one, shared term reinforced the impression that this was a multi-partner, multi-stakeholder movement. Finally, a common understanding of the different target audiences—especially care providers and policymakers—who needed to hear the message meant that often, influencers' messages converged or reached the same audience members at different points, reinforcing the message.

Flexibility within the influencers' approaches to their D&A/RMC-related work also supported their awareness raising efforts. By maintaining a constant awareness of the context in which they were working and a willingness to adapt and evolve given that context, the influencers were able to maintain their relevance and level of persuasion regardless of environmental changes. Mechanisms and efforts to allow for tailoring via language (i.e., translating into local languages and commonly understood, contextually-relevant terms, such as "obstetric violence" or "mistreatment" versus "disrespect and abuse")—while still complementing the shared lexicon—and message choice also supported that flexibility. The recognition that culturally appropriate language, materials, and channels must be employed highlights the importance of using the right words—in the right language—to make a message as clear as possible for the target audience. This is a similar finding to that of a recent review of principles and processes of promoting maternal health rights in which the authors describe this "process of vernacularism as being critical for local stakeholders to adopt rights principles" [5]. Several influencers also noted that they used different messages for different audiences. The purpose of this tactic was to ensure that each audience was receiving a message that would resonate most with them given their interests, concerns, prior knowledge, and values. Global health networks may benefit from the finding that while consistency—as noted above—is important for creating a sense of belonging to a larger movement, flexibility is equally as important to ensure that messages, materials, and approaches resonate with the community in which they are shared. The case of RMC is an insightful example of how networks can achieve balance, creating a movement to effect change at both the global and local levels.

Finally, collaboration among the influencers and their individual networks helped synchronize messages and allowed organizations to amplify their reach as well as complement and support shared goals. Organizational buy-in also created opportunities for more individuals to get involved, creating a mutually supportive environment and growing the community of RMC advocates. Every influencer used partnerships to gain access to resources and audiences they could not access alone. Partnerships allowed influencers to leverage the authority of trusted messengers and experts in other organizations as well as to lend individuals the authority of their and others' backing organizations.

Jeremy Shiffman posits that global health networks face four primary challenges: problem-defining, positioning, coalition-building, and governance [7]. The RMC Global Council's use of consistent messaging and a shared language with room for tailoring to specific contexts helped to overcome Shiffman's first two challenges, and the council's partnerships helped to overcome the challenge of coalition-building. Indeed, all of these factors may have also been supported by the strength of the existing maternal health network: both Shiffman and Smith (2016) note that the network of global health actors driving the maternal health agenda can be considered among the more successful examples of global health networks of the past few decades thanks to concerted efforts to clearly define the problem and agree on a position [3, 4, 7].

The findings of this case study should be considered in light of some methodological limitations. First, it relied solely on the recollections of individuals who acted as influencers and the influenced individuals, which are subject to memory or recall bias. Second, the sample size was limited, particularly in the case of the influenced individuals. Including more influenced individuals could have provided greater insight into how the messages shared by members of the RMC Global Council's resonated in a wider variety of settings (e.g. other countries/regions, different types of organizations). Including more individuals overall—influencers and influenced—could have also provided an even more robust picture of the case, but this study was not designed to test saturation. Third, although the study team made an effort to consider awareness-raising resources from a variety of fields, the process to select the resources ultimately used to build the draft framework was inherently subjective and thus, other relevant theories, tools, or frameworks may have been overlooked. Finally, the data collection tools were structured around the awareness-raising framework, which used a number of communications concepts and terms (e.g. message, tone, communication channel) that seemed unfamiliar or irrelevant to several of the key informants given that their work was not part of a formal communications campaign or strategy. Indeed, one influencer noted that she and her colleagues "never saw [themselves] as raising awareness in the way that communications or advocacy people do" and reiterated throughout her interview that her organization's work was not done with a communications mindset. Although analysis of the key informants' responses showed that many of the respondents were indeed using the concepts included in the framework, the fact that the respondents did not recognize the terms used may have affected their understanding of and responses to the interview questions.

The validated framework describes the strategies and tactics needed for a successful awareness-raising "effort" that entails more than a traditional communications, public information, or advocacy campaign. As the case of D&A/RMC awareness raising demonstrates, not all individuals or organizations commenced their work with the express intention of raising awareness about D&A or RMC; several of the influencers represented research organizations exploring the causes of D&A in order to identify ways to promote RMC. Indeed, only one of the influencer organizations (WRA) we spoke with used a formal tool or theory (SmartChart) to guide their work. Often, raising awareness about D&A/RMC was embedded in research projects, programs, or training sessions on other maternal and newborn health, quality of care, and human rights topics. "Effort" is thus perhaps a more comprehensive term than campaign, and one that allows for the inclusion of a variety of activities and makes the resulting framework relevant for a broader audience. Furthermore, presented thus, this innovative framework outlining key strategies for successful awareness-raising efforts becomes a tool that networks can use to overcome some of the challenges of problem-defining, positioning, and coalition-building.

Conclusion

This case study draws on the FfEC, SmartChart 3.0, and Network Theory to develop a new awareness-raising framework, and, in doing so, provides a fresh, new perspective on each of these existing resources. By linking these three resources together, we have created a robust new framework that allows networks of advocates to approach awareness raising from multiple angles and levels—including policy change, formal communication planning, and strategic partnerships and networks—simultaneously and address issues that others have identified as perennial challenges to networks' success. As others have pointed out, awareness for awareness's sake is not enough [43–45]. Because many of the members of the RMC Global Council were not focused specifically on awareness-raising as an end, but rather, a means to an end (such as informing research findings or policy change), raising awareness of D&A and the need for RMC was an important precursor to empowering women to speak up for themselves, changing laws and policies to promote RMC and protect women's rights, and improving facility conditions and the quality of health care.

Thus, the results of this case study present two opportunities for networks. First, the RMC Global Council can learn from its own success as it strategizes future directions and next steps for ensuring every woman's right to RMC (as well as providers' rights to respectful working conditions). Second, and more broadly, other global health networks—and their respective researchers, program planners, and advocates—can utilize this validated framework, with its clear strategies and tactics, to help plan and evaluate future campaigns designed to raise awareness of neglected issues and in doing so, drive momentum in global health, human rights, and quality of care.

Abbreviations

AMDD: Averting Maternal Death and Disability (Columbia University); D&A: disrespect and abuse during childbirth; FFEC: Framework for Effective Campaigns; RMC: Respectful maternity care; USAID: United States Agency for International Development; WHO: World Health Organization; WRA: White Ribbon Alliance

Acknowledgements

The authors would like to thank all key informants who participated in this study, as well as Dr. Ana Langer (Women and Health Initiative, Harvard T.H. Chan School of Public Health) for supporting the project, Betsy McCallon (White Ribbon Alliance) and Elena Ateva (White Ribbon Alliance) for providing access to the RMC Global Council, and Dr. Shoba Ramanandhan (Dana Farber Cancer Institute) for providing input to the study design and tool development. We would also like to thank Emily Peca and James M. Sherry from the USAID Translating Research into Action (TRAction) project.

Funding

Funding for this study was provided by the Bill & Melinda Gates Foundation.

Authors' contributions

MO'C and RRJ developed the study concept and design. MO'C led the development of the study tools with support from KM and RRJ. MO'C conducted all key informant interviews. MO'C and KM completed the data analysis and developed the final, validated framework. MO'C led the writing with support from KM and oversight from RRJ.

Competing interests

The authors declare they have no competing interests.

References

1. Shiffman J, Quissell K, Schmitz HP, Pelletier DL, Smith SL, Berlan D, Gneiting U, Van Slyke D, Mergel I, Rodriguez M, et al. A framework on the emergence and effectiveness of global health networks. Health Policy Plan. 2016; 31(Suppl 1):i3–16.
2. George AS, Branchini C, Portela A. Do interventions that promote awareness of rights increase use of maternity care services? A Systematic Review. PLoS One. 2015;10(10):e0138116.
3. Smith SL, Shiffman J. Setting the global health agenda: the influence of advocates and ideas on political priority for maternal and newborn survival. Soc Sci Med. 2016;166:86–93.
4. Smith SL, Rodriguez MA. Agenda setting for maternal survival: the power of global health networks and norms. Health Policy Plan. 2016;31(Suppl 1):i48–59.
5. George AS, Branchini C. Principles and processes behind promoting awareness of rights for quality maternal care services: a synthesis of stakeholder experiences and implementation factors. BMC Pregnancy Childbirth. 2017;17(1):264.
6. Sayers R. Principles of awarenes-raising: information literacy, a case study. In. UNESCO Asia and Pacific Regional Bureau for Education: Bangkok, Thailand; 2006.
7. Shiffman J. Four challenges that Global Health networks face. Int J Health Policy Manag. 2017;6(4):183–9.
8. TCC Group: High-Level Notes from the Convening. In: Assessing Policy and Advocacy Efforts: The Road Forward in M&E: 2014; Seattle, Washington; 2014.
9. Hastings MB. Pulling Back the curtain on disrespect and abuse: the movement to ensure respectful maternity care. In. Washington, DC: Health Policy Project; 2015.
10. Geddes J, Humphrey T, Wallace RM: Respectful midwifery care in Malawi: A human rights-based approach. Afr J Midwifery Womens Health 2017, 11(4).
11. Safe Motherhood Network Federation: August 2013 newsletter. In. Nepal; 2013.
12. Islamic Republic of Afghanistan Ministry of Public Health Public Relations Office: Ministry of Public Health holds Respectful Maternity Care Workshop. In. Kabul, Afghanistan; 2016.
13. Zaggi H. In search of enhanced health sector. Independent. Abuja, Nigeria: In; 2013.
14. Ajzen I: From intentions to actions: A theory of planned behavior In: Action control. edn. Heidelberg: Springer Berlin; 1985: 11–39.
15. Prochaska JO, Velicer WF. The transtheoretical model of health behavior change. Am J Health Promot. 1997;12(1):38–48.
16. Bronfenbrenner U: Ecological Models of Human Development. In: International Encyclopedia of Education. Volume 3, 2 edn. Edited by Elsevier; 1994.
17. Bandura A: Health promotion from the perspective of social cognitive theory. Psychol Health 1998, 13(4).
18. United Nations Environment Program: Development of an Awareness Raising Toolkit for Managing Mercury Waste at Household and Community Level: Summary Report. In.; 2011.
19. ELINET: Guide to Literacy Awareness Raising in Europe: Report on ELINET's Awareness Raising Toolkit. In. eli-net.eu: European Literacy Policy Network; 2015.
20. OXFAM. Norwegian Ministry of Foreign Affairs: the change Maker's toolkit: a toolkit for raising awareness on gender roles & women's political participation in the MENA region. In. Oxfam Great Britain: United Kingdom; 2014.

21. World Health Organization: The prevention and elimination of disrespect and abuse during facility-based childbirth. In: WHO Statement. Geneva, Switzerland: World Health Organization; 2015.
22. Miller S, Lalonde A. The global epidemic of abuse and disrespect during childbirth: history, evidence, interventions, and FIGO's mother-baby friendly birthing facilities initiative. Int J Gynaecol Obstet. 2015;131(Suppl 1):S49–52.
23. Bohren MA, Vogel JP, Hunter EC, Lutsiv O, Makh SK, Souza JP, Aguiar C, Saraiva Coneglian F, Diniz AL, Tuncalp O et al: The Mistreatment of Women during Childbirth in Health Facilities Globally: A Mixed-Methods Systematic Review. PLoS Med 2015, 12(6):e1001847; discussion.
24. [http://whiteribbonalliance.org/campaigns2/respectful-maternity-care/].
25. Jewkes R, Abrahams N, Mvo Z. Why do nurses abuse patients? Reflections from south African obstetric services. Soc Sci Med. 1998;47(11):1781–95.
26. Belli LF: La violencia obstétrica: otra forma de violación a los derechos humanos. Revista Redbioética/UNESCO Año 4 2013, 1(7):25–34.
27. Castro R, Erviti J. Violations of reproductive rights during hospital births in Mexico. Health and Human Rights. 2003;7(1):90–110.
28. d'Oliveira AF, Diniz SG, Schraiber LB. Violence against women in health-care institutions: an emerging problem. Lancet. 2002;359(9318):1681–5.
29. Campbell OM, Graham WJ. Lancet maternal survival series steering g: Strategies for reducing maternal mortality: getting on with what works. Lancet. 2006;368(9543):1284–99.
30. Bowser D, Hill K: Exploring Evidence for Disrespect and Abuse in Facility-Based Childbirth: Report of a Landscape Analysis. In. Edited by USAID-TRAction Project: Harvard School of Public Health, University Research Co. LLC; 2010.
31. Bohren MA, Hunter EC, Munthe-Kaas HM, Souza JP, Vogel JP, Gulmezoglu AM. Facilitators and barriers to facility-based delivery in low- and middle-income countries: a qualitative evidence synthesis. Reprod Health. 2014;11(1):71.
32. Khosla R, Zampas C, Vogel JP, Bohren MA, Roseman M, Erdman JN. International human rights and the mistreatment of women during childbirth. Health Hum Rights. 2016;18(2):131–43.
33. Abuya T, Warren CE, Miller N, Njuki R, Ndwiga C, Maranga A, Mbehero F, Njeru A, Bellows B. Exploring the prevalence of disrespect and abuse during childbirth in Kenya. PLoS One. 2015;10(4):e0123606.
34. Kruk ME, Kujawski S, Mbaruku G, Ramsey K, Moyo W, Freedman LP. Disrespectful and abusive treatment during facility delivery in Tanzania: a facility and community survey. Health Policy Plan. 2014.
35. Kujawski S, Mbaruku G, Freedman LP, Ramsey K, Moyo W, Kruk ME. Association between disrespect and abuse during childbirth and Women's confidence in health facilities in Tanzania. Matern Child Health J. 2015; 19(10):2243–50.
36. RMC Global Council: Respectful Maternity Care: Universal Rights of Childbearing Women. In. Edited by Alliance WR. Washington, DC; 2011.
37. Spotlight: White Ribbon Alliance Fosters a Growing Community of Practice to Advance Respectful Maternity Care [https://www.whiteribbonalliance.org/2018/01/31/white-ribbon-alliance-fosters-a-growing-community-of-practice-to-advance-respectful-maternity-care/].
38. Yin RK. Case study research: design and methods. 5th ed. Thousand Oaks, California: Sage Publications; 2013.
39. Weiss JA, Tschirhart M. Public info campaigns as policy instruments. J Policy Anal Management. 1994;13(1):82–119.
40. Spitfire Strategies: Smart Chart 3.0. In. Washington, D.C. : Spitfire Strategies; 2016.
41. Borgatti SP, Halgin DS. On Network Theory. Organ Sci. 2011;22(5).
42. Respectful Maternity Care: The Universal Rights of Childbearing Women. In. Washington, D.C. : White Ribbon Alliance; 2011.
43. Christiano A, Neimand A. Stop raising awareness already. Stanf Soc Innov Rev. Spring 2017;2017.
44. Purtle J, Roman LA. Health awareness days: sufficient evidence to support the craze? Am J Public Health. 2015;105(6):1061–5.
45. Beck J. What good is 'Raising awareness?'. The Atlantic: In; 2015.

18

Mapping the lack of public initiative against female genital mutilation in Denmark

Gro Møller Christoffersen[1], Peter James Bruhn[2*], Rosanna de Neergaard[3], Susanne Engel[4] and Vibeke Naeser[5]

Abstract

Background: Female genital mutilation (FGM) is a harmful practice prevalent in 35 countries, mainly in Africa, as well as in some Middle Eastern countries and a few Asian countries. FGM comprises all procedures that involve partial or complete resection of, or other injury to, external female genitalia for non-medical reasons. The practice of FGM has spread to Western countries due to migration. The European Institute for Gender Equality recommend that FGM be combatted by nationally coordinated efforts through implementation of national action plans, guidelines for professionals as well as comprehensive research in the field. FGM was outlawed in Denmark 2003, but no national actions plan has been implemented. Instead, the task of combatting FGM is currently under the responsibility of local governments in the form of the 98 municipalities. The aim of this study is to investigate the Danish municipalities' efforts to prevent FGM on the local level, and whether these initiatives are in accordance with international recommendations and standards.

Methods: All 98 Danish municipalities were invited to respond to a questionnaire regarding FGM in their respective municipalities. The inclusion process and questionnaire was designed after a pilot study, which included 29 municipalities. The questionnaire consisted of four overall areas of focus: "action plan", "registration", "information material" and "preventive initiatives". Demographic data were gathered from the 2017 census by Statistics Denmark. Risk countries were defined as countries with a tradition for FGM, identified from the 2016 UNICEF definition.

Results: A total of 67 municipalities participated in the study. At the time of census, 1.8% of the Danish population was immigrants with origins in risk countries. A total of 10.4% of the responding municipalities indicated to have implemented a specific action plan against FGM. A total of 7,5% had implemented specific preventive initiatives against FGM. Registration of reported FGM cases were indicated to be performed in 73.1% of the responding municipalities; however, only 17.9% stated to perform registration of FGM specifically as such, and not as general child abuse.

Conclusions: Our study shows that the current situation of FGM registration and prevention being under local administrative responsibility in the 98 Danish municipalities has led to a severe lack of coordinated public initiative against FGM.

Keywords: Female genital mutilation, Female genital cutting, Migrant health, Pricking

* Correspondence: peterjamesbruhn@gmail.com
[2]Department of Surgical Gastroenterology, Copenhagen University Hospital North Zealand, Dyrehavevej 29, 3400 Hillerød, Denmark
Full list of author information is available at the end of the article

Plain English summary

Female genital mutilation (FGM) is a harmful practice where female external genitalia are injured or partly or completely removed due to non-medical reasons. The practice of FGM has spread to European countries with immigration from countries with a tradition for FGM. The European Institute for Gender Equality recommends that FGM should be combatted by nationally coordinated preventive efforts in the form of, among other things, a national action plan. FGM was outlawed in Denmark in 2003, but no national action plan has been implemented. The task of combatting FGM is currently under the responsibility of local governments in the form of the 98 municipalities. We sought to investigate whether FGM is combatted in accordance with international standards on the local level. We invited the Danish municipalities to respond to a questionnaire regarding FGM prevention in their respective municipalities. We also analyzed demographic data regarding distribution of immigrants from countries that practice FGM, across the respective municipalities. We found that only very few Danish municipalities have implemented specific action plans against FGM, or have implemented specific preventive initiatives against FGM. Overall, only very few Danish municipalities live up to international recommendations and standards regarding FGM prevention. Thus, we conclude that the current situation of FGM registration and prevention being under local administrative responsibility in the 98 municipalities has led to a severe lack of coordinated public initiative against FGM in Denmark.

Background

Female genital mutilation (FGM) is a harmful practice prevalent in 35 countries, mainly in Africa, as well as in some Middle Eastern countries and a few Asian countries [1]. The practice is described by the World Health Organization (WHO) as follows: "Female genital mutilation (FGM) comprises all procedures that involve partial or total removal of the external female genitalia, or other injury to the female genital organs for non-medical reasons (...) FGM is recognized internationally as a human rights violation. It reflects deep-rooted inequality between the sexes, and constitutes an extreme form of discrimination against women" [2]. Due to migration over the past decades the practice of FGM has spread to European and other Western countries [3–10]. It has been estimated by the European Parliament that 500,000 women and girls have been subjected to FGM whereas 180,000 girls are in risk of being subjected to FGM [11]; though some argue that this is an under-estimation [4].

Female genital mutilation was outlawed in Denmark in 2003. In 2013, the European Institute for Gender Equality (EIGE) published an official recommendation for Denmark to define and implement a national action plan such as "national guidelines for professionals across a variety of sectors as well as coordination of the effort to combat FGM. Comprehensive and in-depth research in the field is also needed as well as prevalence surveys of FGM in Denmark" [12]. However, several changing governments have not implemented a national action plan to prevent and combat FGM in Denmark. A proposal for a national action plan was drafted by Danish NGOs and a number of individual authors in 2007–2008 and was submitted to the Health Committee of the Parliament in 2009. This action plan was not implemented. Instead, the 98 Danish municipalities individually administrate the responsibility of combatting FGM on a local level.

The lack of political prioritization of the FGM issue in Denmark is unusual in a Nordic context. Finland, Sweden and Norway, along with several other European countries, have implemented comprehensive national and international guidelines to combat FGM [12–17].

In this study, our aim is to investigate the Danish municipalities' initiatives to prevent FGM on the local level, and whether these initiatives are in accordance with international recommendations and standards.

Methods

Questionnaire

In order to gain insight into if and how FGM is combated through public efforts on the local level in the 98 Danish municipalities, a questionnaire was developed. We designed the entirety of the questionnaire, since a validated questionnaire on the subject of FGM prevention on the local governmental level has not yet been published. During the questionnaire design process, we used a checklist proposed by Eysenbach et al. [18]. The questionnaire consisted of four main areas of focus, which we defined as "action plan", "registration of FGM", "information material" and preventive initiatives. These areas of focus were chosen in accordance with the concluding focus points described by EIGE in their 2013 report on the subject of FGM in Denmark, as well as efforts described in other Scandinavian action plans regarding FGM [12, 13, 16]. In those parts of the questionnaire where doubt about terminology could have an impact on answers, the question was supplemented with a definition, so as to ensure measurement validity. An action plan was defined as "A point to point guideline for professionals on how to act when being made aware of a case of FGM or of a girl in potential risk of FGM". Most questions were closed-ended with possible answers being yes/no/do not know. When questions were not close-ended, these could be answered with different given categories or free text (Additional file 1). The questionnaire was answered through a webpage and took few minutes to complete.

Pilot project

A total of 29 municipalities in the Capital Region in Denmark were invited to participate in a pilot project, which consisted of the questionnaire described earlier. The specific department in each of the municipalities with the main responsibility for children, reports of child abuse or likewise, were identified through the respective municipality's website or by telephone. By contacting the general manager with the overall responsibility for the department in question within each municipality, contact information for the individual employee appointed in charge of handling reports of cases of FGM, and with the most adequate knowledge about the particular area, was acquired. The questionnaire was then sent electronically to this person as the potential responder. If the initial contact did not result in a reply, the municipalities were then contacted by telephone or by email once more. The questionnaire was then revised, taking into account the feedback from the 29 municipalities in the pilot project. The revision simply consisted of the addition of a comment field to each question, enabling the respondents to elaborate their answers, if necessary. When revision of the questionnaire was complete, all 98 municipalities were invited to respond to the questionnaire through the process described above. Informed consent for study participation was obtained.

Demographics

Demographic data were gathered from the April 2017 census by Statistics Denmark, using the publicly available Statbank [19]. Data regarding the prevalence of citizens in each municipality originating in countries with tradition of FGM was gathered in order to compare the municipalities participating and not participating in the study, and to evaluate whether a high prevalence of citizens from risk countries was correlated with a higher possibility of having implemented a specific action plans against FGM.

First-generation immigrants are defined as individuals born in a different country than Denmark, and who have achieved status of permanent residents in Denmark at the time of the census. Second-generation immigrants are defined as individuals born in Denmark to two first-generation immigrant parents, and with a status of permanent residency in Denmark at the time of census. Risk countries were defined as countries with a tradition of FGM, and were identified in accordance with the UNICEF definition from 2016 [1], the Embará people of Colombia being excluded due to lack of data regarding the number of people from this ethnic group residing in Denmark. High-risk countries were defined as countries with FGM prevalence above 50%.

Statistics

Quantitative data are presented as frequencies and proportions. Statistical analysis was performed using IBM SPSS Statistics (version 19 for iOS, IBM Corporation, Armonk, NY). Figures were created using GraphPad Prism (version 6 for iOS, GraphPad Software, San Diego, CA).

Results

All 98 municipalities in Denmark were invited to participate in the study by responding to a questionnaire. A total of 67 municipalities participated in the study. The municipalities that did participate in the study had an average of 1.09% of the population with origins in countries with tradition of FGM and a median of 0.86%. The municipalities that did not participate in the study had an average of 1.21% and a median of 0.84%.

Demographics

As of the first of April 2017, a total of 91,121 first- and second-generation immigrants with origins in countries with a tradition of FGM resided in Denmark. This equals 1.8% of Danish population. A total of 41,896 of these were females. A total of 33,198 first- and second-generation immigrants originated from the 12 high-risk countries, comprising 0.7% of the total Danish population. A total of 14,929 of these were females.

The percentage of the population being first- or second-generation immigrants from countries with a tradition of FGM varied within the municipalities from 0% to 4.1% with a median of 0.8%. Only one municipality had 0% of the population originating in countries with a tradition of FGM. The ten municipalities with the highest prevalence of citizens with origins in risk countries were all situated within or in immediate proximity to the three most populated cities in Denmark (Fig. 1).

Questionnaire

Firstly, the municipalities were asked whether they regard FGM as a current problem in their municipality. One (1.5%) municipality regarded FGM as a current problem within its respective municipality, 59 (88%) answered "no" and seven (10.4%) answered "do not know". To the question of whether the municipality currently receives petitions concerning FGM from citizens and social workers, 47 (70.1%) municipalities answered "no", seven (10.4%) municipalities answered "yes" and 13 (19.4%) answered "do not know".

Action plans

A total of seven (10.4%) municipalities stated that they had implemented a specific action plan for cases regarding FGM. Of these seven, one municipality, Copenhagen, made their action plan available upon request, while the

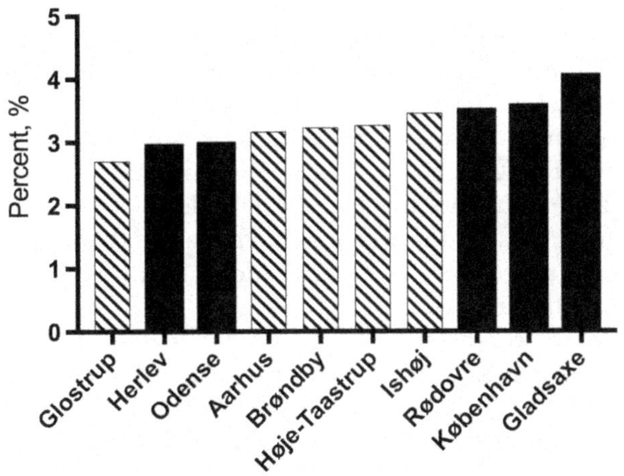

Fig. 1 Prevalence of citizens with origins in risk countries in the ten highest-prevalence municipalities. Municipalities that did not respond to the questionnaire are indicated with shaded bars

remaining six municipalities did not. A total of 57 (85%) municipalities stated that they do not have a specific action plan, while three (4.5%) replied, "do not know".

The municipality of Copenhagen was the only out of the aforementioned ten municipalities with the highest population share of citizens originating in a risk country, to state that they have implemented a specific action plan for combatting FGM.

Of the 57 municipalities where no specific action plan has been implemented, 13 (22.8%) municipalities indicated that FGM is included in other action plans within the given municipality. One municipality stated to be in the process of developing an action plan.

Thus, 46 municipalities (68.7%) indicated that they have not implemented a specific action plan regarding FGM, that FGM currently is not included in other action plans, that they are currently not in the process of developing a specific action plan towards cases of FGM or that they do not know whether an action plan has been implemented in their municipality.

Preventive initiatives

Five (7.5%) municipalities stated that they have developed and implemented preventive initiatives to combat FGM. These municipalities defined their initiatives in the comment field sections as follows: 1) outreach conversations with parents and families in relevant groups; 2) lectures about Danish legislation regarding FGM during Danish language courses for immigrants; 3) preschool interviews with the school nurse, and 4) outreach healthcare visits.

A total of 44 (65.7%) municipalities replied "no" to having implemented preventive initiatives against FGM. Of these, one (2.3%) municipality stated to be in the process of preparing implementation of specific initiatives and preventive work against FGM, whereas 43 (97.7%) municipalities stated not to be. Eighteen (26.9%) municipalities answered "do not know", to whether they had implemented preventive initiatives against FGM.

Registration

A total of 49 (73.1%) municipalities indicated to have implemented routine registration of cases of FGM or suspicion hereof, whereas seven (10.5%) municipalities reported not to perform routine registration, and 11 (16.4%) were unaware if registration is performed. To the question of whether the municipalities register cases of FGM specifically and not under other categories of abuse or violence against children, 12 (17.9%) municipalities answered "yes". A total of 22 (32.8%) municipalities stated to register cases of FGM under other categories concerning abuse or violence towards children. To the question of whether data from these registrations were available upon request, two (3%) municipalities answered "yes". These two municipalities had unfortunately not made this data accessible to the public.

Information material

Five (7.5%) municipalities indicated that they offer booklets or other written information material to the citizens or relevant professionals regarding FGM, while 54 (80.6%) municipalities stated that no information material of any kind had been developed or were available. Eight (11.9%) municipalities responded "do not know" to this question. Of the 10 municipalities with the highest share of citizens from risk countries, one municipality stated to offer information material about FGM to citizens and/or relevant professionals.

Discussion

It was in the light of the fact that Denmark has not yet implemented a coordinated national action plan to combat FGM that we chose to undertake the present study to investigate whether the task of combating FGM was satisfactorily managed on the local level by the 98 Danish municipalities. Other Scandinavian countries have developed and implemented national action plans in order to create national as well as regional foundations for preventing FGM. In Sweden, FGM was prohibited in 1982, and several state prevention programmes was implemented from 1993. A national action plan was established in Sweden in 2003, as well as comprehensive guidelines from The Swedish Board of Health and Welfare to officials in the social sector. Johndottor et al. states that when dealing with cases of FGM, a crucial and facilitating factor is having guidelines so as to achieve knowledge of how to act practically when dealing with victims of FGM [13]. In Norway, a national action plan was developed and implemented in 2000 and a subsequent 3-year national project against FGM was launched in 2001 with continuous evaluations throughout the following years [16].

Our study showed that only 10.4% of the responding municipalities reported to have implemented a specific action plan to combat FGM. Our study also showed that only a small minority of Danish municipalities have implemented specific preventive efforts against FGM, have developed specific registration procedures for cases of FGM and/or have information material available for distribution. Furthermore, there seems to be no relation between the prevalence of immigrants with origins in risk countries and the probability of a certain municipality having implemented a specific action plan to combat FGM. Unfortunately, these facts are not in accordance with recommendations made by international actors in the field. It is recommended to implement a national action plan, and to combat and perform registration of FGM separately from other forms of abuse and violence towards children and adolescents [20–23]. A national action plan will furthermore ensure a consistent and uniform approach to the issue of FGM across municipality boundaries.

A total of seven municipalities reported to have received petitions regarding FGM cases; however, only one municipality stated that they view FGM as a current problem within the municipality. It can only be speculated whether the relatively rare occurrence of FGM petitions in Danish municipalities is a result of a general low incidence of FGM in Denmark, or is a result of a lack of coordinated registration and awareness among front workers.

In England, the introduction of coordinated registration systems in regards to cases of FGM revealed that over 1700 women and girls had undergone FGM and was treated by the NHS between in September 2014. This information was crucial so as to form a picture of the prevalence of FGM in the country and in order to support national prevention programmes [24]. There is currently no such national registration system in Denmark. Our study shows that registration of FGM specifically as such is performed in only 17.9% of Danish municipalities, and that 19.4% were unaware if there had been petitions received regarding FGM in their respective municipalities. These results suggest that Danish municipalities lack the necessary data to draw reliable conclusions as to whether or not FGM is a current problem.

A study by Van Baelen et al. based on demographic data from 2011 estimated that 7910 girls and women living in Denmark had been subjected to FGM before immigration [4]. The current prevalence of girls and women having been, or in risk of being, submitted to FGM in Denmark is unknown. A 2016 study by Ziyada et al. on FGM prevalence in Norway, which has a comparable number to Denmark of immigrants with origins in risk countries, estimated a prevalence of 17,300 girls and women having been subjected to FGM, and a prevalence of 3000–7900 girls in risk of being subjected to FGM [7]. We strongly recommend further investigation into the current prevalence of FGM in Denmark using the definitions, models and methodological approaches as recommended by the 2013 and 2015 EIGE reports [25, 26].

It is a weakness of the study that it does not offer explanations as to the reasons why the respective municipalities have chosen not to implement specific preventive measures or action plans against FGM. It is also a weakness that we did not gather data describing the responders of the questionnaire with regard to their knowledge about FGM, laws and their respective amount of influence within the respective municipalities. Furthermore, it was not possible to externally validate our data collected from the questionnaire, given the fact that there is no existing studies or data sources containing information enabling us to corroborate our findings. It could also be considered a weakness of our study that only 67 of the 98 municipalities responded to the questionnaire. In particular, of the ten municipalities in Denmark with the highest prevalence of immigrants with origins in risk countries, five municipalities did not participate in the study. However, the response rate of 68% is in line with what is considered a successful response rate for an online survey [18, 27–29]. The questionnaire consisted of quite few categories, which limited the extent of the results, but it could also be argued that this was a strength considering the relatively high response rate for an online survey.

Conclusions

In conclusion, our study shows that the current situation of FGM registration and prevention being under local administrative responsibility, has led to a severe lack of coordinated public initiative against FGM in Denmark. Besides the lack of a coordinated, national action plan there seems to be a general lack of public awareness on the issue. In October 2017, the second conviction on FGM in Denmark was given to two parents for having their daughters subjected to FGM abroad. In the High Court of Western Denmark, the President of the court halved the sentence from the District Court from 18 to 9 months of prison, arguing "There has not been provided evidence of the procedure having consequences for the girls including consequences for their sexual health" [30]. This sentence was referred to in the national newspapers, but we have not been able to find any news articles questioning the sentence or the citation of the President of the High Court of Western

Denmark, despite the fact that the international research on FGM has shown all types of FGM to be harmful practices, severely jeopardizing the health of women and girls [1, 31–35].

As such, Denmark does not live up to international recommendations in the field and it should be considered to implement nationally coordinated efforts against FGM such as an elaborate action plan, coordinated data collection and research programs to ensure a consistent approach towards FGM throughout the nation.

Abbreviations

EIGE: European Institute for Gender Equality; FGM: Female genital mutilation; WHO: World Health Organization

Acknowledgements

We would like to acknowledge Lea Leas and Anne Christine Stender Heerdegen for their aid in data collection during the pilot project.

Funding

This study did not receive funding.

Authors' contributions

GC, PB, RN, SE, VN: Study conception and design. GC, PB, SE, VN: Data collection. GC, PB, VN: Data analysis and interpretation. GC, PB, VN: Manuscript preparation. PB, VN: Critical revision. All authors have read and approved the final manuscript.

Competing interests

The authors declare that they have no competing interests.

Author details

[1]University of Copenhagen, Faculty of Health and Medical Sciences, Blegdamsvej 3, 2200 Copenhagen N, Denmark. [2]Department of Surgical Gastroenterology, Copenhagen University Hospital North Zealand, Dyrehavevej 29, 3400 Hillerød, Denmark. [3]Department of Emergency Medicine, Zealand University Hospital Slagelse, Ingemannsvej 50, 4200 Slagelse, Denmark. [4]Department of Culture, Municipality of Sermersooq, Kuussuaq 2, 3900 Nuuk, Greenland. [5]Department of Obstetrics and Gynecology, Zealand University Hospital Næstved, Ringstedgade 61, 4700 Næstved, Denmark.

References

1. UNICEF. Female genital mutilation/cutting: a global concern. New York: United Nations Childrens Fund; 2016.
2. WHO: Female Genital Mutilation Fact Sheet, available at http://www.who.int/mediacentre/factsheets/fs241/en/. Accessed 11 Oct 2016.
3. Farina P, Ortensi LE, Menonna A. Estimating the number of foreign women with female genital mutilation/cutting in Italy. Eur J Pub Health. 2016;26(4):656–61.
4. Van Baelen L, Ortensi L, Leye E. Estimates of first-generation women and girls with female genital mutilation in the European Union, Norway and Switzerland. Eur J Contracept Reprod Health Care. 2016;21(6):474–82.
5. Teixeira AL, Lisboa M. Estimating the prevalence of female genital mutilation in Portugal. Public Health. 2016;139:53–60.
6. Goldberg H, Stupp P, Okoroh E, Besera G, Goodman D, Danel I. Female genital mutilation/cutting in the United States: updated estimates of women and girls at risk, 2012. Public Health Rep. 2016;131(2):340–7.
7. Ziyada MM, Norberg-Schulz M, Johansen REB. Estimating the magnitude of female genital mutilation/cutting in Norway: an extrapolation model. BMC Public Health. 2016;16:110.
8. Dubourg D, Richard F, Leye E, Ndame S, Rommens T, Maes S. Estimating the number of women with female genital mutilation in Belgium. Eur J Contracept Reprod Health Care. 2011;16(4):248–57.
9. Koukkula M, Keskimaki I, Koponen P, Molsa M, Klemetti R. Female genital mutilation/cutting among women of Somali and Kurdish origin in Finland. Birth. 2016;43(3):240–6.
10. Zurynski Y, Phu A, Sureshkumar P, Cherian S, Deverell M, Elliott EJ, for Australian Paediatric Surveillance Unit Female Genital Mutilation Study Steering C. Female genital mutilation in children presenting to Australian paediatricians. Arch Dis Child. 2017;102(6):509–15.
11. European Parliament resolution of 24 March 2009 on combating female genital mutilation in the EU. Available at http://www.europarl.europa.eu/sides/getDoc.do?pubRef=-//EP//NONSGML+TA+P6-TA-2009-0161+0+DOC+PDF+V0//EN. Accessed 2 Oct 2016.
12. EIGE. Study to map the current situation and trends of FGM - country reports. European Union, 2013. Available at http://eige.europa.eu/rdc/eige-publications/study-map-current-situation-and-trends-fgm-country-reports. Accessed 11 Oct 2016.
13. Johnsdotter, Carlbom. FGM in Sweden: Swedish legislation regarding "female genital mutilation" and implementation of the law. 2004 (Research Report in Sociology). Department of Sociology, Lund University.
14. van Kolfschooten F. Dutch government cracks down on female circumcision. Lancet. 2004;363(9420):1531.
15. PM outlines tough new measures to tackle FGM. J Fam Health Care. 2014;24(5):7.
16. The Norwegian Government's International Action Plan for Combating Female Genital Mutilation. 2014. Available at http://www.regjeringen.no/globalassets/upload/kilde/ud/bro/2003/0011/ddd/pdfv/197557-ud_kjonnslemlestelse_eng.pdf. Accessed 9 Oct 2016.
17. Ministry of Social Affairs and Health, Finland, Action Plan for the prevention of circumcision of girls and women 2012–2016. 2012. Available at https://julkaisut.valtioneuvosto.fi/bitstream/handle/10024/73924/URN%3ANBN%3Afi-fe201504226370.pdf?sequence=1%20. Accessed 9 Oct 2016.
18. Eysenbach G. Improving the quality of web surveys: the checklist for reporting results of internet E-surveys (CHERRIES). J Med Internet Res. 2004;6(3):e34.
19. Statistics Denmark census 2017, Statbank. available at http://www.statistikbanken.dk/statbank5a/default.asp?w=1280. Accessed 20 June 2017.
20. Berg K. Female genital mutilation: implications for social work. Soc Work. 1997;65(3):16–26.
21. Royal College of Midwives, Royal College of Nursing, Royal College of Obstetricians andGynaecologists, Equality Now and UNITE. Tackling FGM In The UK: Intercollegiate Recommendations for Identifying, Recording and Reporting. London: Royal College of Midwives, Royal College of Nursing, Royal College of Obstetricians and Gynaecologists, Equality Now and UNITE; 2013.
22. Morgan J. Working towards an end to FGM. Lancet. 2015;385(9971):843–4.
23. Creighton SM, Dear J, de Campos C, Williams L, Hodes D. Multidisciplinary approach to the management of children with female genital mutilation (FGM) or suspected FGM: service description and case series. BMJ Open. 2016;6(2):e010311.
24. Health and Social Care Information Center. Female Genital Mutilation (FGM), September 2014, experimental statistics, available at http://www.digital.nhs.uk/catalogue/PUB15711. Accessed 19 Oct 2016.
25. EIGE. Female genital mutilation in the European Union and Croatia. Lithuania: European Union; 2013.
26. EIGE. EIGE. Estimation of girls at risk of female genital mutilation in the European Union. Lithuania: European Union; 2015.
27. Cook JV, Dickinson HO, Eccles MP. Response rates in postal surveys of healthcare professionals between 1996 and 2005: an observational study. BMC Health Serv Res. 2009;9:160.
28. Fincham JE. Response rates and responsiveness for surveys, standards, and the journal. Am J Pharm Educ. 2008;72(2):43.
29. Asch DA, Jedrziewski MK, Christakis NA. Response rates to mail surveys published in medical journals. J Clin Epidemiol. 1997;50(10):1129–36.
30. Ritzau. Landsret halverer straf til forældre for omskæring af døtre. Berlingske Tidende. October 18th 2017. Available at http://www.b.dk/nationalt/landsret-halverer-straf-til-foraeldre-for-omskaering-af-doetre. Accessed 18 Oct 2017.

31. Ahmed MR, Shaaban MM, Meky HK, Amin Arafa ME, Mohamed TY, Gharib WF, Ahmed AB. Psychological impact of female genital mutilation among adolescent Egyptian girls: a cross-sectional study. Eur J Contracept Reprod Health Care. 2017;22(4):280–5.
32. Berg RC, Underland V. The obstetric consequences of female genital mutilation/cutting: a systematic review and meta-analysis. Obstet Gynecol Int. 2013;2013:496564.
33. Berg RC, Odgaard-Jensen J, Fretheim A, Underland V, Vist G. An updated systematic review and meta-analysis of the obstetric consequences of female genital mutilation/cutting. Obstet Gynecol Int. 2014;2014:542859.
34. Abdulcadir J, Tille JC, Petignat P. Management of painful clitoral neuroma after female genital mutilation/cutting. Reprod Health. 2017;14(1):22.
35. Yassin K, Idris HA, Ali AA. Characteristics of female sexual dysfunctions and obstetric complications related to female genital mutilation in Omdurman maternity hospital, Sudan. Reprod Health. 2018;15(1):7.

19

Exploring perceptions of group antenatal Care in Urban India

R. Rima Jolivet[1*], Bella Vasant Uttekar[2], Meaghan O'Connor[3], Kanchan Lakhwani[2], Jigyasa Sharma[4] and Mary Nell Wegner[1]

Abstract

Background: Making high-quality health care available to all women during pregnancy is a critical strategy for improving perinatal outcomes for mothers and babies everywhere. Research from high-income countries suggests that antenatal care delivered in a group may be an effective way to improve the provision, experiences, and outcomes of care for pregnant women and newborns. A number of researchers and programmers are adapting group antenatal care (ANC) models for use in low- and middle-income countries (LMIC), but the evidence base from these settings is limited and no studies to date have assessed the feasibility and acceptability of group ANC in India.

Methods: We adapted a "generic" model of group antenatal care developed through a systematic scoping review of the existing evidence on group ANC in LMICs for use in an urban setting in India, after looking at local, national and global guidelines to tailor the model content. We demonstrated one session of the model to physicians, auxiliary nurse midwives, administrators, pregnant women, and support persons from three different types of health facilities in Vadodara, India and used qualitative methods to gather and analyze feedback from participants on the perceived feasibility and acceptability of the model.

Results: Providers and recipients of care expressed support and enthusiasm for the model and offered specific feedback on its components: physical assessment, active learning, and social support. In general, after witnessing a demonstration of the model, both groups of participants—providers and beneficiaries—saw group ANC as a vehicle for delivering more comprehensive ANC services, improving experiences of care, empowering women to become more active partners and participants in their care, and potentially addressing some current health system challenges.

Conclusion: This study suggests that introducing group ANC would be feasible and acceptable to stakeholders from various care delivery settings, including an urban primary health clinic, a community-based mother and child health center, and a private hospital, in urban India.

Keywords: Antenatal care, Prenatal care, Group care, Feasibility study, Qualitative methods, India

* Correspondence: rjolivet@hsph.harvard.edu
[1]Maternal Health Task Force, Women & Health Initiative, Department of Global Health and Population, Harvard T.H. Chan School of Public Health, 651 Huntington Avenue, Boston, MA 02115, USA
Full list of author information is available at the end of the article

Plain English summary

Research from high-income countries suggests women who receive antenatal care (ANC) in a group may have better experiences and outcomes of care than those who get ANC through individual visits with a health care provider. However, there are few published studies on group ANC in low- and middle-income countries. In this study, we asked participants to share their views about whether group ANC could work and whether it would be acceptable in Vadodara, India. To conduct the study, we developed a "generic" model of group ANC, and then made sure the content matched the care guidelines from the Indian Ministry of Health and Family Welfare. We demonstrated one session of the group model to doctors, auxiliary nurse midwives, pregnant women, and support persons (mothers-in-law, mothers, husbands). These demonstrations were held in three different locations in Vadodara where ANC is typically provided: a private maternity hospital, a public health clinic, and a community-based mother and child health center. Focus group discussions, interviews, and a survey were used to learn from the participants what they thought about the group model. The feedback received through these methods showed that pregnant women and their families, as well as health care providers and administrators, thought it would be feasible and acceptable to conduct group ANC in Vadodara. Participants suggested ideas to better the chances for success in providing group ANC in this setting, including making sure that there is enough staff and space to support the model.

Background

Making high-quality health care available to all women during pregnancy is a critical strategy for improving perinatal outcomes for mothers and babies everywhere. A recent conceptual framework published by the World Health Organization (WHO) includes provision of appropriate services, assurance of positive experience of care, and effective care delivery by the health system within one comprehensive definition of quality of maternal and newborn care in facilities. The framework emphasizes the importance of three types of outcomes of high quality care: coverage of key practices, health outcomes, and people-centered outcomes. It also calls for innovations in healthcare delivery to meet achieve these outcomes [1].

Group Care in High-income Countries

Many studies from high-income countries have reported positive pregnancy experiences and improved birth outcomes among women receiving antenatal care (ANC) in a group, compared to those receiving traditional one-to-one ANC. In high-income settings, the most widespread model of group ANC with the most extensive evidence base is CenteringPregnancy® which combines clinical care, education, and peer support in one bundled program [2]. A randomized controlled trial of group care in the United States by Ickovics et al. [3] found a 33% decrease in the odds of preterm delivery for women in group care as well as better utilization of ANC, increased prenatal knowledge, increased readiness for labor and delivery, higher satisfaction with care, and higher rates of breastfeeding initiation than women receiving individual ANC. The study also found that there were no differences in the cost of group ANC compared to usual care [3]. Similarly, Earnshaw et al. [4] analyzed data from two separate randomized controlled trials of group ANC and reported that young, urban women in group ANC demonstrated higher levels of engagement and attended more ANC visits than controls. The results of a cluster-randomized controlled trial conducted in 14 urban health centers in the United States demonstrated that women in group ANC delivered significantly fewer infants who were small for gestational age compared to women in traditional ANC [5]. Studies have also demonstrated a significant improvement in appropriate pregnancy weight gain for women in group care compared to individual ANC [6, 7]. However, a Cochrane systematic review of four randomized controlled trials (two in the United States, one in Sweden, and one in Iran) (2015) found no differences in health outcomes between women in group and individual ANC, noting that the review was limited by the small number of trials and participants [8]. The overall positive outcomes reported by group ANC studies conducted in high-income settings suggest that, with some adaptations in the number and content of sessions to meet local guidelines, the group care format might improve quality and experiences of ANC for women in low- and middle-income countries (LMICs) as well.

Group Care in low- and Middle-Income Countries

Although several researchers and programmers are currently exploring the implementation and outcomes of group ANC in LMICs, few studies have been published to date and the body of knowledge on the safety and effectiveness of group ANC in LMICs is limited [9]. Nevertheless, a few small, descriptive studies have assessed perceptions of the acceptability and feasibility of group care among various target audiences in LMICs. Patil et al. [10] assessed the feasibility and acceptability of group ANC with health care providers, decision makers, and women in Malawi and Tanzania, and reported positive responses. Ghani [11] surveyed frontline health workers in Egypt; responses indicated health workers felt the group model would have positive effects on early prevention and detection of complications, patient empowerment, and self-care behaviors, but could face barriers to implementation related to staff training requirements and cost. Arnold et al. [12] surveyed seven male partners of pregnant women who participated in group ANC in Botswana and reported positive responses such as satisfaction with care, increased access to information, and an experience of group care as respectful and sufficiently private.

The few research studies conducted to date that have evaluated the effects of group ANC in LMICs generally report positive results. In Iran, Jafari et al. [13] conducted a cluster-randomized trial of group ANC at 14 health care facilities with a total of 628 participants, 320 of whom received group ANC. The intervention resulted in reductions in the number of low birth-weight babies and preterm births, intrauterine growth restriction and perinatal loss, although none of these findings was statistically significant. Women receiving group care were, however, significantly more likely to take prenatal vitamins and iron, and to be using a contraceptive method at 2 months postpartum. Women receiving group ANC also reported significantly higher satisfaction with the information they received, the relationship with their provider, and the quality of care and service delivery, and scored significantly higher on the Kotelchuck Index assessing adequacy of ANC utilization [13, 14]. The positive outcomes of group ANC reported across settings provide sufficient rationale to explore the potential for this innovation in additional LMIC settings.

This paper describes the results of a qualitative research study conducted in Vadodara, India to explore the feasibility and acceptability of a model of group ANC designed for use in LMICs. By collecting the perspectives of care providers, care managers, and care recipients (pregnant women and their accompanying family members) on the strengths and challenges related to introducing an alternative, evidence-based group model of ANC, we aimed to answer two questions:

1) What are the likely strengths and challenges of implementing an evidence-based model of group ANC in the context of three types of care-delivery settings (private, public, and community-based) in urban India?
2) Are there any context-specific modifications or adaptations that would increase the potential of this model of ANC to: a) be implemented effectively within the local health system; and b) improve patient and provider experiences by responding to specific population health needs or health system problems in Vadodara?

Methods

Study setting and design

This research was conducted in Vadodara, a city located in the western Indian state of Gujarat, with a population of 2.3 million [15]. In Vadodara, pregnant women may receive ANC at a public, district tertiary-care hospital, sub-district hospitals, urban public health clinics (UPHCs), community-based maternal and child health centers (*anganwadis*), and private maternity hospitals. To assess stakeholder perceptions of group ANC within the unique patient populations served by these different types of facilities, we collected data in three settings: a private hospital, a UPHC, and a community-based *anganwadi*. The specific study sites were selected in collaboration with a local representative of the Indian Ministry of Health and Family Welfare (MOHFW), and permission was gained from physicians/administrators in those facilities. The study was carried out collaboratively by a team of researchers from the Centre for Operations Research and Training in Vadodara, and the Harvard T.H. Chan School of Public Health in Boston, MA.

We used a descriptive, qualitative study design to assess the feasibility and acceptability of group ANC to potential stakeholders. Given the novelty of the group ANC model in the study setting, we incorporated a demonstration of one mock session of group ANC into the study design to allow participants to visualize and directly experience the proposed innovation. The demonstration in each setting was followed immediately by data collection using qualitative methods, which are detailed below.

Model

We conducted a systematic review of the published literature and a series of key informant interviews to gather evidence on the components of group antenatal care models in current use in LMICs. Two existing group models emerged as most influential in LMIC settings: nine out of the nineteen unique models identified reportedly drew from CenteringPregnancy® [2] and four out of nineteen reported they were informed by the Home Based Lifesaving Skills (HBLSS) program [16]. We synthesized the data collected through this systematic scoping review and compiled the common elements of the group ANC models reviewed to describe a "generic" model of group ANC specifically for use in LMICs. This evidence review and synthesis is described in Sharma, et al. [9].

We then reviewed the ANC guidelines from the MOHFW and added clinical and educational content to the "generic" model to ensure compliance with the recommended standards of care in the study setting [17, 18]. Two adaptations were made:

1) The number of group sessions was set at four (not inclusive of the initial intake visit): three antenatal sessions and one post-natal care (PNC) session. This number fulfills the Indian MOHFW's minimum recommendation for four antenatal care visits (one intake visit plus three group antenatal visits) and includes the recommended PNC visit at 6 weeks postpartum.
2) The content for each of the four group sessions reflects the clinical care standards found in the most recent MOHFW maternal and newborn health register and guidelines for ANC and skilled attendance at birth.

Participants

Study participants were recruited from two groups of key stakeholders: care receivers and care providers. Care receivers included pregnant women and any support person (e.g. mother, mother-in-law, and husband) whom the women chose to accompany them. Care providers included clinicians who provide ANC (physicians and auxiliary nurse midwives) (ANMs) from each of the study sites and administrators who coordinate the provision of care at these sites. Pregnant women age 18 or older, up to 26 weeks gestation, receiving antenatal care at the study site, and who had attended at least one previous ANC visit during the current pregnancy were eligible to participate. Health care providers were eligible if they were a nurse, midwife, physician, or physician-administrator who was working at the study site and involved in the provision of antenatal care (In the Indian health system, attending physicians often also serve as facility administrators). Physicians and auxiliary nurse midwives from each site were recruited directly by the study team. Pregnant women were recruited by staff at the three study sites using convenience sampling. Each participant was given lunch and compensation for their transportation costs (200 Indian rupees, which is equivalent to approximately $3 US dollars).

Demonstration of the model

We developed an agenda for one mock session of group ANC based on our generic model components tailored to the local context, and used it to demonstrate the model for study participants. The demonstration for the care providers was conducted in English by two members of the Harvard research team (RJ and MO'C) who played the role of group facilitators, with translation into Gujarati from the CORT research team (BU and KL) as needed. A local physician and ANM were recruited to play the roles of the group facilitators during the demonstrations that were conducted for pregnant women and their support persons. These sessions were conducted in the local language (either Gujarati or Hindi) to maximize participants' understanding and participation.

A total of four demonstrations of the group ANC model were conducted: one for providers/administrators (held at a central location), and one at each of the three study sites for women and their family members. Before each demonstration, the study team provided a short introduction to the research study and its aims, requested and collected signed consent, briefly outlined the group ANC model, and clarified that the participants would not be receiving actual clinical care. In the demonstration that was staged for care providers and administrators, participants were asked to play the role of pregnant women so they could observe and experience how care is provided in the group ANC model. The content and format for all four demonstrations was the same and is described in detail in Table 1. During the first 30 min, participants took and recorded their own weight and blood pressure, completed two worksheets about their diet and discomforts during this pregnancy, and saw the clinician in rotation for a brief (mock) physical exam. The co-facilitator opened the group with a short icebreaker. The icebreaker was followed by a facilitated discussion during which participants developed and agreed on shared behavioral norms and guidelines for the group. The rest of the session focused on the interactive learning component of the model: the participants engaged in a facilitated discussion about nutrition during pregnancy and participated in a group activity and discussion of common discomforts and danger signs during pregnancy. The co-leaders guided the discussions and activities using a facilitative leadership style to encourage active participation from the women. The demonstration ended with a short activity in which each participant shared one thing they learned, designed to summarize and close the session.

Data collection

Data was collected through a mix of focus group discussions, in-depth interviews, and a written survey. The questions used to guide the focus group discussions and in-depth interviews were designed to elicit participants' perceptions regarding the feasibility and acceptability of the group ANC model in general, as well as specific elements of the model, and to capture any perceived barriers to implementation along with recommendations for how to overcome them. All physicians participated in an in-depth interview. All ANMs participated in a focus group discussion followed by an individual survey that asked the same questions as those posed in the in-depth interview. The purpose of the survey was to validate the focus group discussion findings and check for any cognitive bias, i.e., groupthink, which may have occurred during the focus group discussion. The pregnant

Table 1 Agenda for Group ANC Session Demonstration

Time	Topic	Leader	Props/Materials	Content
30	Physical self-assessment Psychosocial self-assessment	Co-leader 2 (auxiliary nurse midwife)	1. Digital scale 2. Portable blood pressure cuff 3. Mock flow chart 4. Nutrition worksheet 5. Common discomforts worksheet	• Show each participant how to take their weight and blood pressure and record the results on a mock flow chart. • Distribute two psychosocial self-assessment sheets and provide guidance on how to complete them.
	Provider physical assessment	Co-leader 1 (physician)	1. 1 charpoy and stool 2. 1 Privacy screen or curtain 3. Measuring tape 4. Fetoscope or Doppler 5. Mock chart	• Welcome women individually to the private corner where the clinical exam will take place. • Conduct a mock physical exam with each woman. • Ascertain that privacy and confidentiality are maintained.
10	Opening ice-breaker	Co-leader 2	Soft ball	• Explain the game whose aim is for everyone to introduce themselves and learn the names of others in the group. • Lead the game; help ensure everyone participates.
10	Group guidelines	Co-leader1 Co-leader 2	1. Flip chart or white board 2. Markers	• Facilitate a discussion to help the group develop its own guidelines for group conduct that is comfortable for everyone. Help the group brainstorm, offering probes. • Ask a volunteer to write the group's agreements on a flip chart, and tell the group that these guidelines will be on display during all their group sessions. • Tell the group that all members and any visitors will be asked to sign a confidentiality agreement.
30	Group discussion	Co-leader 1 Co-leader 2	Nutrition worksheet	• Use the worksheet to lead a facilitated discussion on nutrition. • Offer discussion prompts, e.g. "Does anyone know which of the foods here are high in calcium? Why is calcium important in pregnancy? What can you do if you don't like any of those foods?" • Acknowledge each participant's comment or question, refer back to the group for further reflection and discussion, then summarize or expand on the discussion. • Once the topic has been exhausted or it is time to move on, wrap up the discussion, ensuring that participants' questions have been answered satisfactorily.
10	Group learning activity	Co-leader 1 Co-leader 2	1. Common discomforts worksheet 2. Green light/red light paddles	• Use the green light/red light paddles to stimulate group discussion about common discomforts during pregnancy, share ways to address them, and discuss when a symptom should be considered a danger sign.
10	Closing ritual/activity	Co-leader 2 Co-leader 1	Yarn ball and scissors	• Explain the closing ritual designed to encourage participants to recap what they learned in the group, illustrate the connections that were made, and end the session.

women and their support persons were randomly assigned to either a focus group discussion or an in-depth interview. The only non-random assignments were to ensure that women and their support persons were not assigned to the same focus group discussion; this separation was made to avoid courtesy and other biases resulting from any potential power imbalances between women and their support persons or other factors. All focus group discussions and in-depth interviews were recorded and transcribed in Gujarati, and then translated into English. English translations were reviewed to identify themes, coded, and analyzed using Atlas.ti, version 8 software (Berlin, Germany, 2017). Themes were extracted from the participants' responses to each question in the focus group discussion, in-depth interview, and survey, and are presented below in the order they were asked. Codes were derived from the research questions and emerged from the collected data. They were color-coded and categorized into themes, and illustrative quotes were selected to represent each emergent theme. Some further quotes were selected to add in-depth understanding and capture variations in responses.

Results

Participants

There were 13 participants in the demonstration for care providers: five physicians, seven ANMs and one *anganwadi* worker. Thirty-eight individuals participated in the demonstration for care receivers: 29 pregnant women and nine support persons. The support persons included three mothers, one mother-in-law, and five husbands. Of the 29 pregnant women, nine were from a private hospital, 10 from a UPHC, and 10 from an *anganwadi*; 12 of the 29 women were primiparous and the remainder were multiparous.

Reflections on current ANC in Vadodara

Study participants were asked to share their perceptions of the strengths and challenges of the one-on-one model of ANC currently in place in Vadodara.

A typical ANC visit and goals for care

Participants were asked to describe a typical ANC visit and reflect on the goals for care during antenatal visits. Providers reported that a typical ANC visit includes confirmation of pregnancy (during the first ANC visit), lab tests, basic health measurements (weight, blood pressure, fundal height), and risk assessment to check for maternal and fetal wellbeing. In general, providers agreed that, in addition to the aforementioned physical exam and laboratory tests, ANC should include education on nutrition and self-care during pregnancy, and they emphasized the importance of attending all four recommended ANC visits. They reported that ANC services are typically provided by a physician with help from a staff nurse (in tertiary settings), an ANM or an accredited social health activist (ASHA) (in public facilities), or a second physician or medical assistant (in private hospitals). The schedule of visits is determined based on the woman's gestational age upon entry into care; she is advised to return for her next visit at least once per trimester during her pregnancy. The public facility providers reported a range of 10–40 ANC cases per day, with higher volume on days when specialty care is available or when a dedicated obstetric clinic (such as Pradhan Mantri Surakshit Matritva Yojana, or PMSMY [17]) is being held. The private hospital providers reported 20–25 cases per day on average.

Pregnant women's responses describing a typical ANC visit were congruous with those of providers, and mentioned physical exam, laboratory testing, as well as education on nutrition or recommended changes in activities of daily living. While women mentioned similar information and services that should be offered during each ANC visit as the providers did, many women also noted ($n = 14$) that assurance from the doctor was critical for wellbeing. Most pregnant women ($n = 16$) reported that ANC was provided either by a physician alone or a physician in combination with a staff nurse ($n = 13$). Pregnant women reported wait times ranging from 15 min to 4 hours. Women who had attended the ANC clinic at the tertiary hospital reported that the entire process (wait time plus visit) could take up to 6 hours. The majority of the pregnant women ($n = 24$) reported visiting more than one facility for ANC during their pregnancy: UPHCs were generally used to confirm the pregnancy and higher-level public facilities (hospitals) were used to address any complications. Women also noted that they would change facilities if they moved from their in-laws' home to their natal home. In Vadodara, and India more broadly, many women adhere to the custom of *sava-mahina*: a woman experiencing her first pregnancy (although occasionally during subsequent pregnancies as well) will live primarily at her parents' home and only return to her in-laws' home 6 weeks after delivery. This custom can affect facility choice.

Strengths and challenges of the current model

Participants were asked about their views on the strengths of the current model of ANC in Vadodara. Providers cited outreach efforts that allowed them to provide access to care for more women, expanded service capacity (more facilities are able to do more advanced laboratory tests), the convenience that electronic health records in the urban primary health centers provide particularly for the management of high-risk pregnancies, and the provision of free services (e.g. delivery services, iron and calcium tablets) in public facilities. One physician remarked, "The current model is good in all ways, like we give tablets free of cost, all services are free of cost. Besides, we give all guidance based on the [MOHFW] guideline which is fully authorized and prepared by experts."

When asked explicitly about any challenges perceived with the current model of ANC, the majority of providers ($n = 8$) and women ($n = 26$) did not report any challenges or frustrations. However, some providers noted frustration with a shortage of personnel at their facilities ($n = 2$) as well as problems with time management given the high volume of their caseloads ($n = 3$); this was noted as a problem particularly at the UPHCs where ANC is provided at the same time as the general outpatient clinic day (OPD). A provider from a UPHC stated, "I have to see 40 to 50 [OPD] patients and around 15 ANC [patients] in three and a half hours. [It is] ...not only pregnant women—I have other patients also to whom I am not able to give sufficient time." For their part, women expressed their dislike for the long wait times but also noted they were used to it.

Reflections on the group ANC model

Following questions about the current model of ANC in Vadodara, participants were asked to share their reflections about what they had just seen and experienced during the group ANC demonstration.

Physical assessment

Participants were asked what they thought about the physical assessment component of the group ANC demonstration. Both providers and pregnant women were generally comfortable with all aspects of the physical assessment, including the time and attention given to each woman's "belly check," and having that exam done in a private area within the group space. Providers reported that they thought doing the clinical checkup in the group space worked well and would be feasible in their respective facilities. They also felt it was possible to maintain privacy and confidentiality despite being in a shared space. One physician and two ANMs noted they liked the low mat for women's exams on the floor (versus an exam table) as it was easier for the pregnant women to get onto it. Regarding the checkup in the group space, one physician stated, "Yes, it is good, it is in the corner, so women don't feel shy. All the patients are checked so they know that everybody is going to be checked, all enjoyed the process."

The majority of women ($n = 17$) also agreed that the checkup in the group space worked well and was done in a way that maintained their privacy and confidentiality. One woman explained, "It was good, [the doctor] was talking all the time and I did not feel that... there was lots of noise in the room or that she was not able to listen to what I said. I did not feel anything like that. She talked softly yet I did not feel that I was in the same room [with everyone else]." However, three women, two of whom were from the private clinic and one from a public site, expressed discomfort with having their checkup done in the group space and stated that they would have preferred a private room.

Self-assessment

Participants were asked their opinions on the self-assessment components of the group ANC model. Overall, the self-assessment activities were well received by all participants. In general, providers felt that having the women take their own blood pressure (BP) and weight measurements was a novel idea, and helped women pay more attention and develop a feeling of ownership of their health information. One physician explained, "When [the women] measured their own weight they felt that they also can do something. There is empowerment of women. Because they had first time taken BP machine in hand. As we just taught them, they themselves used it so they felt happy from inside." Another physician noted, "That was a great idea I think, because when we tell them that your BP is this much, we don't know whether it registers with them or not. Here when they did [it] on their own, they notice their BP more. And peers are doing the same thing so they compare with them."

The pregnant women also enjoyed taking their own BP and weight, noting that it made them pay closer attention to what the numbers meant and how those numbers can affect their health. According to one woman, "It was good we weighed ourselves and wrote in the report [worksheet] ourselves. We got to know how to check BP. I liked that I measured my BP on my own; in the hospital, we would not come to know [that information] as provider would just write it on their own. They do not tell us, so we do not realize." The majority of the providers ($n = 10$) also felt that the self-assessment worksheets worked well. While they did express concerns that some women—particularly in less literate communities—may need assistance with completing the worksheets, they were confident that overall, women would get used to it and, when necessary, they could receive help. None of the women reported any difficulty or discomfort with the self-assessment worksheets used during the demonstration, even though a few had required assistance from their peers or the co-facilitator to complete the written worksheets.

Peer support and education

Participants were asked for their opinions about the learning component of the group ANC demonstration. Providers and pregnant women responded positively to the group discussion and group activities. The providers were highly enthusiastic about the peer support and education aspects of the model. They felt that group ANC could accomplish all of the goals of high-quality ANC while also providing more time for counseling and learning. Providers appreciated the interactive learning style that the discussion promoted. The physician who acted as a group leader for the demonstrations noted her surprise at how willing the women were to engage in the discussion: "Initially I was little skeptical whether I would be able to get answers [from the women]. But when we finally tried it, lot of information came from them, especially in the private [hospital] the level of knowledge was too good [meaning "very good"]. Even in the public [settings], in slums, though knowledge was not so much, we could encourage women to talk and many of the answers came from them."

The women also reportedly enjoyed the discussion and stated that it gave them the opportunity to learn from the provider as well as each other. One pregnant woman explained, "Everyone gets chance to speak [and] due to that, a good atmosphere is also created. If only the service provider speaks, after sometime it feels like a lecture. As everyone speaks and shares their experience, we get to learn from that also. If I'm not suffering at present but some other lady is suffering and I hear her experiences, and after some time if I have a similar problem then I will remember about the discussion at that time." Another pregnant woman noted that the group discussion was helpful for participants who were shy; although they did not speak up themselves, they had the chance to learn from others who might be going through similar situations.

Both providers and pregnant women also felt that the group activity was an effective, entertaining way to learn about information related to pregnancy (in the demonstration the topic was common discomforts and danger signs). Providers liked that the activity was fun and interactive while still being informative. One demonstrator remarked, "[This activity was a] good one. You learn when you are having fun. I didn't find that women were getting bored or were in hurry, everyone was pretty attentive. I could see that they were happy playing games and learning. It is a better way of teaching." The same demonstrator noted that she had been worried that women might copy one another's answers or could be unwilling to share personal information about discomforts but that the women proved otherwise, offering their original thoughts and experiences.

The pregnant women also reported positive feedback on the group activity. One woman said that she preferred it to a one-on-one meeting with the physician: "If we all are together we do enjoy having fun (*masti ho jaati hai)* and we also learn. We like to learn more in the form of games rather than sitting alone, waiting for the doctor; that I don't like."

Other aspects of the model

Participants were asked for feedback on other aspects of the model, including a set schedule of visits and the duration of each session. Five providers expressed concerns about introducing a set schedule of visits for group ANC. Three providers were worried about what would happen if they were called away to attend an emergency during a scheduled group sessions. They also expressed concern about women forgetting pre-scheduled sessions. Pregnant women, on the other hand, expressed a preference for the idea of a set schedule of appointments, and thought it would allow them to better manage their time. One woman explained: "That would be good that in advance we know the schedule, so we can finish other work and come."

When asked for their opinions on the length of the group sessions (90–120 min), providers stated that it would be feasible and acceptable in each of their settings, although some thought it might present a challenge to manage OPD patients at the same time. Still, they reported that they would appreciate the increased efficiency of seeing 10–12 ANC patients in that period of time. However, providers from public facilities believed that 120 min would likely be necessary in settings serving less educated women in order to allow more time for discussion. A provider commented, "Initially again, I was doubtful that women will be ready to spend two hours, but we didn't feel any time that any one of them was bored or was not attentive or was in a hurry to go home. In fact, I had an experience that they wanted to keep on talking. I didn't feel that anyone felt like leaving even when session was over. I think if they have a good experience they would take out time." And, "In a way we see, group ANC is good. Together for all 10 women, physical checkups are done and their BP, weight, etc. is completed in one and half hour to two hours. Otherwise in individual visit women come one by one so our lot of time goes in that. If we call women together, it will save our time, and they will get to know each other."

Overall, pregnant women expressed satisfaction with the proposed session duration of 90–120 min because it was spent actively participating, rather than simply waiting to see the doctor. One woman remarked, "It is better to come over here rather than watching TV at home, at least by coming here we felt good and learnt something new." In their focus group discussion, all of the husbands ($n = 5$) also agreed with that sentiment.

Solutions to potential barriers

Participants were asked to identify any potential barriers to implementation in their setting, and to share their ideas about solutions that could help overcome those barriers. Providers made several concrete suggestions:

a) Conduct sessions in the afternoons as most women are occupied with chores and household responsibilities in the mornings
b) In addition to grouping women by similar gestational age, be sure to organize groups based on a common language (demonstration sessions showed that not all women attending a facility in Vadodara speak the same language)
c) To ensure consistency of leadership, if one group leader is unable to join a session due to an unforeseen event, ensure that the co-facilitator, who

is familiar with the group and its concerns, is available to lead the session

d) To ensure continuity of care, if a pregnant woman is unable to join a session due to an unforeseen event, ensure that she can schedule an individual ANC visit so that her care is not interrupted
e) Consider engaging an additional support person (not clinical staff) at the facility to manage the logistical aspects of the group (i.e. scheduling, pre-session reminders to the women)
f) Engage leadership at a higher level in the (public) system to help support the implementing facilities and their staff

The providers from the public facilities felt that support from leadership at the health system level would be essential to the successful implementation of the group model. One ANM explained: "Yes, we can do [group ANC] but we need support for that. Meeting space for all the people, making groups [with a] minimum [of] 8–12 women."

Three pregnant women felt that pre-session reminders (phone call or text) would help group ANC participants remember to attend each group visit, and one woman suggested that it might be helpful to have a physiotherapist join the sessions.

The potential barriers to implementing group ANC in Vadodara as well as the concrete solutions offered to overcome them, while hypothetical, provide useful insights and suggestions grounded in knowledge of an urban health system in the Indian context that should be tested through implementation research.

Discussion

To our knowledge, this is the first study to evaluate the feasibility and acceptability of group ANC in India and the first study in Asia to evaluate a group model for pregnant women that includes a clinical care component. The findings provide evidence to support the rationale for future studies designed to evaluate the effects of group ANC on health outcomes, experiences of care, and system performance in India. The results of this qualitative assessment of stakeholders' perceptions about the potential feasibility and acceptability of introducing group ANC in India were positive following participation in a demonstration of one mock session of the model.

While some participants expressed initial skepticism about the group model in concept, after participating in the demonstration the reaction of both providers and recipients of care was generally enthusiastic. Overall, pregnant women who participated were more open to the novel experience. Ultimately, both groups of participants saw group ANC as a vehicle for delivering more comprehensive ANC services, improving experiences of care, empowering women to become more active partners and participants in their care, and potentially addressing some current health system challenges. For example, both women and providers felt that group ANC might help to reduce wait times for women while care providers and administrators also expressed optimism that group ANC could improve patient retention in facilities. Care administrators identified patient retention as a priority goal as well as a challenge in Vadodara. The feedback gathered through the various qualitative methods also suggests some concrete system requirements that, if met, could help to ensure effective implementation of this model.

This study has some limitations. Due to resource and time constraints, we were only able to demonstrate one session of the full four-session model and participants' responses and perceptions may have been different following a longer exposure to the model. Our study had a relatively small number of participants although the number was likely adequate given the qualitative methods used; however, we cannot fully ascertain the adequacy of the sample size as our study was not designed to test saturation. Our study instruments (focus group discussion guides, in-depth interview guides, and written survey) were not validated prior to use in this study. In addition, because the researchers were involved in the model demonstration as well as the data collection, there is a possibility of social desirability bias in the responses. Finally, because our study was conducted only in three urban facilities, the outcomes may not be transferable to other settings. Future research on group ANC in India could assess its feasibility and acceptability in a broader variety of settings, and evaluate outcomes of the model in both rural and urban facilities.

Our research complements and builds on the small but growing evidence base of studies assessing the feasibility of group ANC in LMICs. Similar to the findings of the three studies published to date that have collected stakeholder responses to group ANC [10–12], our research also recorded positive responses from study participants. The results of our study provide support for testing the group ANC model in urban India, as they indicate that the model would be both possible and welcome in this setting. We also gathered some specific suggestions to improve the feasibility of implementing group ANC in urban India. These include ensuring adequate staffing ratios to handle the volume and range of patients presenting to the clinics who are not enrolled in group ANC; hiring dedicated personnel to help with group ANC logistics and scheduling; giving attention to the space requirements for effective group ANC; and initiation of a system of appointment reminders for women. These insights could be useful to others planning to implement the model in similar LMIC settings.

This study is particularly timely given the recently updated WHO ANC recommendations (2016), which identify group ANC as a health systems intervention with the potential to improve the utilization and quality of ANC. The WHO report offers the following context-specific research recommendation:

> "Group antenatal care provided by qualified health-care professionals may be offered as an alternative to individual antenatal care for pregnant women in the context of rigorous research, depending on a woman's preferences and provided that the infrastructure and resources for delivery of group antenatal care are available" [1].

Conclusions

This qualitative research study collected the perceptions of care providers, care administrators, pregnant women and their family support persons to assess the feasibility and acceptability of a model of group ANC that was developed through a systematic scoping review of group care in LMICs. It demonstrates positive responses from stakeholders of all types in a variety of care delivery settings following active participation in a demonstration of the model. It provides specific feedback from participants on each of the major components of the group care model: physical assessment, active learning, and peer support. It suggests concrete ways to facilitate the introduction of the group ANC model in urban India and to overcome potential system barriers to implementation.

Abbreviations

ANC: Antenatal care; ANM: Auxiliary nurse midwife; ASHA: Accredited social health activist; BP: Blood pressure; CORT: Centre for operations research and training; LMICs: Low- and middle-income countries; MOHFW: Ministry of Health and Family Welfare; OPD: Out-patient clinic day; PMSMY: Pradhan mantri surakshit matritva yojana; PNC: Postnatal care; UPHC: Urban primary care clinic; WHO: World Health Organization

Acknowledgements

The authors would like to thank the following people for their contributions to the development of the research study described in this paper and for their support during its implementation: Ana Langer, Maternal Health Task Force, Women & Health Initiative, Harvard T.H. Chan School of Public Health; M.E. Khan, CORT; Sandhya Barge, CORT; Jashoda Sharma, CORT; Shoba Ramanadhan, Harvard Catalyst consultant; and the two individuals who acted as co-facilitators in the demonstrations of the group ANC model that were conducted with the study participants.

Funding

Funding for this study was provided by the John D. and Catherine T. MacArthur Foundation. The funding body had no role in the design of the study or the collection, analysis, and interpretation of data or in writing the manuscript.

Authors' contributions

RRJ, MO'C, and MNW developed the concept and study design. RRJ, BVU, MO'C, JS, and KL participated in the conception, design, analysis and/or interpretation of data. RRJ and BVU served as primary investigators and project directors in the US and India, respectively. MO'C and KL served as research coordinators and project managers in the US and India, respectively. BVU and MO'C managed the IRB applications, with inputs from other members of the team, in the US and India, respectively. RRJ, MO'C, JS, BVU and KL contributed to the development of the demonstration model, and the study instruments. RRJ, BVU, MO'C and KL participated in the model demonstration. BVU and KL led participant and demonstrator recruitment, selection of study sites, carried out the data collection, transcribed and translated the data into English, and analyzed the results. All authors participated in writing the manuscript by reviewing drafts and approving the final version.

Competing interests

The authors declare that they have no competing interests.

Author details

[1]Maternal Health Task Force, Women & Health Initiative, Department of Global Health and Population, Harvard T.H. Chan School of Public Health, 651 Huntington Avenue, Boston, MA 02115, USA. [2]Centre for Operations Research and Training, 402 Woodland Apartment, Race Course Circle, Vadodara, Gujarat 390 007, India. [3]Maternal Health Task Force, Women & Health Initiative, Harvard T.H. Chan School of Public Health, 651 Huntington Avenue, Boston, MA 02115, USA. [4]Department of Global Health and Population, Harvard T. H. Chan School of Public Health, 677 Huntington Ave, Boston, MA 02115, USA.

References

1. WHO Recommendations on Antenatal Care for a Positive Pregnancy Experience. Geneva: World Health Organization; 2016.
2. Rising SS. Centering pregnancy: an interdisciplinary model of empowerment. J Nurse Midwifery. 1998;43(1):9.
3. Ickovics JR, Kershaw TS, Westdahl C, Magriples U, Massey Z, Reynolds H. Rising SS: group prenatal care and perinatal outcomes: a randomized controlled trial. Obstet Gynecol. 2007;110(2 Pt 1):330–9.
4. Earnshaw VA, Rosenthal L, Cunningham SD, Kershaw T, Lewis J, Rising SS, Stasko E, Tobin J, Ickovics JR. Exploring group composition among young, urban women of color in prenatal care: implications for satisfaction, engagement, and group attendance. Womens Health Issues. 2016;26(1):110–5.
5. Ickovics JR, Earnshaw V, Lewis JB, Kershaw TS, Magriples U, Stasko E, Rising SS, Cassells A, Cunningham S, Bernstein P, et al. Cluster randomized controlled trial of group prenatal care: perinatal outcomes among adolescents in new York City health centers. Am J Public Health. 2016; 106(2):359–65.
6. Magriples U, Boynton MH, Kershaw TS, Lewis J, Rising SS, Tobin JN, Epel E, Ickovics JR. The impact of group prenatal care on pregnancy and postpartum weight trajectories. Am J Obstet Gynecol. 2015;213(5): 688 e681–9.
7. Tanner-Smith EE, Steinka-Fry KT, Gesell SB. Comparative effectiveness of group and individual prenatal care on gestational weight gain. Matern Child Health J. 2014;18(7):1711–20.
8. Catling CJ, Medley N, Foureur M, Ryan C, Leap N, Teate A, Homer CS. Group versus conventional antenatal care for women. Cochrane Database Syst Rev. 2015;2:CD007622.
9. Sharma J, O'Connor M, Jolivet RR. Group antenatal care in low- and middle-income countries: a systematic evidence synthesis. Reprod Health. 2018; 15(1):38. https://doi.org/10.1186/s12978-018-0476-9.
10. Patil CL, Abrams ET, Klima C, Kaponda CP, Leshabari SC, Vonderheid SC, Kamanga M, Norr KF. CenteringPregnancy-Africa: a pilot of group antenatal care to address millennium development goals. Midwifery. 2013;29(10):1190–8.
11. Ghani RMA. Perception toward conducting the centering pregnancy model in the Egyptian teaching hospitals: a step to improve the quality of antenatal care. Eur J Biol Med Sci Res. 2014;2(2):45–54.

12. Arnold J, Morgan A, Morrison B. Paternal perceptions of and satisfaction with group prenatal Care in Botswana. Online J Cult Competence Nurs Healthc. 2014;4(2):17–26.
13. Jafari F. Maternal and neonatal outcomes of group prenatal care: a new experience in Iran. Early Hum Dev. 2010;86:S140.
14. Jafari F, Eftekhar H, Mohammad K, Fotouhi A. Does group prenatal care affect satisfaction and prenatal care utilization in Iranian pregnant women? Iran J Public Health. 2010;39(2):52–62.
15. Population of Vadodara. 2017. http://indiapopulation2017.in/population-of-vadodara-2017.html. Accessed 28 Mar 2018.
16. Buffington ST, Sibley LM, Beck DR, Armbruster DA. Home based life saving skills - second edition. Silver Spring: American College of Nurse-Midwives; 2010.
17. Maternal Health Division. Pradhan Mantri Surakshit Matritva Abhiyan. New Delhi: Ministry of Health and Family Welfare, Government of India; 2016.
18. Maternal Health Division. Guidelines for antenatal care and skilled attendance at birth by ANMs/LHVs/SNs. New Delhi: Ministry of Health and Family Welfare, Government of India; 2010.

20

The correlation between raised body mass index and assisted reproductive treatment outcomes

Prasanna Raj Supramaniam[1*], Monica Mittal[1], Enda McVeigh[2] and Lee Nai Lim[1]

Abstract

Background: Public funding for fertility services within the United Kingdom is limited, and therefore, strict guidance exists regarding who can be offered treatment under the National Health Service (NHS). Body mass index (BMI) is a universal criteria adopted by both the public and private sector.

This study addresses an important aspect of the impact of a raised BMI on fertility treatment outcomes. We standardise the analysis of the data by only including studies incorporating the WHO BMI criteria; the current reference point for clinicians and clinical commissioning groups in ascertaining which group of patients should receive treatment. This study is an update of the previous systematic review performed in 2010, with the inclusion of a larger number of cycles from central databases such as the Society for Assisted Reproductive Technology (SART).

Methods: An electronic literature search was conducted through the Cochrane, Medline and Embase libraries. Data extraction for each outcome measure was pooled and expressed as an odds ratio with 95% confidence intervals. Where clinical heterogeneity was evident, the random effects model was used to calculate the risk ratio and a fixed effects model was used for the remaining studies. A p value < 0.05 was considered statistically significant.

Results: A total of 49 studies have been identified and included in this systematic review. Overweight and obese (BMI ≥ 25 kg/m^2) women have a statistically significant lower live birth rate (OR 0.81, 95% CI 0.74–0.89, $p < 0.00001$) following Assisted Reproductive Technology (ART) when comparisons are drawn to women with a normal BMI. An increase is also demonstrated in the number of miscarriages experienced by women with a BMI ≥ 30 kg/m^2 (OR 1.52, 95% CI 1.28–1.81, $p < 0.00001$).

Conclusion: Although this review concludes that a clear impact of BMI on ART outcomes is demonstrated, there remains questions as to the pathophysiology underlying these differences. This review supports the government's stringent criteria regarding BMI categories under which NHS funding is made available for ART, through a clear description of poor reproductive outcomes in women with a BMI ≥ 30 kg/m^2.

Keywords: Body mass index (BMI), Assisted reproductive technology (ART), Overweight, Obese

* Correspondence: prasannaraj@doctors.org.uk

[1]Oxford University Hospitals NHS Foundation Trust, John Radcliffe Hospital, Headley Way, Headington, Oxford OX3 9DU, UK

Full list of author information is available at the end of the article

Plain English summary

This study highlights the impact of an overweight or obese female partner on fertility treatment outcomes, in particular focusing on IVF. Women who are overweight or obese have been shown to be less likely to have a life birth outcome from an IVF cycle. They are also more likely to suffer from early miscarriages whilst undergoing fertility treatments.

Main manuscript

The correlation between raised body mass index and assisted reproductive treatment outcomes: A systematic review and meta-analysis of the evidence.

Background

Obesity is a major challenge for today's clinicians. In 2016, the World Health Organisation (WHO) [1] stated that a staggering 39% of adults aged > 18 years fell into the overweight category, of which 40% were accounted for by women. Furthermore, 13% of the adult population were documented to be obese, with women accounting for 15% (WHO Global Health Observatory Data 2016). A raised body mass index (BMI) has been linked to a number of medical comorbidities, as well as being implicated in having a detrimental impact on the reproductive capacity of women in particular. Women who fall into high BMI categories can present with hypothalamic-pituitary ovarian dysfunction and thus, low fecundity rates. In 2011, Rittenberg et al., [2] concluded that women with a BMI ≥ 25.0 kg/m^2 had a lower live birth rate through assisted reproductive treatments (ART) compared with women of a normal BMI. This has been further supported by multiple large studies evaluating the impact of BMI on ART outcomes.

The WHO classification of BMI is widely referred to, and provides standardisation for comparison of research outcomes. A documented BMI of 18.5–24.9 kg/m^2 is considered normal and healthy and the preferred range. A BMI of 25–29.9 kg/m^2 refers to overweight and a BMI ≥ 30 kg/m^2 is considered obese. The latter range is further subdivided into Class 1 (30.0–34.9 kg/m^2), Class 2 (35.0–39.9 kg/m^2) and Class 3 (≥ 40.0 kg/m^2).

This paper, considers the current evidence regarding the impact of raised BMI on outcomes following ART treatment. A systematic review and meta-analysis of the available evidence will help provide or refute the current recommendations from the government regarding the allocation of resources for fertility treatment.

Methods

Search strategy

Literature searches were conducted through the Cochrane, Embase and Medline libraries (1966–2017). The medical subject headings (MeSH) were generated for two categories: 1. Body mass index (BMI, overweight, obesity); 2. in vitro fertilisation (IVF)/ intracytoplasmic sperm injection (ICSI) (embryo, embryo transfer, ART). All identified papers were reviewed by two authors (PRS and MM) independently. All discrepancies, regarding inclusion or exclusion of the data were discussed with a final decision mutually agreed upon.

Study inclusion and exclusion criteria

All relevant published studies reporting on the effects of BMI on IVF and ICSI pregnancy outcomes were included. Studies that reported donor cycles, conception by natural cycles, intrauterine insemination, waist hip ratio, and non-WHO classification of BMI were excluded. In addition, studies reporting on the effects of paternal body mass index on IVF/ ICSI outcomes were also excluded.

Outcome measures

The primary outcome measure assessed was live birth rate following an IVF/ ICSI cycle. Secondary outcome measures included: clinical pregnancy rate; and, miscarriage rate. The presence of a gestational sac on an ultrasound scan at least four weeks following on from an embryo transfer was used as confirmation for a clinical pregnancy. The clinical pregnancy rate was calculated per IVF/ ICSI cycle. For the purpose of this review, miscarriage was defined as pregnancy loss ≤ 20 weeks gestation. The miscarriage rate was calculated per clinical pregnancy.

Statistical analysis

Data extraction for each outcome measure was pooled and expressed as an odds ratio (OR) with a 95% confidence interval (CI). Clinical heterogeneity (I^2) [3] was considered significant when the I^2 value was < 50%. Where clinical heterogeneity was evident, the random effects model (DerSimonian and Laird, 1986) was used to calculate the risk ratio, and clinical heterogeneity was explored by comparing the variation in studies, such as, study design, study quality and interventions. Particular care was taken to further evaluate studies with similar first authors to avoid heterogeneity in the study population. For the remaining pooled data, the fixed effect model [4] was used to calculate the risk ratio. Statistical analysis was performed using the RevMan 5.3 software. A p value < 0.05 was considered statistically significant.

Results

The search strategy yielded 7458 electronic citations (Fig. 1). Of this, 2830 were removed secondary to duplications. Titles and abstracts were reviewed for the remaining 4628 publications. After screening of the titles and abstracts, 4508 publications were further excluded.

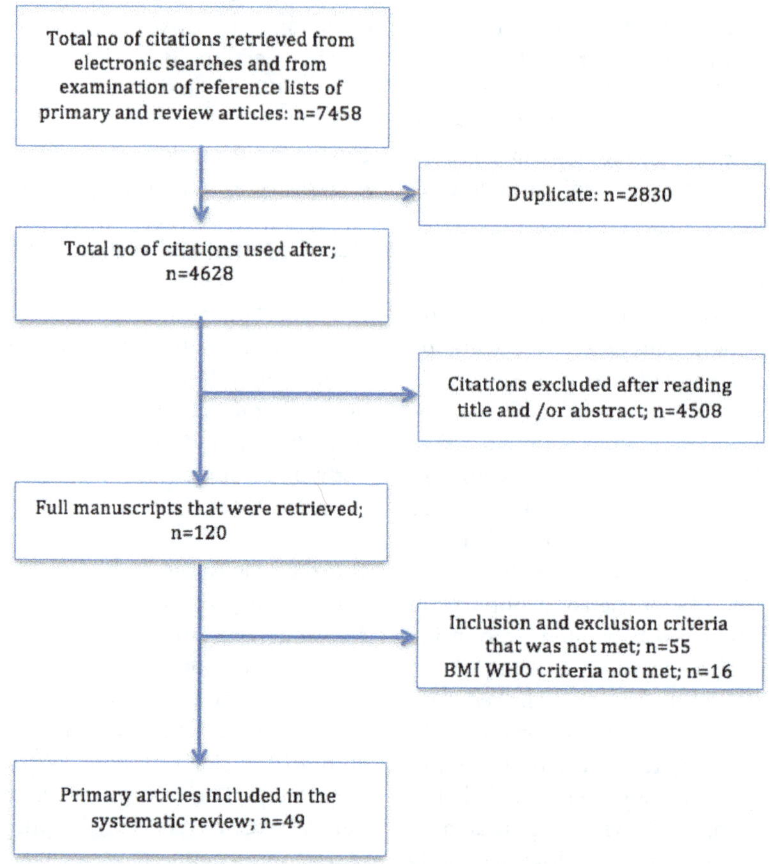

Fig. 1 Flow chart for literature search and study selection

Full manuscripts were obtained for the remaining 120 articles. A further 16 articles were excluded as they did not use the WHO classification for BMI categories. A further 55 articles were excluded as per the inclusion exclusion criteria. The remaining 49 articles met all requirements and were included in this systematic review and meta-analysis (Table 1).

Primary outcome measure

Life birth rate per IVF/ ICSI cycle

In women with a BMI ≥25 kg/m^2 versus BMI < 25 kg/m^2, a total of 14 studies were pooled and a statistically significant reduction in the live birth rate (OR 0.81, 95% CI 0.74–0.89, $p < 0.00001$; Fig. 2a) was seen. There was significant heterogeneity between the included studies ($I^2 = 65\%$).

A total of 11 studies compared women with a normal BMI against those who were overweight (BMI 25–29.9 kg/m^2). An analysis of the pooled data showed a statistically significant reduction in the live birth rate in women with a BMI 25–29.9 (OR 0.92, 95% CI 0.86–0.97, $p = 0.005$; Fig. 2b). No significant heterogeneity ($I^2 = 18\%$) was documented.

Data for women with a normal BMI versus BMI ≥ 30 kg/m^2 came from the pooling of 10 studies. The live birth rate for women with a BMI ≥30 kg/m^2 was statistically significantly lower than for women with a normal BMI (OR 0.81, 95% CI 0.79–0.82, $p < 0.00001$; Fig. 2c). No significant heterogeneity ($I^2 = 0\%$) was detected in the data source.

Secondary outcome measures

Clinical pregnancy rate

A total of 37 studies were pooled for BMI < 25 kg/m^2 versus BMI ≥25 kg/m^2. A statistically significant reduction in the clinical pregnancy rate was demonstrated for women with a BMI ≥25 kg/m^2 (OR 0.82, 95% CI 0.77–0.88, $p < 0.00001$; Fig. 3a). However, there was significant heterogeneity ($I^2 = 58\%$, p < 0.00001) between the studies analysed.

A statistically significant reduction in the clinical pregnancy rate was demonstrated for women with a BMI between 25 and 29.9 kg/m^2 when compared to women with a normal BMI (19 studies pooled, OR 0.89, 95% CI 0.84–0.94, $p < 0.00001$; Fig. 3b). No significant heterogeneity ($I^2 = 31\%$) was seen between the studies.

Table 1 Details of included studies

Study	Methodology (population size)	Intervention	Exclusion Criteria	BMI Categories (kg/m^2) and numbers	Outcome Measures
Fedorcsak et al. 2000 [8] (1996–1998)	Retrospective Cohort study (383 women)	IVF/ICSI	12 patients excluded as incomplete data	< 25.0 (304 women) ≥25.0 (79 women)	Live birth rate Fertilization rate No of oocytes retrieved Abortion rate
Wittemer et al. 2000 [9] (1997–1998)	Retrospective study (398 women)	IVF/ICSI	None stated	< 20.0 (87 women) 20.0–25.0 (222 women) ≥ 25.0 (89 women)	Pregnancy rate Delivery rate Miscarriage rate
Wang et al. 2000 [10] (1987–1998)	Retrospective study (3586 women)	IVF/ICSI and GIFT	None stated	< 20.0 (441 women) 20.0–24.9 (1910 women) 25.0–29.9 (814 women) 30.0–34.9 (304 women) ≥35.0 (117 women)	Probability of achieving at least one pregnancy
Loveland et al. 2001 [11] (1997–1999)	Retrospective study (139 women / 180 cycles)	IVF	Women > 40 years of age, blastocyst or frozen embryo transfer, donor cycles	≤25 (70 women / 87 cycles) > 25 (69 women / 93 cycles)	Number of oocytes Clinical pregnancy rate Spontaneous abortion Ongoing pregnancy rate
Wang et al. 2001 [12] (1987–1999)	Cohort study (1018 women)	IVF/ICSI/ GIFT	Women whose BMI or PCOS status was not assessed	< 20.0 (112 women) 20.0–24.9 (509 women) 25.0–29.9 (231 women) 30.0–34.9 (116 women) ≥35.0 (50 women)	Spontaneous abortion
Wang et al. 2002 [13] (1987–1999)	Retrospective analysis (2349 women)	IVF/ICSI/ GIFT	Ectopic pregnancy, late pregnancy, women whose BMI was measured >/= 1 year before pregnancy	< 18.5 (70 women) 18.5–24.9 (1508 women) 25–29.9 (503 women) 30–34.9 (198 women) ≥35 (70 women)	Spontaneous miscarriage
Winter et al. 2002 [14] (1994–1999)	Cohort (1123 women / 1196 cycles)	IVF/ICSI/ GIFT		< 18.5 (26 women) 18.5–25.0 (701 women) 25.1–30.0 (243 women) 30.1–35.0 (107 women) > 35.0 (46 women)	Early pregnancy loss
Doody et al. 2003 [15] (2000–2003)	Retrospective analysis (822 retrievals)	IVF/ICSI	Donor cycles, age > 40 years	< 25 (460 women) 25–29.9 (194 women) 30–34.9 (89 women) > 35 (79 women)	Pregnancy rate Implantation rate No of oocytes No of embryos transferred Ongoing pregnancy rate
Fedorcsak et al. 2004 [16] (1996–2002)	Retrospective Study (2660 women / 5019 cycles)	IVF/ICSI	None stated	< 18.5 (76 women/136 cycles) 18.5–24.9 (1839 women/ 3457 cycles) 25.0–29.9 (504 women/ 963 cycles) ≥30.0 (241 women/ 463 cycles)	No of oocytes collected No of embryo transferred No of embryo transfers No of biochemical pregnancies Early pregnancy loss Miscarriage (6–12 weeks), (> 12 weeks) Ectopic pregnancy Stillbirth Live birth rate Dose of FSH Duration of FSH
Ryley et al. 2004 [17]	Retrospective study (6827 cycles)	IVF	Women with BMI > 40	< 20.0 (466 cycles) 20.0–24.9 (3605 cycles) 25.0–29.9 (1632 cycles) 30.0–34.9 (724 cycles) =35 (400 cycles)	Clinical pregnancy rate No of oocytes
Van Swieten et al. 2005 [18]	Observational (162 women/ 288 cycle)	IVF/ICSI	None stated	< 25 (101 women) 25–30 (32 women) > 30 (29 women)	Fertilisation rate No oocytes retrieved Clinical pregnancy rate Abortion rate

Table 1 Details of included studies *(Continued)*

Study	Methodology (population size)	Intervention	Exclusion Criteria	BMI Categories (kg/m^2) and numbers	Outcome Measures
Hammadeh et al. 2005 [19]	Prospective (52 women)	IVF	None stated	≤25.0 (28 women) > 25.0 (24 women)	Pregnancy rate
Dechaud et al. 2006 [20]	Prospective study (573 women/ 789 cycles)	IVF/ICSI	Women with a history of uterine surgery, hydrosalpinges evidenced by ultrasonography, three or more failed attempts at IVF, frozen-thawed cycles, women undergoing pre-implantation diagnosis and those using a protocol other than the long protocol	< 20 (186 women/ 264 cycles) 20–25 (283 women/ 394 cycles) 25–30 (68 women/ 83 cycles) ≥30 (36 women/ 48 cycles)	Duration of ovarian stimulation Dose of FSH Implantation rate No of oocytes Fertilization rate Clinical pregnancy rate Miscarriage rate
Dokras et al. 2006 [21] (1995–2005)	Retrospective Study (1293 women)	IVF/IVF with ICSI	Women > 38 years of age, day 2 transfer cycles, cryopreserved embryo transfers, donor oocyte cycle, gamete intrafallopian transfer and zygote intrafallopian transfer cycles	< 25 (683 women) 25–29.9 (295 women) 30.0–39.9 (236 women) ≥40 (79 women)	No of follicles aspirated Fertilization rate No of embryo(s) transferred Clinical pregnancy rate Miscarriage rate Delivery rate Days of stimulation
Mitwally et al. 2006 [22]	Cohort (183 cycles)	IVF	None stated	< 25.0 (102 cycles) ≥25.0 (81 cycles)	Clinical pregnancy rate
Metwally 2007 [23] (2001–2006)	Retrospective analysis (426 women)	IVF/ICSI	Cycles on women whose BMI was unrecorded	19–24.9 (241 women) 25–29.9 (113 women) ≥30 (72 women)	Fertilization rate Clinical pregnancy rate Dose of FSH Duration of FSH No of oocytes collected
Esinler et al. 2008 [24]	Retrospective Study (775 women/ 1113 cycles)	ICSI	Freeze-thaw cycles, female age > 40, presence of PCOS, history of irregular menstrual cycle and suspected poor ovarian response	18.5–24.9 (451 women/ 627 cycles) 25.0–29.9 (222 women/ 339 cycles) ≥30.0 (102 women/ 147 cycles)	Clinical pregnancy rate Fertilization rate No of miscarriages No of oocytes Dose of FSH Duration of FSH
Martinuzzi et al. 2008 [25] (2004–2006)	Retrospective study (417 women)	IVF	Women > 36 years of age, cycle day-3	< 18.5 (21 women) 18.5–24.9 (267 women) 25.0–29.9 (77 women) ≥30 (52 women)	No of oocytes Fertilization rate Implantation rate Clinical pregnancy rate Ongoing pregnancy rate
Moini et al. 2008 [26] (2002–2003)	Cross-sectional study (287 women)	IVF/ICSI	Women who did not have polycystic ovary syndrome, age > 40 years, BMI < 20, women with hypo/ hyperthyroidism, hyperprolactinemia and diabetes type 1	20–25 (133 women) 25.1–30 (117 women) > 30 (37 women)	No of oocytes No of transferred embryos Clinical pregnancy rate Miscarriage rate
Sneed et al. 2008 [27] (2005–2006)	Retrospective analysis (1273 women)	IVF	Frozen cycles, donor oocyte or gestational surrogacy cycles, age > 44 years	< 18.5 (28 women) > 18.5–24.9 (613 women) > 25–29.9 (325 women) > 30 (307 women)	No of oocytes No of embryo transfers Fertilization rate Implantation rate Spontaneous abortion Clinical pregnancies Live birth rate
Ozgun et al. 2009 [28] (2006–2007)	Prospective study (604 women)	ICSI	Women > 42 years old, medical co-morbidities such as diabetes mellitus, hyper or hypothyroidism, basal FSH > 15 IU/L, thawed embryo transfer cycles, history of prior ovarian surgery, poor responders, couples with more than one etiology for their infertility	< 18.5 (10 women) 18.5–24.9 (232 women) 25–29.9 (229 women) 30–35.9 (111 women) ≥36 (22 women)	No of Pregnancy Total FSH dosage

Table 1 Details of included studies *(Continued)*

Study	Methodology (population size)	Intervention	Exclusion Criteria	BMI Categories (kg/m^2) and numbers	Outcome Measures
Sathya et al. 2010 [29]	Retrospective study (308 women)	IVF	Women > 40 years of age, FSH > 10 mIU/ml	< 25 (88 women) 25–30 (147 women) > 30 (73 women)	No of embryos transferred Clinical pregnancy rate Missed abortion rate Multiple pregnancy rate Ectopic pregnancy rate Implantation rate Gonadotrophin dosage
Zhang et al. 2010 [30] (2002–2008)	Retrospective study (2628 women)	IVF/ICSI	Patients with severe endometriosis (III and IV stage) diagnosed by laparoscopy, more than two failed previous attempts, preimplantation diagnosis cycles, frozen thawed cycles, protocols other than the long protocol	18.5–24.9 (2222 women) 25.0–29.9 (379 women) ≥30.0 (27 women)	No of oocytes Fertilization rate Pregnancy rate Early pregnancy loss rate Ectopic pregnancy Miscarriage rate Live birth rate Days of FSH stimulation Dosage of FSH stimulation Ongoing pregnancy rate
Bellver et al. 2010 [31] (2001–2007)	Retrospective study (6500 cycles)	IVF/ICSI	None stated	< 20 (669 women / 1070 cycles) 20–24.9 (2620 women/ 3930 cycles) 25–29.9 (676 women/ 1081 cycles) ≥ 30 (262 cycles/ 419 cycles)	Total dose of gonadotrophin No of oocytes Fertilization rate No of embryos transferred Implantation rate Pregnancy rate Clinical pregnancy rate Clinical and global miscarriage rate Live birth rate
Vilarino et al. 2010 [32] (2008)	Retrospective (208 cycles/ 191 women)	IVF/ICSI	Frozen and donor oocyte-derived cycles	< 25 (137 cycles) ≥25 (71 cycles)	Fertilisation rate No of transferred embryos Pregnancy rate Early pregnancy loss Clinical miscarriage rate Ectopic pregnancy Live birth rate Dosage of FSH
Farhi et al. 2010 [33] (2006–2007)	Retrospective study (233 women/ 233 cycles)	IVF	Women ≥38 years of age, other than 2 high-quality embryos, ≥3 previous IVF attempts, women with hydrosalpinx, fibroid uterus, congenital uterine anomaly and chronic illness	≤25.0 (160 women) > 25.0 (73 women)	Live birth rate Pregnancy rate No of oocytes Fertilization rate
Davies et al. 2010 [34] (2008–2009)	232 cycles	IVF	Donor egg, gestational carrier and pre-implantation genetic diagnosis cycles	< 25.0 (176 cycles) > 25.0 (56 cycles)	Fetal heartbeat rates
Funabiki et al. 2011 [35] (2006–2010)	Retrospective study (859 women)	IVF	None stated	< 18.5 (152 women) 18.5–25.0 (648 women) ≥25.0 (59 women)	Pregnancy rate Ongoing pregnancy rate Miscarriage rate No of oocytes
Hill et al. 2011 [36]	Prospective study (117 women)	IVF	Women > 42 years of age, patients with elevated FSH levels (≥12 mIU/mL)	< 25.0 (58 women) ≥25.0 (59 women) < 30.0 (96 women) ≥30.0 (21 women)	Live birth rate Pregnancy rate Implantation rate No of oocytes No of embryo transferred Days of stimulation

Table 1 Details of included studies *(Continued)*

Study	Methodology (population size)	Intervention	Exclusion Criteria	BMI Categories (kg/m^2) and numbers	Outcome Measures
Pinborg et al. 2011 [37] (2005–2006)	Cohort study (487 women/ 1417 cycles)	IVF/ ICSI/ FET	Patients undergoing intrauterine insemination cycles, patients with an existing child from fertility treatment, couples who had adopted a child in the 12th month follow-up period and couples who had no treatment during the first 12 months of follow up	< 18.5 (20 women) 18.5–24.9 (305 women) 25.0–29.9 (103 women) ≥30.0 (59 women)	Fertilization rate No of oocytes Biochemical pregnancy rate Ectopic pregnancy rate Ongoing pregnancy rate Miscarriage rate Live birth rate Dose of gonadotrophin stimulation
Parker et al. 2011 [38] (2010–2011)	Retrospective study (995 patients)	IVF/ICSI	None stated	< 18.5 (18 women) 18.5–24.9 (475 women) 25–29.9 (241 women) > 30 (221 women)	No of oocytes Clinical pregnancy rate Implantation rate Ongoing pregnancy rate Total FSH dosage No of embryo transferred
Rittenberg et al. 2011 [39] (2006–2010)	Cohort Study (413 women)	IVF/ICSI	Women > 40 years, BMI < 18.5, BMI > 35, pre-implantation genetic diagnosis, donor oocyte or embryos frozen for fertility preservation prior to cancer therapy cycles, mullerian duct anomalies, monozygotic twin gestations	18.5–24.9 (192 women) ≥25 (133 women)	Oocyte fertilisation rate No of oocytes Clinical pregnancy rate Live birth rate Miscarriage rate Duration of stimulation
Singh et al. 2011 [40] (2008–2010)	Retrospective Study (328 women/ 342 cycles)	IVF/ICSI	Women with confounding factors for poor response, endometrial pathologies, hydrosalpinx, ≥3 previous failed attempts, frozen thawed cycles	< 18.5 (26 women) 18.5–24.9 (141 women) 25–29.9 (131 women) > 30 (18 women)	Fertilisation rate Pregnancy rate Total dose of FSH Total days of stimulation No of oocytes retrieved Fertilization rate Clinical pregnancy rate
Luke et al. 2011 [41] (2007–2008)	Historical cohort study (152,500 cycles)	IVF	Women whose height and weight were not recorded, gestational carrier cycles, research or embryo banking with no outcome reported	< 18.5 (4254 cycles) 18.5–24.9 (86,860 cycles) 25–29.9 (35,452 cycles) 30.0–34.9 (15,406 cycles) 35.0–39.9 (6920 cycles) 40.0–44.9 (2513 cycles) 45.0–49.9 (805 cycles)	Pregnancy rate Fetal death or stillborn
Chavarro et al. 2012 [42] (2004–2011)	Prospective study (170 women/ 233 cycles)	IVF/ICSI	Women < 18 and > 45 years of age	< 20 (22 women) 20–22.4 (47 women) 22.5–24.9 (42 women) 25–29.9 (35 women) ≥30 (24 women)	Clinical pregnancy rate Total gonadotrophin dose Fertilization rate Clinical pregnancy rate Live birth rate
Galal et al. 2012 [43]	Prospective cohort (220 women)	ICSI	None stated	< 25.0 (110 women) > 25.0 (110 women)	No of oocytes Fertilization rate Clinical pregnancy rate No of embryos transferred
Werner et al. 2012 [44] (2008–2012)	Retrospective study (355 women)	IVF	None stated	< 18.5 (13 women) 18.5–24.9 (209 women) 25.0–29.9 (88 women) > 30.0 (45 women)	Pregnancy rate Clinical implantation rate Sustained implantation rate
Zander-Fox et al. 2012 [45] (2006–2007)	Retrospective study (2089 cycles)	IVF/ICSI	Women > 38 years of age, natural and donor cycles	18.5–24.9 (1065 cycles) 25.0–29.9 (486 cycles) 30.0–34.9 (244 cycles) 35.0–39.9 (144 cycles) ≥40.0 (118 cycles)	No of oocytes Fertilisation rate Live delivery Clinical pregnancy No of oocytes
Ozgun et al. 2012 [46] (2005–2010)	Retrospective cohort (935 women)	ICSI	No exclusion criteria	< 18.5 (18 women) 18.5–24.9 (398 women) 25–29.9 (355 women) ≥30 (164 women)	Clinical pregnancy rateNo of oocytes Miscarriage rate Total gonadotrophin dose

Table 1 Details of included studies *(Continued)*

Study	Methodology (population size)	Intervention	Exclusion Criteria	BMI Categories (kg/m^2) and numbers	Outcome Measures
Ramezanzadeh et al. 2012 [47] (2010–2011)	Prospective study (236 women)	IVF	Male factor infertility according to the WHO criteria, presence of systemic disease, age < 18 years or > 40 years and donor oocytes	< 25 (93 women) 25–30 (94 women) > 30 (49 women)	No of oocytes Fertilization rate No of embryo transferred Biochemical pregnancies Clinical pregnancy rate Implantation rate
Moragianni et al. 2012 [48] (2007–2008)	Retrospective cohort study (4609 women)	IVF/ IVF-ICSI	Women < 20 years and > 47 years of age, donor oocytes, gestational surrogacy, cryopreserved embryos or those that lacked BMI documentation	< 18.5 (92 women) 18.5–24.99 (2605 women) 25.0–29.99 (1027 women) 30.00–34.99 (477 women) 35.00–39.99 (275 women) > 40.0 (133 women)	No of oocytes retrieved Duration of stimulation Total dosage of gonadotrophin No of embryo transferred Implantation Clinical pregnancy Biochemical pregnancy Global miscarriage Ectopic pregnancy Live birth Multiple birth
Bailey et al. 2014 [49] (2001–2010)	Retrospective Cohort Study (79 women / 101 cycles)	IVF/ICSI	Women < 40 years of age, height and weight measurements > 3 months from the start of cycle, in-vitro maturation, FSH > 10 mIU/mL, uncontrolled thyroid disease, history of chemotherapy or radiation exposure, recurrent pregnancy loss, uterine factor, balanced translocation in either partner, surgically documented endometriosis or pelvic adhesions, history of pelvic inflammatory disease, adenomyosis and submucosal myoma	18.7–24.9 (51 cycles) 25.0–29.9 (19 cycles) ≥30.0 (31 cycles)	Chemical pregnancy Miscarriage Clinical Pregnancy Live Birth rate Duration of stimulation of gonadotrophin Dosage of gonadotrophin No of oocytes retrieved
Schliep et al. 2014 [50] (2005–2010)	Prospective Cohort Study (721 women)	IVF/ICSI	Men with non-obstructive azoospermia	< 18.5 (32 women) 18.5–24.9 (407 women) 25–29.9 (147 women) 30–34.9 (72 women) ≥35 (63 women)	Fertilization rate Pregnancy rate Live birth rate
Cai et al. 2017 [51] (2013–2014)	Retrospective Cohort Study (4401 women / 4798 fresh transfer cycles	IVF/ICSI	Mild stimulation cycles, natural cycles and luteal-phase stimulation cycle, patients with diabetes, glucose intolerance and thyroid abnormality	< 18.5 (886 cycles) 18.5–24.9 (3642 cycles) ≥25 (670 cycles)	Fertilization rate Live birth rate Miscarriage rate Dosage of gonadotrophin
Ozekinci et al. 2015 [52] (2008–2013)	Retrospective Cohort Study (298 women)	IVF-ICSI	Underweight women, women > 38 years of age, transfer of > 2 embryos, frozen cycles	18.5–24.9 (164 cycles) 25–29.9 (70 cycles) ≥30 (64 cycles)	Dosage of gonadotrophin Duration of stimulation
Caillon et al. 2015 [53] (2006–2009)	Retrospective study (582 women)	IVF-ICSI	Underweight women	18.5–24.9 (409 women) ≥25 (149 women)	Dosage of gonadotrophin Implantation rate Miscarriage rate Live birth rate
Provost et al. 2016 [54] 2008–2010	Retrospective Cohort Study (239,127 cycles)	IVF	Women with a height < 48 in. and weight < 70 pounds	< 18.5 (7149 cycles) 18.5–24.9 (134,588 cycles) 25–29.9 (54,822 cycles) 30–34.9 (24,922 cycles) 35–39.9 (11,747 cycles) 40–44.9 (4084 cycles) 45–49.9 (1292 cycles) > 50 (463 cycles)	Implantation rate Clinical pregnancy rate Miscarriage rate Live birth rate
Russo et al. 2017 [55] 2010–2014	Retrospective Cohort Study (520 women)	Not specified	Congenital uterine anomalies, endometrial polyps, intrauterine synechiae, adenomyosis, intra-cavity fibroids, hydrosalpinges, donor cycles, poor quality embryos, cleavage stage embryos, and women > 40 years	< 20 (51 women) 20–24.9 (294 women) 25–29.9 (64 women) 30–39.9 (58 women) ≥40 (54 women)	Miscarriage rate Clinical pregnancy rate Live birth rate Dosage of gonadotrophin

Table 1 Details of included studies *(Continued)*

Study	Methodology (population size)	Intervention	Exclusion Criteria	BMI Categories (kg/m^2) and numbers	Outcome Measures
Christensen et al. 2016 [56] (1999–2009)	Retrospective Cohort Study (5342 cycles)	IVF/ICSI	Missing information on BMI or treatment type, premature ovulation before oocyte retrieval, intrauterine insemination cycles	< 18.5 (158 cycles) 18.5–24.9 (3539 cycles) 25–29.9 (1171 cycles) ≥30 (474 cycles)	Dosage of gonadotrophin Clinical pregnancy rate

BMI Body Mass Index, *IVF* in vitro fertilization, *ICSI* intracytoplasmic sperm injection, *OHSS* ovarian hyperstimulation syndrome, *GIFT* gamete intra-Fallopian transfer, *HCG* human chorionic gonadotrophin, *FSH* follicle stimulation hormone

Pooled analysis from 18 studies demonstrated a statistically significant reduction in the clinical pregnancy rate for women with a BMI ≥30 kg/m^2 when compared to women with a normal BMI (OR 0.80, 95% CI 0.74–0.87, $p < 0.00001$; Fig. 3c). There was no significant heterogeneity ($I^2 = 32\%$) present between the studies.

Miscarriage rate

An increased risk of miscarriage is demonstrated in women with a BMI ≥25 kg/m^2 when compared to women with a BMI < 25 kg/m^2 (26 studies pooled, OR 1.30, 95% CI 1.15–1.48, $p < 0.0001$; Fig. 4a). However, significant heterogeneity ($I^2 = 53\%$, $p = 0.0001$) was seen between the studies.

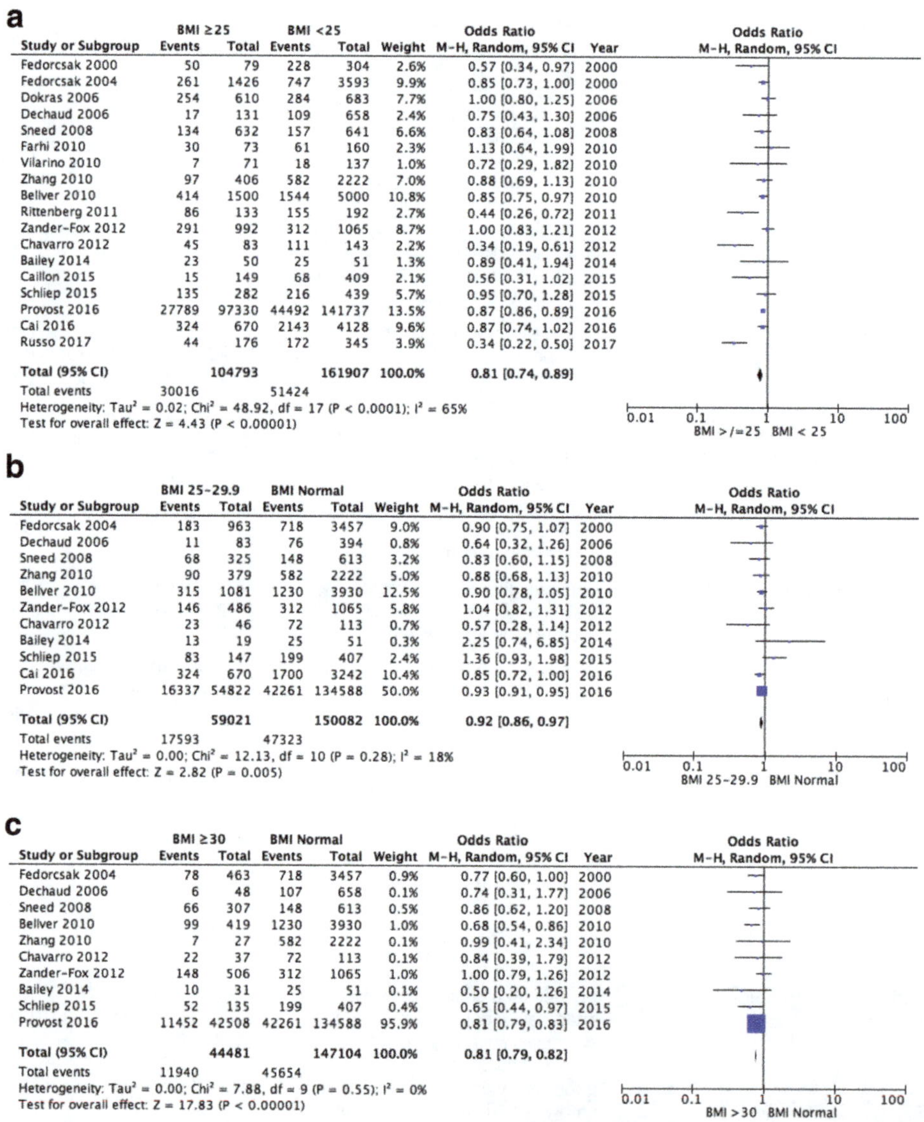

Fig. 2 Meta-analysis of live-birth rate: (**a**) BMI ≥25 kg/m^2 versus BMI < 25 kg/m^2; (**b**) Normal BMI versus BMI 25–29.9 kg/m^2; (**c**) Normal BMI versus BMI ≥30 kg/m^2

a

Study or Subgroup	BMI ≥25 Events	BMI ≥25 Total	BMI <25 Events	BMI <25 Total	Weight	Odds Ratio M-H, Random, 95% CI	Year
Wang 2000	499	1232	1116	2351	6.2%	0.75 [0.66, 0.87]	2000
Wittemer 2000	20	70	60	255	1.1%	1.30 [0.72, 2.35]	2000
Loveland 2001	24	93	42	87	1.0%	0.37 [0.20, 0.70]	2001
Doody 2003	127	362	195	460	3.3%	0.73 [0.55, 0.98]	2003
Ryley 2004	739	2756	1283	4071	7.0%	0.80 [0.72, 0.89]	2004
Hammadeh 2005	8	24	13	28	0.3%	0.58 [0.19, 1.78]	2005
Van Swieten 2005	20	61	46	101	0.9%	0.58 [0.30, 1.13]	2005
Mitwally 2006	28	81	52	102	1.1%	0.51 [0.28, 0.93]	2006
Metwally 2007	51	185	73	241	1.9%	0.88 [0.57, 1.34]	2006
Dokras 2006	295	610	320	683	4.5%	1.06 [0.85, 1.32]	2006
Dechaud 2006	17	131	109	658	1.3%	0.75 [0.43, 1.30]	2006
Sneed 2008	166	632	185	641	4.0%	0.88 [0.69, 1.12]	2008
Moini 2008	30	154	39	133	1.3%	0.58 [0.34, 1.01]	2008
Davies 2010	21	56	101	176	1.0%	0.45 [0.24, 0.83]	2010
Vilarino 2010	16	71	36	137	0.9%	0.82 [0.42, 1.60]	2010
Zhang 2010	134	406	754	2222	4.3%	0.96 [0.77, 1.20]	2010
Farhi 2010	16	73	29	160	0.8%	1.27 [0.64, 2.52]	2010
Bellver 2010	616	1500	2243	5000	6.8%	0.86 [0.76, 0.96]	2010
Sathya 2010	90	220	38	88	1.5%	0.91 [0.55, 1.50]	2010
Rittenberg 2011	124	133	181	192	0.5%	0.84 [0.34, 2.08]	2011
Funabiki 2011	11	34	117	332	0.7%	0.88 [0.41, 1.87]	2011
Parker 2011	222	462	234	493	3.8%	1.02 [0.79, 1.32]	2011
Pinborg 2011	105	435	213	746	3.5%	0.80 [0.61, 1.04]	2011
Hill 2011	31	59	28	58	0.8%	1.19 [0.57, 2.45]	2011
Werner 2012	93	133	149	222	1.7%	1.14 [0.72, 1.81]	2012
Ramezanzadeh 2012	47	190	30	93	1.3%	0.69 [0.40, 1.19]	2012
Chavarro 2012	63	83	124	143	0.8%	0.48 [0.24, 0.97]	2012
Ozgun 2012	124	519	128	416	3.3%	0.71 [0.53, 0.94]	2012
Galal 2012	58	110	75	110	1.3%	0.52 [0.30, 0.90]	2012
Zander-Fox 2012	354	992	385	1065	5.3%	0.98 [0.82, 1.17]	2012
Bailey 2014	25	50	29	51	0.7%	0.76 [0.35, 1.66]	2014
Schliep 2015	149	282	242	439	3.1%	0.91 [0.68, 1.23]	2015
Ozekinci 2015	40	134	52	164	1.5%	0.92 [0.56, 1.50]	2015
Provost 2016	34872	97330	53704	141737	8.6%	0.92 [0.90, 0.93]	2016
Cai 2016	376	670	2451	4128	5.6%	0.88 [0.74, 1.03]	2016
Christensen 2016	353	1645	949	3697	6.3%	0.79 [0.69, 0.91]	2016
Russo 2017	44	176	172	345	2.1%	0.34 [0.22, 0.50]	2017
Total (95% CI)		**112154**		**172025**	**100.0%**	**0.82 [0.77, 0.88]**	
Total events	40008		65997				

Heterogeneity: Tau² = 0.01; Chi² = 85.35, df = 36 (P < 0.00001); I² = 58%
Test for overall effect: Z = 5.82 (P < 0.00001)

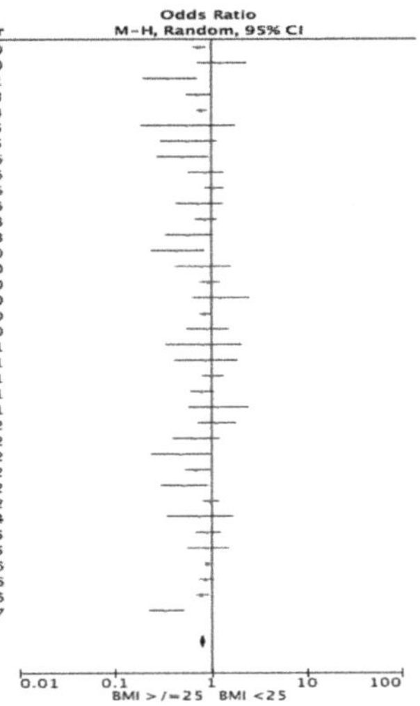

b

Study or Subgroup	BMI 25–29.9 Events	BMI 25–29.9 Total	BMI Normal Events	BMI Normal Total	Weight	Odds Ratio M-H, Random, 95% CI	Year
Wang 2000	342	814	917	1910	8.1%	0.78 [0.66, 0.93]	2000
Ryley 2004	450	1632	1130	3605	11.0%	0.83 [0.73, 0.95]	2004
Dechaud 2006	11	83	76	394	0.7%	0.64 [0.32, 1.26]	2006
Metwally 2007	34	113	73	241	1.3%	0.99 [0.61, 1.61]	2006
Moini 2008	25	117	39	133	0.9%	0.65 [0.37, 1.17]	2008
Sneed 2008	106	325	221	613	3.5%	0.86 [0.65, 1.14]	2008
Bellver 2010	457	1081	1761	3930	10.4%	0.90 [0.79, 1.03]	2010
Zhang 2010	125	379	754	2222	4.9%	0.96 [0.76, 1.21]	2010
Pinborg 2011	68	257	199	702	2.8%	0.91 [0.66, 1.26]	2011
Parker 2011	121	241	219	475	3.0%	1.18 [0.86, 1.61]	2011
Chavarro 2012	34	46	83	113	0.5%	1.02 [0.47, 2.23]	2012
Zander-Fox 2012	385	1065	182	486	5.3%	0.95 [0.76, 1.18]	2012
Ozgun 2012	87	355	123	398	2.8%	0.73 [0.53, 1.00]	2012
Werner 2012	58	88	142	209	1.1%	0.91 [0.54, 1.55]	2012
Schliep 2015	89	147	225	407	2.1%	1.24 [0.85, 1.82]	2015
Ozekinci 2015	22	70	52	164	0.9%	0.99 [0.54, 1.80]	2015
Christensen 2016	247	1171	905	3539	8.5%	0.78 [0.66, 0.91]	2016
Cai 2016	376	670	1928	3242	8.0%	0.87 [0.74, 1.03]	2016
Provost 2016	20175	54822	51009	134588	24.1%	0.95 [0.93, 0.97]	2016
Total (95% CI)		**63476**		**157371**	**100.0%**	**0.89 [0.84, 0.94]**	
Total events	23212		60038				

Heterogeneity: Tau² = 0.00; Chi² = 26.16, df = 18 (P = 0.10); I² = 31%
Test for overall effect: Z = 3.92 (P < 0.0001)

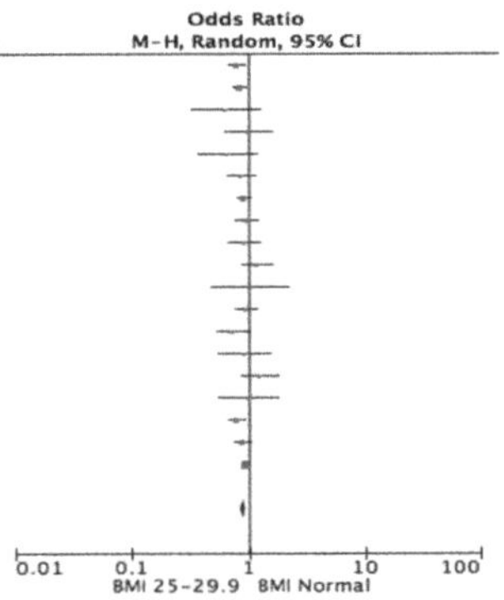

c

Study or Subgroup	BMI ≥30 Events	BMI ≥30 Total	BMI Normal Events	BMI Normal Total	Weight	Odds Ratio M-H, Random, 95% CI	Year
Wang 2000	157	421	917	1910	8.7%	0.64 [0.52, 0.80]	2000
Ryley 2004	289	1124	1130	3605	13.2%	0.76 [0.65, 0.88]	2004
Metwally 2007	17	72	73	241	1.6%	0.71 [0.39, 1.31]	2006
Dechaud 2006	6	48	76	394	0.8%	0.60 [0.25, 1.46]	2006
Moini 2008	5	37	39	133	0.6%	0.38 [0.14, 1.04]	2008
Sneed 2008	80	307	175	618	5.2%	0.89 [0.65, 1.22]	2008
Zhang 2010	9	27	754	2222	0.9%	0.97 [0.44, 2.18]	2010
Bellver 2010	159	419	1761	3930	9.2%	0.75 [0.61, 0.93]	2010
Parker 2011	101	221	219	475	4.9%	0.98 [0.71, 1.36]	2011
Pinborg 2011	37	178	199	702	3.4%	0.66 [0.45, 0.99]	2011
Chavarro 2012	29	37	83	113	0.8%	1.31 [0.54, 3.18]	2012
Werner 2012	35	45	142	209	1.0%	1.65 [0.77, 3.53]	2012
Ozgun 2012	37	164	123	398	3.0%	0.65 [0.43, 0.99]	2012
Zander-Fox 2012	172	506	385	1065	8.4%	0.91 [0.73, 1.14]	2012
Schliep 2015	60	135	225	407	3.5%	0.65 [0.44, 0.96]	2015
Ozekinci 2015	18	64	52	164	1.4%	0.84 [0.45, 1.59]	2015
Christensen 2016	106	474	905	3539	8.1%	0.84 [0.67, 1.05]	2016
Provost 2016	14697	42508	51009	134588	25.3%	0.87 [0.85, 0.89]	2016
Total (95% CI)		**46787**		**154713**	**100.0%**	**0.80 [0.74, 0.87]**	
Total events	16014		58267				

Heterogeneity: Tau² = 0.01; Chi² = 25.08, df = 17 (P = 0.09); I² = 32%
Test for overall effect: Z = 5.47 (P < 0.00001)

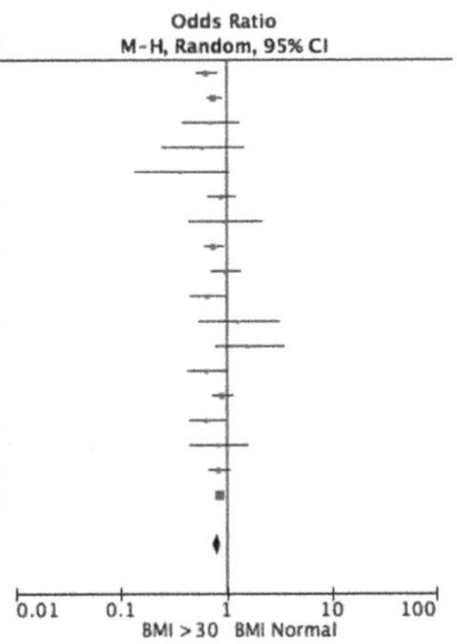

Fig. 3 Meta-analysis of clinical pregnancy rate: (**a**) BMI ≥25 kg/m^2 versus BMI < 25 kg/m^2; (**b**) Normal BMI versus BMI 25–29.9 kg/m^2; (**c**) Normal BMI versus BMI ≥30 kg/m^2

Women with a BMI 25–29.9 kg/m^2 were also more likely to have a miscarriage when compared to women with a normal BMI (18 studies pooled, OR 1.15 95% CI 1.05–1.26, $p = 0.002$; Fig. 4b). There was no significant clinical heterogeneity ($I^2 = 16\%$) in this group.

The risk of miscarriage is further increased in women with a BMI ≥30 kg/m^2 when compared to women who fall into a normal BMI category (17 studies pooled, OR 1.52, 95% CI 1.28–1.81, $p < 0.00001$; Fig. 4c). No significant heterogeneity ($I^2 = 46\%$) was demonstrated between the studies.

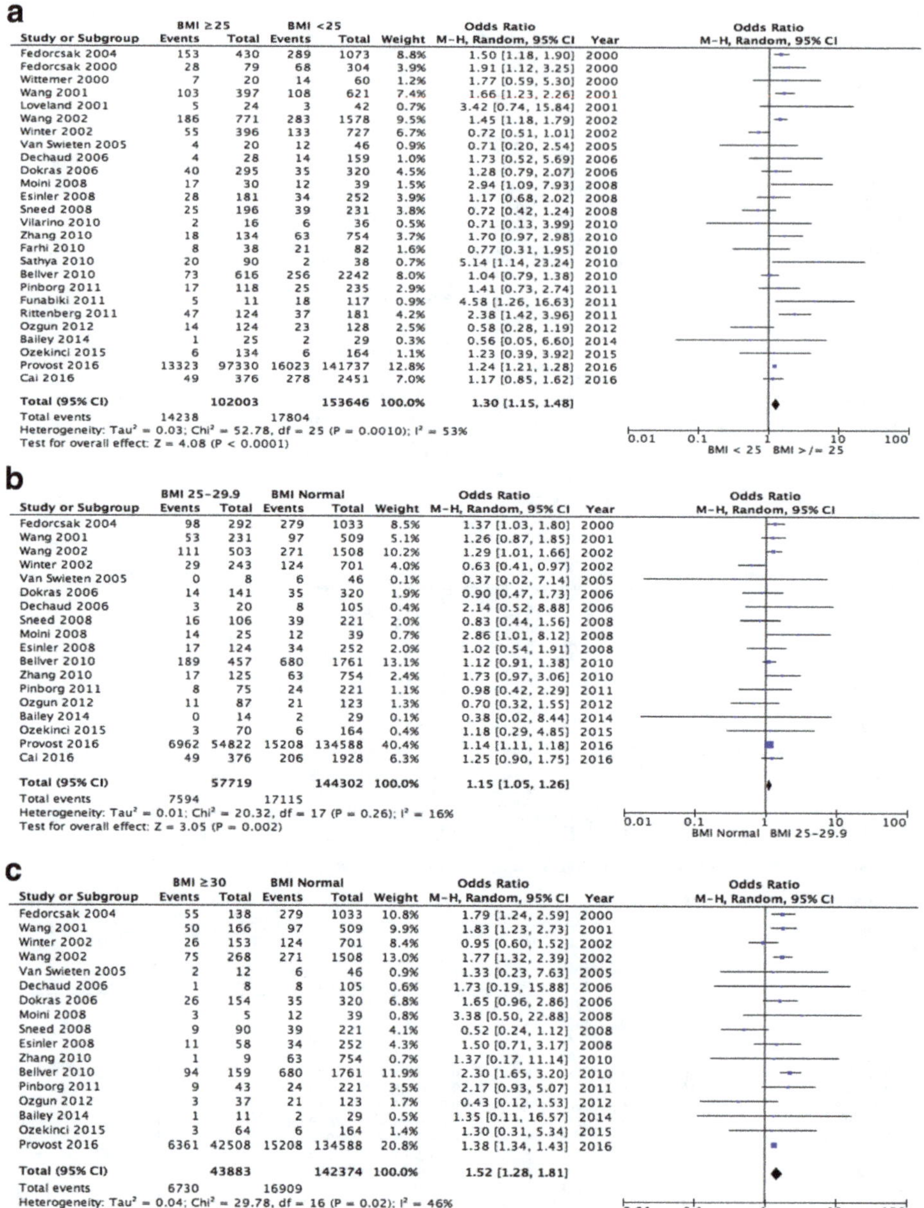

Fig. 4 Meta-analysis of miscarriage rate: (**a**) BMI ≥25 kg/m^2 versus BMI < 25 kg/m^2; (**b**) Normal BMI versus BMI 25–29.9 kg/m^2; (**c**) Normal BMI versus BMI ≥30 kg/m^2

Dosage of gonadotrophin stimulation

Women with a BMI ≥25 kg/m^2 required significantly larger total gonadotrophin dosages than women with a BMI < 25 kg/m^2 (15 studies pooled, weighted mean difference [WMD] 196.03iu, 95% CI 131.91–260.16, $p < 0.00001$; Fig. 5a). However, significant heterogeneity ($I^2 = 75\%$, $p < 0.00001$) was present between the studies.

Women with a BMI 25–29.9 kg/m^2 were demonstrated to require significantly higher total gonadotrophin dosages than women with a normal BMI (12 studies pooled, WMD 83.67iu, 95% CI 24.54–142.80, $p = 0.006$; Fig. 5b). However, significant heterogeneity ($I^2 = 80\%$, $p < 0.00001$) existed between the studies.

Furthermore, increased total dosages of gonadotrophin was documented for women with a BMI ≥30 kg/m^2 when compared to women whose BMI fell into the normal category (13 studies pooled, WMD 363.58iu, 95% CI 252.99–474.17, $p < 0.00001$; Fig. 5c). However, significant heterogeneity ($I^2 = 81\%$, $p < 0.00001$) was present between the studies.

a

Study or Subgroup	BMI ≥25 Mean	BMI ≥25 SD	BMI ≥25 Total	BMI <25 Mean	BMI <25 SD	BMI <25 Total	Weight	Mean Difference IV, Random, 95% CI	Year
Dechaud 2006	2,344	897	131	2,046	879	658	6.4%	298.00 [130.35, 465.65]	2006
Metwally 2007	1,986	200	185	1,797	227	241	10.9%	189.00 [148.36, 229.64]	2006
Esinler 2008	2,921	1,199	486	2,517	1,057	627	7.6%	404.00 [269.06, 538.94]	2008
Ozgun 2009	2,765	1,158	519	2,342	1,038	416	7.4%	423.00 [282.02, 563.98]	2009
Zhang 2010	2,727	1,049	406	2,587	933	2222	8.6%	140.00 [30.84, 249.16]	2010
Sathya 2010	2,680	996	220	2,491	1,058	88	4.0%	189.00 [-68.27, 446.27]	2010
Bellver 2010	2,265	874	1500	2,178	918	5000	10.7%	87.00 [35.97, 138.03]	2010
Farhi 2010	2,462	1,219	73	2,085	1,032	160	2.9%	377.00 [54.87, 699.13]	2010
Vilarino 2010	1,494	489	71	1,545	481	137	7.4%	-51.00 [-190.37, 88.37]	2010
Luke 2011	3,467.1	2,279.5	61386	3,446.7	20,538	91114	7.6%	20.40 [-114.17, 154.97]	2011
Singh 2011	2,892	962	149	2,577	1,053	167	4.8%	315.00 [92.82, 537.18]	2012
Moragianni 2012	2,989	1,834	1912	2,835	1,921	2697	8.6%	154.00 [44.39, 263.61]	2012
Chavarro 2012	1,987	896	59	1,701	989	111	3.4%	286.00 [-7.46, 579.46]	2012
Bailey 2014	2,049	1,176	50	1,755	1,008	51	1.9%	294.00 [-133.53, 721.53]	2014
Caillon 2015	2,314	703.6	149	2,146	659.8	409	7.8%	168.00 [38.18, 297.82]	2015
Total (95% CI)			**67296**			**104098**	**100.0%**	**196.03 [131.91, 260.16]**	

Heterogeneity: $Tau^2 = 9358.56$; $Chi^2 = 56.00$, $df = 14$ ($P < 0.00001$); $I^2 = 75\%$
Test for overall effect: $Z = 5.99$ ($P < 0.00001$)

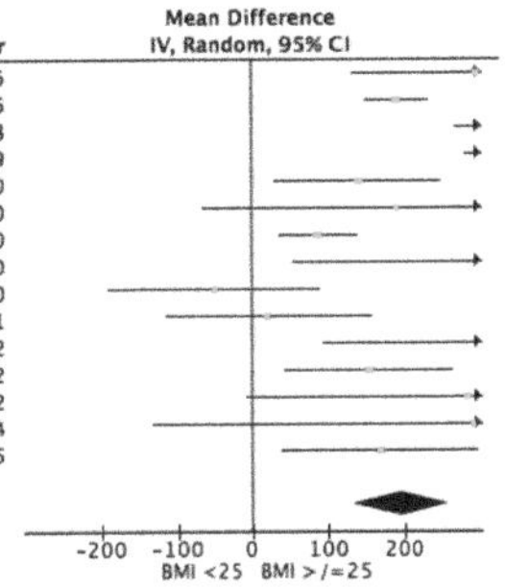

b

Study or Subgroup	BMI 25-29.9 Mean	BMI 25-29.9 SD	BMI 25-29.9 Total	BMI Normal Mean	BMI Normal SD	BMI Normal Total	Weight	Mean Difference IV, Random, 95% CI
Bailey 2014	1,305	545.5	19	1,755	1,008	51	2.2%	-450.00 [-819.72, -80.28]
Bellver 2010	2,215.4	859.2	1081	2,176.9	919.9	3930	13.8%	38.50 [-20.24, 97.24]
Chavarro 2012	1,867	913	35	1,746.3	993.8	89	2.2%	120.70 [-245.52, 486.92]
Dechaud 2006	2,281	967	83	2,047	888	394	4.8%	234.00 [8.24, 459.76]
Esinler 2008	2,779.1	1,160.1	339	2,516.5	1,057.2	627	7.9%	262.60 [113.95, 411.25]
Luke 2011	3,434	2,517	35452	3,458	21,031	86860	8.3%	-24.00 [-166.29, 118.29]
Metwally 2007	1,970.8	239.6	113	1,979.1	227.3	241	14.1%	-8.30 [-60.98, 44.38]
Moragianni 2012	3,014	2,044.5	1027	2,844.9	1,918.8	2605	8.1%	169.10 [23.96, 314.24]
Ozekinci 2015	2,015	968	70	1,859	1,065	164	3.5%	156.00 [-123.27, 435.27]
Ozgun 2012	2,661	1,136	355	2,344	1,918.8	2605	8.5%	317.00 [177.74, 456.26]
Singh 2011	9.92	1.66	131	10.25	1.79	141	15.9%	-0.33 [-0.74, 0.08]
Zhang 2010	2,688	966	379	2,587	933	2222	10.6%	101.00 [-3.71, 205.71]
Total (95% CI)			**39084**			**99929**	**100.0%**	**83.67 [24.54, 142.80]**

Heterogeneity: $Tau^2 = 5713.28$; $Chi^2 = 54.11$, $df = 11$ ($P < 0.00001$); $I^2 = 80\%$
Test for overall effect: $Z = 2.77$ ($P = 0.006$)

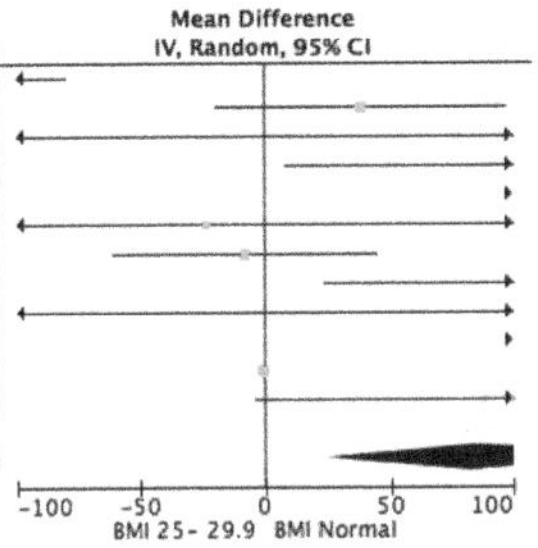

c

Study or Subgroup	BMI ≥30 Mean	BMI ≥30 SD	BMI ≥30 Total	BMI Normal Mean	BMI Normal SD	BMI Normal Total	Weight	Mean Difference IV, Random, 95% CI	Year
Dechaud 2006	2,454	757	48	2,047	888	394	8.2%	407.00 [175.59, 638.41]	2006
Metwally 2007	2,009	109	72	1,797	227	241	12.5%	212.00 [173.85, 250.15]	2006
Esinler 2008	3,248	1,255	147	2,517	1,057	627	8.5%	731.00 [511.90, 950.10]	2008
Sathya 2010	2,658	887	73	2,490	1,058	88	6.6%	168.00 [-132.44, 468.44]	2010
Bellver 2010	2,395	899	419	2,177	920	3930	11.7%	218.00 [127.24, 308.76]	2010
Zhang 2010	3,272	1,798	27	2,587	933	2222	2.2%	685.00 [5.69, 1364.31]	2010
Luke 2011	3,507.7	1,907.6	25644	3,458	21,031	86860	10.5%	49.70 [-92.10, 191.50]	2011
Moragianni 2012	2,959	1,554	885	2,845	1,919	2605	10.9%	114.00 [-12.15, 240.15]	2012
Chavarro 2012	2,163	860	24	1,746	994	89	4.8%	417.00 [15.72, 818.28]	2012
Singh 2011	3,150	520	18	2,567	1,088	141	6.6%	583.00 [283.07, 882.93]	2012
Ozgun 2012	2,991	1,175	164	2,344	1,022	398	8.8%	647.00 [441.04, 852.96]	2012
Bailey 2014	2,505	1,230	31	1,755	1,008	51	3.4%	750.00 [236.18, 1263.82]	2014
Ozekinci 2015	2,455	1,343	64	1,859	1,065	164	5.3%	596.00 [228.81, 963.19]	2015
Total (95% CI)			**27616**			**97810**	**100.0%**	**363.58 [252.99, 474.17]**	

Heterogeneity: $Tau^2 = 25006.12$; $Chi^2 = 64.21$, $df = 12$ ($P < 0.00001$); $I^2 = 81\%$
Test for overall effect: $Z = 6.44$ ($P < 0.00001$)

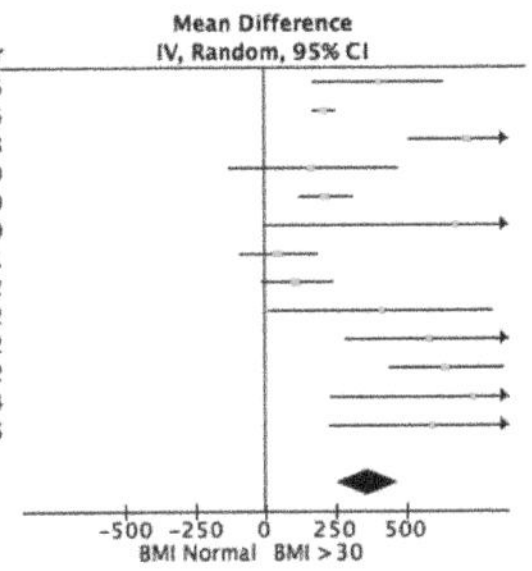

Fig. 5 Meta-analysis of total gonadotrophin dose: (**a**) BMI ≥25 kg/m^2 versus BMI < 25 kg/m^2; (**b**) Normal BMI versus BMI 25–29.9 kg/m^2; (**c**) Normal BMI versus BMI ≥30 kg/m^2

Duration of gonadotrophin stimulation

No significant difference in duration of stimulation therapy was documented between women with a BMI < 25 kg/m^2 or ≥25 kg/m^2 (13 studies pooled, WMD 0.10, 95% CI -0.10-0.31, $p = 0.32$; Fig. 6a), however significant heterogeneity ($I^2 = 95\%$, $p < 0.00001$) existed between the included studies.

Furthermore, no significant difference was seen for duration of gonadotrophin stimulation between women with a BMI 25–29.9 kg/m^2 versus a normal BMI (8 pooled studies, WMD 0.02, 95% CI -0.10-0.13, $p = 0.79$, $I^2 = 48\%$; Fig. 6b) or for women with a BMI ≥30 kg/m^2 versus a normal BMI (12 pooled studies, WMD 0.12 95% CI -0.24-0.47, $p = 0.52$; Fig. 6c), however significant heterogeneity ($I^2 = 96\%$, $p < 0.00001$) was noted between the studies for the latter comparison.

Discussion

Public funding for fertility services within the United Kingdom is limited, and therefore, strict guidance exists regarding who can be offered treatment under the National Health Service (NHS). Body mass index (BMI) is a universal criteria adopted by both the public and private sector. This study addresses an important aspect of the impact of a raised BMI on fertility treatment outcomes.

We standardise the analysis of the data by only including studies incorporating the WHO BMI criteria; the current reference point for clinicians and clinical commissioning groups in ascertaining which group of patients should receive treatment. This study is an update of the previous systematic review performed in 2010, with the inclusion of a larger number of cycles from central databases such as the Society for Assisted Reproductive Technology (SART).

This systematic review and meta-analysis has clearly highlighted the negative impact of a raised BMI on the outcomes following ART treatment, with documented lower success rates and higher rates of miscarriages as well as higher total dosage of gonadotrophin usage with

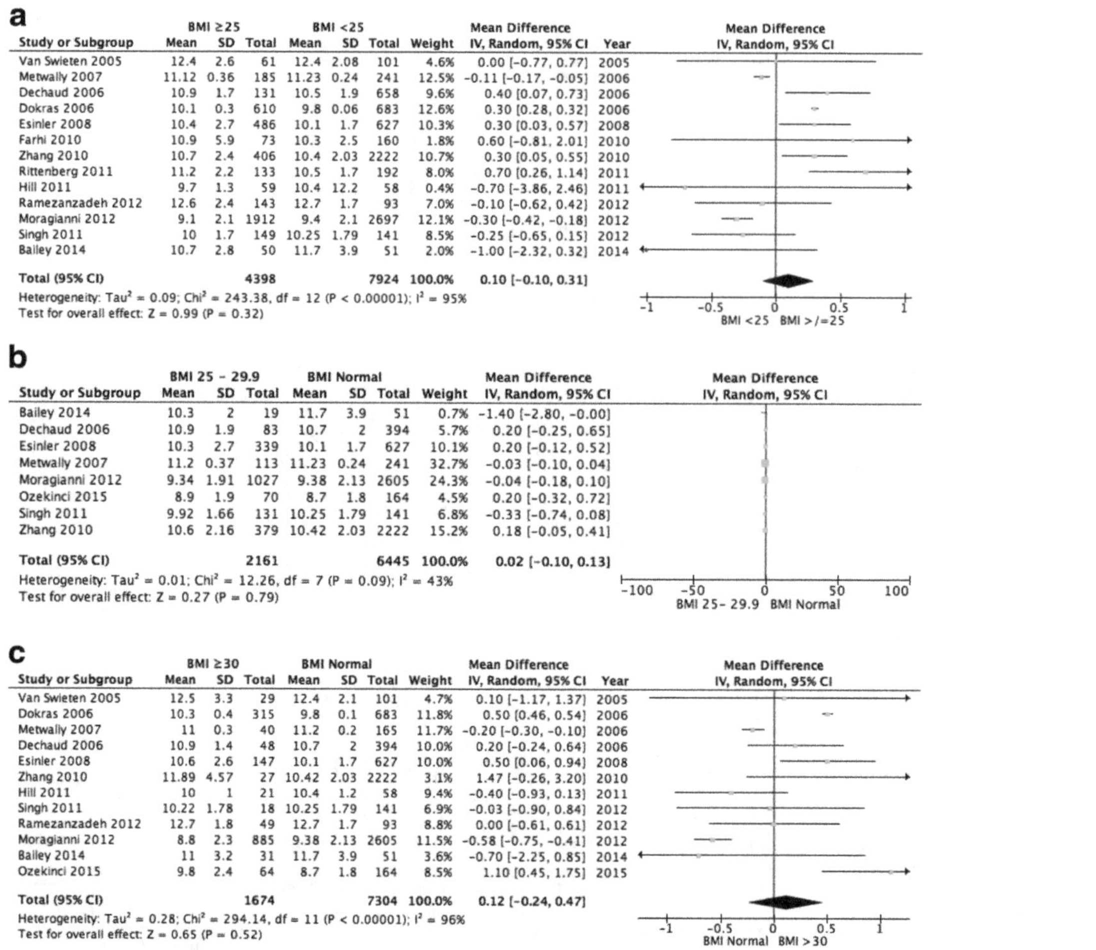

Fig. 6 Meta-analysis of duration of gonadotrophin stimulation: (**a**) BMI ≥25 kg/m^2 versus BMI < 25 kg/m^2; (**b**) Normal BMI versus BMI 25–29.9 kg/m^2; (**c**) Normal BMI versus BMI ≥30 kg/m^2

no effect on the duration of stimulation. The latter may have been balanced by higher dosages of treatment which can also have a cost implication. However, as most studies have included a BMI category of < 25 kg/m^2, which would also include underweight women with a BMI < 18 kg/m^2, the detrimental effects of which have been addressed in a number of previous studies, a risk of bias cannot be confidently excluded. This has been addressed through the inclusion of studies allowing for a sub-group analysis of women with a normal BMI with overweight and obese women.

The presented data is able to demonstrate statistical significance with low clinical heterogeneity for a number of factors reflective of success through ART treatment. Despite this, caution is advised for interpretation of the presented information as only a few of the included studies controlled for confounding factors such as age, smoking and duration of infertility. In order to reduce further clinical heterogeneity, studies not incorporating the WHO classification for BMI and paternal BMI were excluded.

The included studies were considered relevant if they conformed to the WHO classification of BMI, despite this, a considerable amount of methodological and clinical heterogeneity existed. The level of statistical heterogeneity for the primary outcome measure live birth rate and secondary outcome measures clinical pregnancy rate and miscarriage rate were limited. However, despite a significant increase in total gonadotrophin dosage requirements with increasing BMI categories, the studies demonstrated significant statistical heterogeneity, limiting their value.

The presented data can act as an aid in the counselling of subjects secondary to a clear impact on ART outcomes being demonstrated across all BMI categories. The evidence supports the government's stringent allocation of funding when resources are significantly limited.

A raised BMI impacts reproductive health at the pre and post embryological stage of development, affecting oocyte quality and the endometrial environment [2].

A recent meta-analysis and systematic review by Best et al., [5] has demonstrated that weight loss can improve pregnancy rate and ovulatory status with a trend favouring spontaneous conception. However, these effects have not been seen through ART. Of note, miscarriage rates were unaltered with a change in weight.

Besides the reproductive health effects of a raised BMI, clinicians should also be aware of the increased rate of pregnancy complications such as pregnancy induced hypertension, pre-eclampsia and gestational diabetes in women with a raised BMI. Women are also at an increased risk of an emergency caesarean section with increasing BMI [6, 7].

A holistic approach should be used when counselling patients seeking ART treatments using an open discussion method to inform patients of the effects of raised BMI on ART and obstetric care. This will allow couples to make an informed decision and to take ownership of their well-being.

Conclusion

This systematic review and meta-analysis further emphasises the negative impact of a raised BMI on ART outcomes. However, the underlying pathophysiology is beyond the scope of this systematic review and will need to be evaluated in future studies. The quality of this systematic review would be further improved if future study designs included the WHO classification of BMI and controlled for confounding variables.

Abbreviations

ART: Assisted reproductive technology; BMI: Body Mass Index; FSH: Follicle stimulation hormone; GIFT: Gamete intra-Fallopian transfer; HCG: Human chorionic gonadotrophin; ICSI: Intracytoplasmic sperm injection; IVF: In vitro fertilization; MeSH: Medical subject headings; NHS: National Health Service; OHSS: Ovarian hyperstimulation syndrome; SART: Society for Assisted Reproductive Technology

Authors' contributions

PRS and MM analyzed and interpreted the data. LNL developed the initial idea. EM and LNL oversaw the progress of the manuscript. All authors read and approved the final manuscript.

Competing interests

The authors declare that they have no competing interests.

Author details

[1]Oxford University Hospitals NHS Foundation Trust, John Radcliffe Hospital, Headley Way, Headington, Oxford OX3 9DU, UK. [2]Nuffield Department of Women's and Reproductive Health, University of Oxford, Level 3, Women's Centre, John Radcliffe Hospital, Oxford OX3 9DU, UK.

References

1. WHO. Obesity and overweight. Geneva: World Health Organization. Fact Sheet 311. Available from http://www.who.int/mediacentre/factsheets/fs311/en/.
2. Rittenberg V, Seshadri S, Sunkara SK, Sobaleva S, Oteng-Ntim E, El-Toukhy T. Effect of body mass index on IVF treatment outcome: an updated systematic review and meta-analysis. Reprod BioMed Online. 2011;23(4):421–39.
3. Higgins JPT, Thompson SG. Quantifying heterogeneity in a meta-analysis. Stat Med. 2002;21(11):1539–58.
4. Mantel N, Haenszel W. Statistical aspects of the analysis of data from retrospective studies of disease. J Natl Cancer Inst. 1959;22:719–48.
5. Best D, Avenell A, Bhattacharya S. How effective are weight-loss interventions for improving fertility in women and men who are overweight or obese? A systematic review and meta-analysis of the evidence. Hum Reprod Update. 2017;23(6):681–705.
6. Aly H, Hammad T, Nada A, Mohamed M, Bathgate S, El-Mohandes A. Maternal obesity, associated complications and risk of prematurity. J Perinatol. 2010;30(7):447–51.
7. Bhattacharya S, Campbell DM, Liston WA, Bhattacharya S. Effect of body mass index on pregnancy outcomes in nulliparous women delivering singleton babies. BMC Public Health. 2007;7:168.
8. Fedorcsak P, et al. Obesity is a risk factor for early pregnancy loss after IVF or ICSI. Acta Obstet Gynecol Scand. 2000;79(1):43–8.
9. Wittemer C, et al. Does body mass index of infertile women have an impact on IVF procedure and outcome? J Assist Reprod Genet. 2000;17(10):547–52.
10. Wang JX, Davies M, Norman RJ. Body mass and probability of pregnancy during assisted reproduction treatment: retrospective study. Br Med J. 2000;321(7272):1320–1.
11. Loveland JB, et al. Increased body mass index has a deleterious effect on in vitro fertilization outcome. J Assist Reprod Genet. 2001;18(7):382–6.
12. Wang JX, Davies MJ, Norman RJ. Polycystic ovarian syndrome and the risk of spontaneous abortion following assisted reproductive technology treatment. Hum Reprod. 2001;16(12):2606–9.
13. Wang X, Davies J, Norman J. Obesity increases the risk of spontaneous abortion during infertility treatment. Obes Res. 2002;10(6):551–4.
14. Winter E, Wang J, Davies MJ, Norman RJ. Early pregnancy loss following assisted reproductive technology treatment. Hum Reprod. 2002;12:3220–3.
15. Doody KM, Langley MT, Marek DE, Nackley AC, Doody KJ. Morbid obesity adversely impacts outcomes with IVF. Fertility Sterility. 2003;80:S160.
16. Fedorcsák P, Dale PO, Storeng R, Ertzeid G, Bjercke S, Oldereid N, Omland AK, Abyholm T, Tanbo T. Impact of overweight and underweight on assisted reproduction treatment. Hum Reprod. 2004;19(11):2523–8.
17. Ryley DA, Bayer SR, Eaton J, Zimon A, Klipstein S, Reindollar. Influence of body mass index (BMI) on the outcome of 6,827 IVF cycles. Fertil Steril. 2004;82(Supplement 2):S38–9.
18. Van ECAM, et al. Obesity and clomiphene challenge test as predictors of outcome of in vitro fertilization and intracytoplasmic sperm injection. Gynecol Obstet Investig. 2005;59(4):220–4.
19. Hammadeh ME, Sykoutris A, Amer AS, Schmidt. Relationship between body mass index (BMI) and plasma lipid concentration and their effect on IVF/ICSI outcome. Fertil Steril. 2005;84(Supplement 1):S422.
20. Dechaud H, et al. Obesity does not adversely affect results in patients who are undergoing in vitro fertilization and embryo transfer. European Journal of Obstetrics Gynecology and Reproductive Biology. 2006;127(1):88–93.
21. Dokras A, et al. Obstetric outcomes after in vitro fertilization in obese and morbidly obese women. Obstet Gynecol. 2006;108(1):61–9.
22. Mitwally MF, Leduc MM, Ogunleye O, Albuarki H, Diamond MP, Abuzeid M. The effect of body mass index (BMI) on the outcome of IVF and embryo transfer in women of different ethnic backgrounds. Fertility Sterility. 2006;86:S68–9.
23. Metwally M, Cutting R, Tipton A, Skull J, Ledger WL, Li TC. Effect of increased body mass index on oocyte and embryo quality in IVF patients. Reprod BioMed Online. 2007;15:532–8.
24. Esinler I, Bozdag G, Yarali H. Impact of isolated obesity on ICSI outcome. Reprod BioMed Online. 2008;17(4):583–7.
25. Martinuzzi K, et al. Elevated body mass index (BMI) does not adversely affect in vitro fertilization outcome in young women. J Assist Reprod Genet. 2008;25(5):169–75.
26. Moini A, et al. The effect of body mass index on the outcome of IVF/ICSI cycles in non polycystic ovary syndrome women. International Journal of Fertility and Sterility. 2008;2(2):82–5.

27. Sneed ML, et al. Body mass index: impact on IVF success appears age-related. Hum Reprod. 2008;23(8):1835–9.
28. Ozgun MT, et al. The influence of body mass index on FSH dose and pregnancy rate in women undergoing ICSI-embryo transfer. Journal of the Turkish German Gynecology Association. 2009;10(1):1–5.
29. Sathya A, et al. Effect of body mass index on in vitro fertilization outcomes in women. Journal of Human Reproductive Sciences. 2010;3(3):135–8.
30. Zhang D, et al. Overweight and obesity negatively affect the outcomes of ovarian stimulation and in vitro fertilisation: a cohort study of 2628 Chinese women. Gynecol Endocrinol. 2010;26(5):325–32.
31. Bellver J, et al. Female obesity impairs in vitro fertilization outcome without affecting embryo quality. Fertil Steril. 2010;93(2):447–54.
32. Vilarino Lima F, et al. Body mass index and fertility: is there a correlation with human reproduction outcomes? Gynecol Endocrinol. 2011;27(4):232–6.
33. Farhi J, et al. High-quality embryos retain their implantation capability in overweight women. Reprod BioMed Online. 2010;21(5):706–11.
34. Davies D, et al. Are the negative effects of being overweight on reproductive potential evident in FET cycles? Reprod BioMed Online. 2010; 20(Supplement S2):S58.
35. Funabiki M, et al. The influence of body mass index (BMI) on pregnancy outcomes among Japanese infertile women. Fertil Steril. 2011;96(3 Supplement 1):S115.
36. Hill MJ, Hong S, Frattarelli JL. Body mass index impacts in vitro fertilization stimulation. ISRN Obstetrics and Gynecology. 2011;2010:1–5.
37. Pinborg A, et al. Influence of female bodyweight on IVF outcome: a longitudinal multicentre cohort study of 487 infertile couples. Reprod BioMed Online. 2011;23(4):490–9.
38. Parker K, et al. Does body mass index (BMI) affect IVF outcomes? Fertil Steril. 2011;96(3 Supplement 1):S124.
39. Rittenberg V, Sobaleva S, et al. Influence of BMI on risk of miscarriage after single blastocyst transfer. Hum Reprod. 2011;26(10):2642–50.
40. Singh N, et al. Correlation of body mass index with outcome of in vitro fertilization in a developing country. Arch Gynecol Obstet. 2012;285(1):259–63.
41. Luke B, et al. Female obesity adversely affects assisted reproductive technology (ART) pregnancy and live birth rates. Hum Reprod. 2011;26(1): 245–52.
42. Chavarro JE, et al. Body mass index and short-term weight change in relation to treatment outcomes in women undergoing assisted reproduction. Fertil Steril. 2012;98(1):109–16.
43. Galal AF, Elhelaly DN. Higher body mass index significantly affects intracytoplasmic sperm injection success rate. Fertil Steril. 2012;97(3 Supplement 1):S9–S10.
44. Werner M, et al. Body mass index (BMI) does not impact endometrial receptivity in fresh IVF cycles: evaluation of implantation rates (IR) and ongoing pregnancy rates (PR) following the transfer of euploid blastocysts. Fertil Steril. 2012;98(3 Supplement 1):S286–7.
45. Zander-Fox DL, et al. Does obesity really matter? The impact of BMI on embryo quality and pregnancy outcomes after IVF in women aged <38 years. Aust N Z J Obstet Gynaecol. 2012;52(3):270–6.
46. Ozgun MT, et al. Effect of body mass index on the risk of miscarriage after ICSI. Int J Gynecol Obstet. 2012;119:S535.
47. Ramezanzadeh F, et al. Impact of body mass index versus physical activity and calorie intake on assisted reproduction outcomes. European Journal of Obstetrics Gynecology and Reproductive Biology. 2012;163(1):52–6.
48. Moragianni VA, Jones SML, Ryley DA. The effect of body mass index on the outcomes of first assisted reproductive technology cycles. Fertil Steril. 2012; 98(1):102–8.
49. Bailey AP, et al. Effect of body mass index on in vitro fertilization outcomes in women with polycystic ovary syndrome. Am J Obstet Gynecol. 2014; 211(2):163.e1–6.
50. Schliep KC, et al. Effect of male and female body mass index on pregnancy and live birth success after in vitro fertilization. Fertil Steril. 2015;103(2):388–95.
51. Cai J, Liu L, Zhang J, Qiu H, Jiang X, Li P, Sha A, Ren J. Low body mass index compromises live birth rate in fresh transfer in vitro fertilization cycles: a retrospective study in a Chinese population. Fertility Sterility. 2017;107(2): 422–9.
52. Ozekinci M, Seven A, Olgan S, Sakinci M, Keskin U, Akar ME, Ceyhan ST, Ergun A. Does obesity have detrimental effects on IVF treatment outcomes? BMC Womens Health. 2015;15:61. https://doi.org/10.1186/s12905-015-0223-0.
53. Caillon H, Fréour T, Bach-Ngohou K, Colombel A, Denis MG, Barrière P, Masson D. Effects of female increased body mass index on in vitro fertilization cycles outcome. Obesity Research & Clinical Practice. 2015;9: 382–8.
54. Provost MP, Acharya KS, Acharya CR, Yeh JS, Steward JG, Eaton JL, Goldfarb JM, Muasher SJ. Pregnancy outcomes decline with increasing body mass index: analysis of 239,127 fresh autologous in vitro fertilization cycles from the 2008-2010 Society for Assisted Reproductive Technology registry. Fertil Steril. 2016;105(3):663–9.
55. Russo M, Ates S, Shaulov T, Dahan MH. Morbid obesity and pregnancy outcomes after single blastocyst transfer: a retrospective, north American study. J Assist Reprod Genet. 2017; https://doi.org/10.1007/s10815-017-0883-9.
56. Christensen MW, Ingerslev HJ, Degn B, Kesmodel US. Effect of female body mass index on oocyte quantity in fertility treatments (IVF): treatment cycle number is a possible effect modifier. A Register-Based Cohort Study PLoS ONE. 2016;11(9):e0163393. https://doi.org/10.1371/journal.

21

Sexual and reproductive health behavior and unmet needs among a sample of adolescents living with HIV in Zambia

Sumiyo Okawa[1*], Sylvia Mwanza-Kabaghe[2,3], Mwiya Mwiya[3], Kimiyo Kikuchi[4], Masamine Jimba[1], Chipepo Kankasa[3] and Naoko Ishikawa[5]

Abstract

Background: Adolescents living with HIV face challenges, such as disclosure of HIV status, adherence to antiretroviral therapy, mental health, and sexual and reproductive health (SRH). These challenges affect their future quality of life. However, little evidence is available on their sexual behaviors and SRH needs in Zambia. This study aimed at assessing their sexual behaviors and SRH needs and identifying factors associated with marriage concerns and a desire to have children.

Methods: This cross-sectional study was conducted at the University Teaching Hospital from April to July 2014. We recruited 200 adolescents aged 15–19 years who were aware of their HIV-positive status. We collected data on their first and recent sexual behavior, concerns about marriage, and desire to have children. We used the Generalized Linear Model to identify factors associated with having concerns about marriage and desire to have children. We performed thematic analysis with open-ended data to determine their perceptions about marriage and having children in the future.

Results: Out of 175 studied adolescents, 20.6% had experienced sexual intercourse, and only 44.4% used condoms during the first intercourse. Forty-eight percent had concerns about marriage, and 87.4% desired to have children. Marriage-related concerns were high among those who desired to have children (adjusted relative risk [ARR] = 2.51, 95% CI = 1.02 to 6.14). Adolescents who had completed secondary school were more likely to desire to have children (ARR = 1.35, 95% CI = 1.07 to 1.71). Adolescents who had lost both parents were less likely to want children (ARR = 0.80, 95% CI = 0.68 to 0.95). Thematic analysis identified that major concerns about future marriage were fear of disclosing HIV status to partners and risk of infecting partners and/or children. The reasons for their willingness to have children were the desire to be a parent, having children as family assets, a human right, and a source of love and happiness.

Conclusions: Zambian adolescents living with HIV are at risk of engaging in risky sexual relationships and have difficulties in meeting needs of SRH. HIV care service must respond to a wide range of needs.

Keywords: HIV, Adolescents, Sexual behavior, Sexual and reproductive health, Zambia

* Correspondence: sumiyo@m.u-tokyo.ac.jp
[1]Department of Community and Global Health, Graduate School of Medicine, The University of Tokyo, Tokyo, Japan
Full list of author information is available at the end of the article

Plain English summary

Adolescents living with HIV face difficulties including sexual and reproductive health (SRH). Physical growth and psychosocial development during adolescence could complicate the challenges. This study examined these adolescents' sexual behaviors, needs, and concerns regarding SRH in Zambia.

This cross-sectional study was conducted at the University Teaching Hospital from April to July 2014. We collected data from 200 adolescents aged 15–19 years who were aware of their HIV-positive status and analyzed their sexual behavior and SRH needs with focus on whether they have concerns about marriage and desires for having children and the details of concerns and the reasons for desires.

Out of 175 adolescents, 20.6% had experienced sexual intercourse, 48.8% had concerns about their marriage, and 87.4% desired to have children. Adolescents who desired to have children were more likely to have concerns about marriage (ARR = 2.51). Adolescents who had completed secondary school were more likely to desire to have children (ARR = 1.35). Adolescents who had lost both parents were less likely to want children (ARR = 0.80). Major concerns about future marriage identified by the adolescents were fear of disclosing HIV status to partners and risk of infecting partners and/or children. The main reasons for their willingness to have children were the desire to be a parent, having children as family assets, a human right, and a source of love and happiness.

In conclusion, Zambian adolescents living with HIV have unmet needs regarding SRH. HIV care for adolescents should respond to a wide range of needs.

Background

Human immunodeficiency virus (HIV) care and antiretroviral therapy (ART) services have significantly reduced AIDS-related deaths [1]. Adolescents are defined as those aged 10–19 years by the World Health Organization (WHO) [2]. They are one of the vulnerable populations affected by HIV. In 2015, 1.8 million adolescents were living with HIV, and this number is still growing globally [3]. About half of them contracted HIV infections from their mothers [4], and HIV is the second most common cause of death among them [5]. Even though they are living with HIV, they are healthier and live longer than those in previous decades. However, staying healthy remains a great challenge due to delayed diagnosis, limited access to treatment, adherence to lifelong treatment, and chronic complications caused by treatment [6, 7].

Adolescents living with HIV face challenges such as recognition of HIV status, adherence to ART, mental health, and sexual and reproductive health (SRH) [8–11]. Rapid physical and psychosocial development throughout adolescence [5] could complicate such challenges. In addition, delayed puberty onset is commonly observed among perinatally-infected adolescents, which can result in low self-image, depression, and reproductive consequences [12]. For example, they make themselves targets for sexual abuse or they may easily engage in sexual intercourse to prove their worth. However, little evidence is available on sexual behaviors of adolescents living with HIV. In high-income counties, 27–46% of adolescents and young adults (ages 13–24) living with HIV have experienced sexual intercourse [13–16]. In low- and middle-income countries, it is less prevalent; for example, 25% of Ugandan adolescents and young adults (ages 11–21) and 5% of Thai adolescents (ages 11–18) living with HIV have experienced sexual intercourse [17, 18].

HIV infection affects primary needs of SRH during adolescence and adulthood. The WHO's definitions of sexual health and reproductive health emphasize "having pleasurable and safe sexual experiences, free of coercion, discrimination and violence" [19] and "having the capability to reproduce and the freedom to decide if, when and how often to do so" [20]. Although they are basic human needs, it would be difficult for people living with HIV to meet these needs. Adolescents may experience various threats such as the risk of HIV transmission to partners, difficulties in disclosing HIV status to an intimate partner, managing subsequent rejection by partners, and optimal and consistent use of condoms [21, 22]. They may be particularly vulnerable to the risk of unsafe sexual activity due to peer pressure, poverty, stigma about HIV, ignorance by sexual partners, and alcohol consumption [17].

Despite multiple barriers to meeting their SRH needs, most adolescents living with HIV, at least in the United States, intended to have children [14]. Although few studies have assessed adolescents' fertility intention in African countries, the rates of fertility intention among male and female adults were ranged between 37 and 51%, and the fertility intention was higher among those who were younger, had fewer children, were taking ART, and perceived themselves to have good health status [23–25]. However, the majority have not discussed their fertility intentions with health care workers [23, 25]. This implies that information and counselling on safe and timely pregnancy and childbirth are not widely provided to adolescents and adults living with HIV in African countries. The WHO has published two guidelines to promote client-friendly SRH services and respond to the complex needs of SRH and rights for adolescents living with HIV [2, 26]. However, little evidence is available to understand adolescents' needs regarding intimate relationships, sexual behavior, marriage, and fertility intention in African countries.

The republic of Zambia has been affected by a high burden of HIV. In 2016, an estimated 12.4% of the adult population was living with HIV while 11,000 adolescents were newly infected [3]. The majority of young adolescents contracted HIV through mother-to-child transmission [27] whereas older adolescents are more likely to get HIV infection through sexual transmission or other routes [4]. Major adolescent health issues in the country are lack of knowledge about HIV, early initiation of sexual intercourse, sexually transmitted diseases, and teenage pregnancy [28, 29]. Qualitative studies have identified the difficulties of disclosing HIV status to a partner [30] and the unmet needs for information on HIV and SRH among adolescents living with HIV [31]. More than 870 health care facilities provided HIV care and treatment services across the country [32], and 67% of adults and 52% of children were receiving ART in 2016 [3]. The University Teaching Hospital is the central hospital in the capital city of Lusaka, which houses the Paediatric and Adult Centers of Excellence in HIV care and treatment. Although HIV care and treatment services have become widely available in the country, the existing services do not address challenges and needs of adolescents adequately. Particularly, limited evidence is available on sexual behaviors and SRH needs, and the quality of care in this area remains underdeveloped. We conducted this study to assess sexual behavior and SRH needs among adolescents living with HIV in Zambia and to identify factors associated with having concerns about marriage and desire to have children.

Methods

Study design and setting

We conducted this cross-sectional study at the Paediatric HIV Centre of Excellence and the Adult HIV Centre of Excellence at the University Teaching Hospital from April to July 2014. The two centres are the national referral centres and the model hospitals for adolescent HIV care and treatment services. The two centres equip various specialists and infrastructure to provide care, laboratory test, treatment, counselling, social welfare services, and support peer group activities. The Paediatric Centre provides the services to children and adolescents and transfers them to the Adult Centre when they turn 16 years old. The Adult Centre provides continuous care and treatment service to the adolescents. Health care workers routinely offer information on SRH to all the adolescents aged 10 years or older when they attend their routine clinical reviews. For adolescents who reported risky sexual behaviors during a regular clinical review, health care workers provided counselling services on the details of SRH and family planning methods, gave them condoms, and suggested that they go for a free counselling and testing service for HIV with their partners.

Participants

The eligible study participants were adolescents aged 15–19 who were aware of their HIV status prior to the survey. Those aged 10–14 years were excluded from the study as SRH is a sensitive topic in Zambian culture, and it was deemed inappropriate to involve young adolescents in sexuality-related research.

We estimated a sample size of 165 to detect the association between educational experience and desire to have children based on a previous study that reported 55% prevalence of fertility intention among those with primary school education or higher and 32% among those with less than primary school education [25] using 5% of alpha, 80% of power, and 10% of potential missing data. However, we recruited 200 adolescents as the reference study used for the sample size estimation mainly targeted adults living with HIV. We did not use random sampling because reliable data of the target population and their contact information were not available during the study. We had a three-month data collection period to enroll at least 200 adolescents in the study as adolescent clients had review appointments every 3 months. We recruited the eligible adolescents when they came to the hospital for a clinical review appointment. Before recruiting adolescents, the research assistants asked health care workers or parents/primary caregivers to confirm the eligibility of the selected adolescents.

Data collection

We used a self-administered structured questionnaire for data collection. The questionnaire included basic characteristics of the participating adolescents, their sexual behavior, SRH issues, concerns about future marriage, and desire for having children, based on existing literature [14, 21, 22, 30, 31]. We developed the questionnaire in English because the study sample used English daily. Before the survey, we conducted a pre-test of the questionnaire to assess their English literacy, edited the questionnaire using simple English, and confirmed that the majority could self-administer the questionnaire. We trained research assistants who were peer educators working for adolescents' HIV care program at the study site. During the survey, respondents could ask the same-gender trained research assistants to help read-out in English or provide verbal translation into local language. Those who could not administer the questionnaire had an interview with the same-gender trained research assistants and responded everything except questions about sexual behavior.

Basic information included the adolescents' gender, age, level of education, survival statuses of parents, and status of taking ART. Regarding sexual behaviors, we first asked whether an adolescent had ever had sexual intercourse. For those who had experienced sexual intercourse, we asked for details about the first sexual intercourse including their age, the partners' age at that time, whether they had been aware of their HIV status, used a condom, and whether they were forced to have sexual intercourse. We also collected information on sexual experience in the preceding 12 months. For those who had had sexual intercourse during that period, we asked whether they disclosed their HIV status to their partner, knew their partners' HIV status before the intercourse, used a condom, and ever asked their partner to take an HIV test. We also asked for information about SRH including whether they had disclosed their HIV status to their intimate partners, who they were comfortable talking to about SRH issues, and whether they had learned about prevention of HIV infection with an intimate partner, the risk of infecting an intimate partner with HIV, how to disclose HIV status to others, and how to develop intimate relationships.

The study outcomes were having concerns (or anxieties) about marriage and a desire to have children in the future. First, we provided a structured question "Do you have any concerns about marriage?" in the questionnaire, and then asked to administer their specific concerns with a single English sentence. In the same way, we asked another structured question "Do you want to have children in the future?" followed by asking their reasons for wanting children.

Data analyses

For quantitative data, we first compared the distributions of background characteristics of the adolescents, their sexual behavior, and SRH issues using chi-square test. We then identified factors associated with having concerns about marriage and desire to have children by using the Generalized Linear Model. We included age, gender, education level, survival statuses of their parents, having someone to talk to about SRH issues, and having learned about four topics on SRH as independent variables of the models which were selected based on the existing literature [14, 23, 31, 33] and estimated crude and adjusted relative risks (RRs). We excluded missing data from the analyses and reported the number of respondents who declined to answer questions in the tables. We analyzed all the quantitative data using Stata (version 13.1).

For qualitative data, we performed thematic analysis to identify patterns of concerns about marriage and reasons they desired to have children. We followed the six phases in the data analysis process suggested by Braun [34]: (1) "familiarizing yourself with your data," (2) "generating initial codes," (3) "searching for themes," (4) "reviewing themes," (5) "defining and naming themes," and (6) "producing the report." Two authors (SO, KK) worked on Phases (1) and (2) independently and reviewed and discussed all codes to enhance reliability of the analyses. After that, the two authors conducted Phases (3), (4), and (5). Finally, SO conducted Phase (6). We manually analyzed all the qualitative data.

Ethical considerations

We obtained ethical approval from the Biomedical Research Ethics Committee of the University of Zambia and the Institutional Ethics Committee of National Center for Global Health and Medicine, Japan. We obtained written informed consent from all participants and written assent from parents or primary caregivers of adolescents aged 15, 16, and 17 years. We anticipated that adolescents may feel pressured to participate in the study as we recruited them at the hospital where they were receiving care. In addition, they may hesitate to respond about sexual behavior if they suspect the individual data could be shared with the hospital staff. To address these potential issues, we informed each adolescent about voluntary participation without any harm if they avail of care in the future and confidentiality in data management.

Results

We recruited 200 eligible adolescents in the study. We excluded two adolescents who withdrew during the survey and 15 adolescents who did not respond about their sexual behavior due to limited English literacy or voluntarily declined to answer. We excluded eight from the dataset because they were outside of the eligible criteria for age, although we asked their age at recruitment. Finally, we included the data of 175 adolescents in the analysis. Seventy-two (41.1%) were boys, and 103 (58.9%) were girls. Sixty-five percent had lost their fathers and/or mothers, and 94.3% were undergoing ART. No significant gender differences were found in the distributions of the basic characteristics (Table 1).

Table 2 shows the sexual behaviors of the adolescents. Thirty-six adolescents (20.6%) had ever experienced sexual intercourse with a mean age of 16.2 (SD 1.0) years among boys and 15.7 (SD 2.0) years among girls at the first intercourse ($p = .51$). Girls were more likely to have an older-aged partner than were boys ($p < .01$). Although 55.6% were already aware of their HIV status at the first intercourse, at least 33.3% did not use a condom. Only girls ($n = 4$) reported that their first sexual intercourse was forced. In the last 12 months prior to the survey, 22 adolescents (12.6%) reported having had sexual intercourse. Of the 22 adolescents, girls were more likely to disclose their HIV status to their partners ($p = .01$) and to know their partner's HIV status ($p = .05$) before engaging in the sexual relationship.

Table 3 shows the SRH issues of the adolescents. About half (48.8%) reported that they had concerns about marriage, and 87.4% desired to have children in the future with no significant gender differences. Twenty percent had disclosed their HIV status to their partners at least once. Higher proportions of the adolescents had learned about the prevention of HIV infection to a

Table 1 Basic characteristics of participants (n = 175)

	Total		Boys		Girls		
	n = 175		n = 72		n = 103		
	n	(%)	n	(%)	n	(%)	p
Age							
15 years	23	(13.1)	7	(9.7)	16	(15.5)	0.28
16 years	42	(24.0)	23	(31.9)	19	(18.5)	
17 years	38	(21.7)	13	(18.1)	25	(24.3)	
18 years	42	(24.0)	17	(23.6)	25	(24.3)	
19 years	30	(17.1)	12	(16.7)	18	(17.5)	
Educational experience							
Incomplete primary school	26	(14.9)	11	(15.3)	15	(14.6)	0.93
Completed primary school	88	(50.3)	35	(48.6)	53	(51.1)	
Completed secondary school or higher	61	(34.9)	26	(36.1)	35	(34.0)	
Parental survival status							
Both parents are alive	61	(34.9)	30	(41.7)	31	(30.1)	0.09
Mother was dead	34	(19.4)	13	(18.1)	21	(20.4)	
Father was dead	35	(20.0)	17	(23.6)	18	(17.5)	
Both parents were dead	45	(25.7)	12	(16.7)	33	(32.0)	
Currently taking ART							
Yes	165	(94.3)	70	(97.2)	95	(92.2)	0.16
No	10	(5.7)	2	(2.8)	8	(7.8)	

partner (82.9%) and the risk of HIV transmission to a partner (74.3%) compared with those who had learned about how to disclose their HIV status to others (58.9%) and how to develop intimate relationships (49.7%).

Table 4 shows the factors associated with having concerns about marriage (n = 168). Adolescents who wanted to have their own children were more likely to have concerns about their future marriage compared with those who did not desire to have children (Adjusted RR [ARR] = 2.51, 95% CI = 1.02 to 6.14). Table 5 shows the factors associated with desiring to have children (n = 175). The adolescents who had completed secondary school or higher were more likely to desire to have children than those who had not completed primary school (ARR = 1.35, 95% CI = 1.07 to 1.71). Adolescents whose parents were both dead were less likely to desire to have children compared with those whose parents were both alive (ARR = 0.80, 95% CI = 0.68 to 0.95).

Table 6 shows the adolescents' concerns or anxieties about future marriage. Out of 82 adolescents who reported that they were concerned about future marriage (Table 3), 63 (76.8%) described the specific concerns. The four major themes that emerged were: disclosing HIV status to partner, options in marriage, HIV transmission to partner and children. Adolescents were anxious about how to disclose HIV status to their intimate partners and their reactions afterwards: *"I wouldn't know how to tell him my HIV status if he is not HIV infected"* (Girl, age 15); *"If the person who will want to marry me finds out that I am HIV positive, he will change his mind about marrying me"* (Girl, age 17). Adolescents also worried about the risk of HIV transmission to their partners and children: *"Will I have to risk her health just for a child? If not, will she have to carry the burden with me?"* (Boy, age 19); *"Is there medicine that can reduce the risk of the baby contracting HIV from the mother?"* (Girl, age 17). To avoid infecting partner and children, some adolescents also considered remaining single or marrying a partner also living with HIV: *"I sometimes think it's better to remain single forever"* (Girl, age 18); *"I think I will have a wife who is (HIV) positive"* (Boy, age 17).

Table 7 shows the reasons why adolescents desired to have children. Out of 153 adolescents who showed the desires to have children in Tables 3, 102 (66.7%) explained the reasons. From the thematic analysis, four major reasons emerged: desire for parenting, children as family assets, positive perception on children, and natural matter. Some adolescents wished to become a parent: *"I want to know how it feels to be a mother"* (Girl, age 18). They expected to have children as household assets: *"I want them to help me when I get old"* (Girl, age 15); *"I want my family name to continue"* (Boy, age 17). Some adolescents showed their love for children and regarded children as sources of happiness

Table 2 Sexual behavior (n = 175)

	Total		Boys		Girls		
	n	(%)	n	(%)	n	(%)	p
First sexual experience							
Ever had sexual intercourse							
Yes	36	(20.6)	15	(20.8)	21	(20.4)	0.90
No	133	(76.0)	54	(75.0)	79	(76.7)	
Declined to answer	6	(3.4)	3	(4.2)	3	(2.9)	
Age at the first sexual intercourse (n = 21)	16.0	(1.6)	16.2	(1.0)	15.7	(2.0)	0.51
Partner's age at the first sexual intercourse (n = 19)	18.4	(3.0)	16.2	(2.6)	20.4	(1.8)	< 0.01
Already aware of HIV status (n = 36)							
Yes	20	(55.6)	6	(40.0)	14	(66.7)	0.19
No	11	(30.6)	7	(46.7)	4	(19.1)	
Declined to answer	5	(13.9)	2	(13.3)	3	(14.3)	
Used condom at first sexual intercourse (n = 36)							
Yes	16	(44.4)	6	(40.0)	10	(47.6)	0.77
No	12	(33.3)	6	(40.0)	6	(28.6)	
Declined to answer	8	(22.2)	3	(20.0)	5	(23.8)	
First sexual intercourse was forced (n = 36)							
Yes	4	(11.1)	0	(0.0)	4	(19.1)	0.17
No	25	(69.4)	11	(73.3)	14	(66.7)	
Declined to answer	7	(19.4)	4	(26.7)	3	(14.3)	
Sexual experience in the last 12 months							
Had sexual intercourse (n = 175)							
Yes	22	(12.6)	7	(9.7)	15	(14.6)	0.49
No	149	(85.1)	64	(88.9)	85	(82.5)	
Declined to answer	4	(2.3)	1	(1.4)	3	(2.9)	
Disclosed HIV status to partner in advance (n = 22)							
Yes	11	(50.0)	1	(14.3)	10	(66.7)	0.01
No	8	(36.4)	3	(42.9)	5	(33.3)	
Declined to answer	3	(13.6)	3	(42.9)	0	(0.0)	
Already knew partner's HIV status (n = 22)							
Yes	10	(45.5)	1	(14.3)	9	(60.0)	0.05
No	12	(54.6)	6	(85.7)	6	(40.0)	
Used condom (n = 22)							
Yes	12	(54.6)	5	(71.4)	7	(46.7)	0.53
No	6	(27.3)	1	(14.3)	5	(33.3)	
Declined to answer	4	(18.2)	1	(14.3)	3	(20.0)	
Asked partner for HIV testing (n = 22)							
Yes	7	(31.8)	1	(14.3)	6	(40.0)	0.38
No	9	(40.9)	3	(42.9)	6	(40.0)	
Declined to answer	6	(27.3)	3	(42.9)	3	(20.0)	

and joy in their lives: *"A child will bring happiness to me and my family"* (Girl, age 17). They also saw children as a blessing: *"Children all are wonderful gifts from God"* (Girl, age 19). Some adolescents stated that having children is a natural outcome of marriage and a human right: *"I am a human being and have the right to have a child. My (HIV-positive) status does not matter"* (Girl, age 17).

Table 3 Sexual and reproductive health needs

	Total		Boys		Girls		
	n	(%)	*n*	(%)	*n*	(%)	*p*
Have concerns about marriage (*n* = 168)							
Yes	82	(48.8)	31	(45.6)	51	(51.0)	0.49
No	86	(51.2)	37	(54.4)	49	(49.0)	
Desire to have children (*n* = 175)							
Yes	153	(87.4)	65	(90.3)	88	(85.4)	0.34
No	22	(12.6)	7	(9.7)	15	(14.6)	
Ever disclosed HIV status to an intimate partner (*n* = 172)							
Yes	35	(20.4)	14	(19.7)	21	(20.8)	0.48
No	71	(41.3)	33	(46.5)	38	(37.6)	
Never had an intimate partner	66	(38.4)	24	(33.8)	42	(41.6)	
Person to talk about SRH issues							
Friend	32	(18.3)	8	(11.1)	24	(23.3)	0.31
Mother	29	(16.6)	12	(16.7)	17	(16.5)	
Peers living with HIV	17	(9.7)	7	(9.7)	10	(9.7)	
Health care worker	7	(4.0)	2	(2.8)	5	(4.9)	
Other	64	(36.6)	32	(44.4)	32	(31.1)	
Nobody	26	(14.9)	11	(15.3)	15	(14.6)	
Education topics on HIV and SRH ever learned							
Preventing HIV transmission to partner							
Yes	145	(82.9)	60	(83.3)	85	(82.5)	0.89
No	30	(17.1)	12	(16.7)	18	(17.5)	
Risk of HIV transmission to partner							
Yes	130	(74.3)	52	(72.2)	78	(75.7)	0.60
No	45	(25.7)	20	(27.8)	25	(24.3)	
How to disclose HIV status to others							
Yes	103	(58.9)	40	(55.6)	63	(61.2)	0.46
No	72	(41.1)	32	(44.4)	40	(38.8)	
How to develop intimate relationships							
Yes	87	(49.7)	42	(58.3)	45	(43.7)	0.06
No	88	(50.3)	30	(41.7)	58	(56.3)	

Table 4 Factors associated with having concerns about marriage (*n* = 168)

	cRR	(95%CI)	aRR	(95%CI)
Age	0.99	(0.88–1.12)	1.11	(0.96–1.29)
Gender				
Boy	0.89	(0.65–1.24)	0.85	(0.62–1.15)
Girl	1.00		1.00	
Educational experience				
Incomplete primary school	1.00		1.00	
Completed primary school	1.55	(0.89–2.71)	1.50	(0.86–2.60)
Completed secondary school or higher	1.22	(0.67–2.23)	0.97	(0.51–1.83)
Parental survival status				
Both parents are alive	1.00		1.00	
Mother was dead	0.85	(0.55–1.32)	0.82	(0.53–1.27)
Father was dead	0.91	(0.60–1.37)	0.93	(0.64–1.35)
Both parents were dead	0.74	(0.48–1.13)	0.73	(0.48–1.12)
Have someone to talk about SRH issues				
Yes	1.20	(0.73–1.98)	1.25	(0.78–2.01)
No	1.00		1.00	
Learned about HIV and SRH				
0–3 items	1.00		1.00	
4 items	0.78	(0.55–1.12)	0.80	(0.55–1.17)
Want to have my children				
Yes	2.64	(1.08–6.43)	2.51	(1.02–6.14)
No	1.00		1.00	

Age is a continuous variable. cRR and aRR mean the crude and adjusted relative risk

Discussion

Twenty percent of the adolescents in our sample had experienced sexual intercourse, and at least 30% of them did not use a condom during the first intercourse. Nearly half of the adolescents expressed concerns about their future marriage. In contrast, the majority of them desired to have their own children in the future. Those who desired to have children were more likely to worry about their marriage. To the best of our knowledge, this is the first quantitative evidence built on the existing study findings in Zambia [30, 31].

Adolescents in the study were less likely to have had sexual intercourse (20.6%) compared with the adolescents (ages 15–19) in the national representative data (49.1% among girls and 47.7% among boys) [29]. Similarly, in the United States, perinatally HIV-infected youths were less likely to practice sexual intercourse compared with uninfected youths [35]. However, it should be highlighted that sexually active adolescents in this study engaged in risky sexual intercourse; nearly 30% did not use a condom during their first intercourse and recent intercourse. Moreover, sexual intercourse commonly took place without recognizing the HIV status, particularly among HIV-positive boys and their partners. In addition, girls had relatively older partners and tended to have forced intercourse. This indicates that girls could be particularly vulnerable to control by their partners' demands for unprotected intercourse. Both girls and boys were sexually active, but the

Table 5 Factors associated with desiring to have children ($n = 175$)

	cRR	95%CI	aRR	95%CI
Age	1.01	(0.97–1.05)	0.97	(0.92–1.03)
Gender				
Boy	1.06	(0.95–1.18)	1.02	(0.92–1.14)
Girl	1.00		1.00	
Educational experience				
Incomplete primary school	1.00		1.00	
Completed primary school	1.11	(0.88–1.39)	1.17	(0.94–1.45)
Completed secondary school or higher	1.24	(0.99–1.54)	1.35	(1.07–1.71)
Parental survival status				
Both parents are alive	1.00		1.00	
Mother was dead	0.90	(0.77–1.04)	0.88	(0.76–1.03)
Father was dead	0.93	(0.82–1.06)	0.92	(0.81–1.05)
Both parents were dead	0.82	(0.69–0.97)	0.80	(0.68–0.95)
Have someone to talk about SRH issues				
Yes	1.10	(0.90–1.34)	1.10	(0.90–1.34)
No	1.00		1.00	
Learned about HIV and SRH				
0–3 items	1.00		1.00	
4 items	1.02	(0.90–1.14)	1.00	(0.88–1.15)

Age is a continuous variable. cRR and aRR mean the crude and adjusted relative risk

process or context of engaging in sexual relationships was not the same.

Adolescents' concerns about marriage were not related only to marriage. Their concerns were widely associated with intimate relationships—namely, disclosing their HIV status to partners, potential rejection afterwards, and the risk of HIV transmission. This indicates that adolescents were facing a dual pressure with rejection and infection in intimate relationships. Similar findings have been reported in Canada, the United States, and Rwanda [21, 22, 36]. Most adolescents in this study had learned about the risk of HIV transmission and the preventive methods, but they had limited information on the ways to develop intimate partnerships and disclose HIV status to others. In addition, health care workers were less utilized as primary counsellors or advisors for their SRH issues. Health care workers should make further effort to develop a better relationship with adolescents and provide them with comprehensive information on SRH.

Table 6 Concerns about future marriage

Main theme	Sub-theme
Disclosing HIV status to partner	Do not know how to disclose my HIV status to partner
	Concern about partner"s reaction after disclosing my HIV status
Options in marriage	Not getting married may be better
	HIV-positive partner may be suitable
HIV transmission to partner	Don"t know how to protect partner from HIV infection
	Concern about the risk of HIV transmission to partner
HIV transmission to children	Don"t know how to protect children from HIV infection
	Concern about the risk of HIV transmission to children

Out of 82 adolescents who had concerns about future marriage, 63 (76.8%) provided open-ended answers to explain the specific concerns or anxieties

Table 7 Reasons that adolescents desire to have children

Main theme	Sub-theme
Desire for parenting	Desire for becoming a parent
	Desire for taking care of children
Children as family assets	Children as my caretakers
	Children as the successors of family
Positive perception on children	Love for children
	Happiness brought by children
	Blessing from God
Natural matter	Natural outcome of marriage
	Human right

Out of 153 adolescents who desired to have children in the future, 102 (66.7%) explained the reasons

Most of the adolescents expressed the desire to have children. They felt that having children has an important meaning in their adulthood. It means that they can achieve their dreams and happiness, secure family assets, and that it is human nature and their right. On the other hand, they were afraid of HIV transmission to their children and had insufficient knowledge about prevention of mother-to-child transmission. Similarly, in the United States and Rwanda, a strong fear of mother-to-child transmission was associated with lower intention to have children [14, 36]. In this study, adolescents who had lost both parents were less likely to desire to have their own children. Loss of parents is linked to multiple negative consequences: psychological distress, caretaking responsibility for younger siblings, dropping out of school, and vulnerability to sexually transmitted diseases and early pregnancy [33, 37, 38]. Due to such childhood experiences and uncertain life expectancy due to being affected by HIV, orphaned adolescents may have a lower motivation to have their own children. Adolescents who completed secondary education had a higher intention to have children. Educational experience is known as a protective factor against health risks in adolescence [39]. On the other hand, those who did not complete primary education had a passive desire for having children. This may indicate that they had limited access to information and/or low literacy about SRH. Orphaned or low-educated adolescents need special support for their pro-active choice of future pregnancy and childbirth.

Adolescents showed unmet SRH needs about intimate and sexual relationships, marriage, pregnancy, and childbirth. However, the current HIV care and treatment services for adolescents do not fully respond to their needs. The health care workers must make more efforts to reach all adolescents regardless of their gender, socio-economic status (e.g. family structure, educational level), and childhood background. Education and counselling should primarily emphasize basic prevention of HIV transmission for safe sexual relationships while considering gender sensitivity and vulnerability. In addition, information on the benefits and risks of disclosing HIV status to a partner should be provided. Follow-up counselling after self-disclosure is also essential for those in psychological distress facing negative outcomes of disclosure. To respond to the complicated SRH needs of adolescents, training on adolescent-centered SRH care should be offered to health care workers. In addition, many Zambians experience the first marriage and pregnancy in late adolescence or early adulthood. It will be beneficial for adolescents to discuss and prepare for safe pregnancy and childbirth in collaboration with family planning and prevention of mother-to-child transmission of HIV programs.

This study has several limitations. First, the generalizability of the study findings is limited as we conducted the study at a tertiary hospital in the national capital with no comparison groups. Second, convenience sampling for recruiting study participants at regular clinical reviews may have contributed to selection bias, because adolescents with no access or no compliance with care were not included in the study, but they would have different patterns of sexual behaviors and different needs regarding SRH. Third, we did not collect data on marital status or route of HIV transmission, which could influence to sexual behavior. Further studies at multiple sites with various target populations would be recommended, and sub-group analysis by geographical area, compliance with care, marital status, and the routes of HIV transmission could provide the study results more clearly. Third, we collected information on sensitive issues about sexual behaviors, which may lead to under-reporting and an increase in missing data. Thus, the study findings could be under-estimated and should not be simply compared with results in other settings. The future study needs to use anonymous survey methods, such as computer-assisted survey. Fourth, the small sample size may limit the power to identify significant associations between participants' characteristics and the study outcome. Despite the limitations, this study used quantitative and qualitative data and identified the knowledge gaps in how HIV infection affects current and future SRH and well-being among adolescents.

Conclusions

Zambian adolescents living with HIV were sexually active. In addition, they were highly concerned about future marriage and fertility opportunities due to potential refusal by their partners and the risks of HIV transmission to their partners and children. HIV care and treatment services should cover a wider area of SRH needs and reach all adolescents regardless of their socio-demographic and -economic backgrounds.

Abbreviations

ART: Antiretroviral therapy; HIV: Human immunodeficiency virus; SRH: Sexual and reproductive health; WHO: World Health Organization

Acknowledgements

The authors would like to thank all study participants, research assistants, and health care workers at University Teaching Hospital for supporting this study. We are grateful to Dr. Kenichi Komada for his technical assistance.

Funding

This work was supported by The Grant for National Center for Global Health and Medicine (26–2 and 28–1).

Authors' contributions

SO, NI, SMK, MM, and CK conceived and designed the study and implemented the survey. SO analyzed the quantitative and qualitative data and drafted the manuscript. KK analyzed the qualitative data. NI, SMK, and MJ critically reviewed the manuscript. All authors approved submission of the manuscript.

Consent for publication

Not applicable.

Competing interests

The authors declare that they have no competing interests.

Author details

[1]Department of Community and Global Health, Graduate School of Medicine, The University of Tokyo, Tokyo, Japan. [2]Department of Educational Psychology, Sociology, and Special Education, School of Education, University of Zambia, Lusaka, Zambia. [3]Paediatric HIV Centre of Excellence, University Teaching Hospital, Lusaka, Zambia. [4]Institute of Decision Science for a Sustainable Society, Kyushu University, Fukuoka, Japan. [5]Bureau of International Health Cooperation, National Center for Global Health and Medicine, Tokyo, Japan.

References

1. UNAIDS. The gap report. Geneva: UNAIDS; 2014.
2. WHO. HIV and adolescents: guidance for HIV testing and counselling and care for adolescents living with HIV: recommendations for a public health approach and considerations for policy-makers and managers. Geneva: WHO; 2013.
3. UNAIDS. AIDSinfo. No date. http://aidsinfo.unaids.org/#. Accessed 29 Sep 2017.
4. UNICEF. 2014 annual results report: HIV and AIDS. New York: UNICEF; 2014.
5. WHO. Health for the world's adolescents: a second chance in the second decade. Geneva: WHO; 2014.

6. Ferrand RA, Munaiwa L, Matsekete J, Bandason T, Nathoo K, Ndhlovu CE, et al. Undiagnosed HIV infection among adolescents seeking primary health care in Zimbabwe. Clin Infect Dis. 2010;51(7):844–51.
7. Mofenson LM, Cotton MF. The challenges of success: adolescents with perinatal HIV infection. J Int AIDS Soc. 2013;16:18650.
8. Gray GE. Adolescent HIV–cause for concern in southern Africa. PLoS Med. 2010;7(2):e1000227.
9. Koenig LJ, Nesheim S, Abramowitz S. Adolescents with perinatally acquired HIV: emerging behavioral and health needs for long-term survivors. Curr Opin Obstet Gynecol. 2011;23(5):321–7.
10. Agwu AL, Fairlie L. Antiretroviral treatment, management challenges and outcomes in perinatally HIV-infected adolescents. J Int AIDS Soc. 2013;16:18579.
11. Mellins CA, Malee KM. Understanding the mental health of youth living with perinatal HIV infection: lessons learned and current challenges. J Int AIDS Soc. 2013;16:18593.
12. Williams PL, Abzug MJ, Jacobson DL, Wang J, Van Dyke RB, Hazra R, et al. Pubertal onset in children with perinatal HIV infection in the era of combination antiretroviral treatment. AIDS. 2013;27(12):1959–70.
13. Koenig LJ, Pals SL, Chandwani S, Hodge K, Abramowitz S, Barnes W, et al. Sexual transmission risk behavior of adolescents with HIV acquired perinatally or through risky behaviors. J Acquir Immune Defic Syndr. 2010; 55(3):380–90.
14. Ezeanolue EE, Wodi AP, Patel R, Dieudonne A, Oleske JM. Sexual behaviors and procreational intentions of adolescents and young adults with perinatally acquired human immunodeficiency virus infection: experience of an urban tertiary center. J Adolesc Health. 2006;38:719–25.
15. Wiener LS, Battles HB, Wood LV. A longitudinal study of adolescents with perinatally or transfusion acquired HIV infection: sexual knowledge, risk reduction self-efficacy and sexual behavior. AIDS Behav. 2007;11(3):471–8.
16. Brogly SB, Watts DH, Ylitalo N, Franco EL, Seage GR 3rd, Oleske J, et al. Reproductive health of adolescent girls perinatally infected with HIV. Am J Public Health. 2007;97:1047–52.
17. Bakeera-Kitaka S, Nabukeera-Barungi N, Nostlinger C, Addy K, Colebunders R. Sexual risk reduction needs of adolescents living with HIV in a clinical care setting. AIDS Care. 2008;20(4):426–33.
18. Lolekha R, Boon-Yasidhi V, Leowsrisook P, Naiwatanakul T, Durier Y, Nuchanard W, et al. Knowledge, attitudes, and practices regarding antiretroviral management, reproductive health, sexually transmitted infections, and sexual risk behavior among perinatally HIV-infected youth in Thailand. AIDS Care. 2015;27(5):618–28.
19. WHO. Sexual health. 2017. http://www.who.int/topics/sexual_health/en/. Assessed 20 Dec 2017.
20. WHO. Reproductive health. 2017. http://www.who.int/topics/reproductive_health/en/. Accessed 20 Dec 2017.
21. Fernet M, Wong K, Richard ME, Otis J, Levy JJ, Lapointe N, et al. Romantic relationships and sexual activities of the first generation of youth living with HIV since birth. AIDS Care. 2011;23:393–400.
22. Fair C, Albright J. "Don't tell him you have HIV unless he's 'the one'": romantic relationships among adolescents and young adults with perinatal HIV infection. AIDS Patient Care STDs. 2012;26(12):746–54.
23. Cooper D, Moodley J, Zweigenthal V, Bekker LG, Shah I, Myer L. Fertility intentions and reproductive health care needs of people living with HIV in cape town, South Africa: implications for integrating reproductive health and HIV care services. AIDS Behav. 2009;13(Suppl 1):38–46.
24. Mmbaga EJ, Leyna GH, Ezekiel MJ, Kakoko DC. Fertility desire and intention of people living with HIV/AIDS in Tanzania: a call for restructuring care and treatment services. BMC Public HealthBMC Public Health. 2013;13:86.
25. Kawale P, Mindry D, Stramotas S, Chilikoh P, Phoya A, Henry K, et al. Factors associated with desire for children among HIV-infected women and men: a quantitative and qualitative analysis from Malawi and implications for the delivery of safer conception counseling. AIDS Care. 2014;26(6):769–76.
26. WHO. Consolidated guideline on sexual and reproductive health and rights of women living with HIV. Geneva: WHO; 2017.
27. Menon A, Glazebrook C, Campain N, Ngoma M. Mental health and disclosure of HIV status in Zambian adolescents with HIV infection: implications for peer-support programs. J Acquir Immune Defic Syndr. 2007;46(3):349–54.
28. National AIDS Council, Ministry of Health, Ministry of Community Development Mother and Child Health. Zambia country report: monitoring the declaration of commitment on HIV and AIDS and the Universal access: biennial report. Lusaka: National AIDS Council; 2014.
29. Central Statistical Office (CSO) [Zambia], Ministry of Health (MOH) [Zambia], ICF International. Zambia Demographic and Health Survey 2013--14. Rockville: Central Statistical Office, Ministry of Health, ICF-International; 2014.
30. Mburu G, Hodgson I, Kalibala S, Haamujompa C, Cataldo F, Lowenthal ED, et al. Adolescent HIV disclosure in Zambia: barriers, facilitators and outcomes. J Int AIDS Soc. 2014;17:18866.
31. Hodgson I, Ross J, Haamujompa C, Gitau-Mburu D. Living as an adolescent with HIV in Zambia – lived experiences, sexual health and reproductive needs. AIDS Care. 2012;24(10):1204–10.
32. National HIV, AIDS STI, TB Council. National HIV AIDS strategic framework 2017--2021. Lusaka: National HIV AIDS STI TB Council; 2017.
33. Cluver LD, Orkin M, Gardner F, Boyes ME. Persisting mental health problems among AIDS-orphaned children in South Africa. J Child Psychol Psychiatry. 2012;53(4):363–70.
34. Braun V, Clarke V. Using thematic analysis in Psychology. Qual Res Psychol. 2006;3(2):77–101.
35. Elkington KS, Bauermeister JA, Robbins RN, Gromadzka O, Abrams EJ, Wiznia A, et al. Individual and contextual factors of sexual risk behavior in youth perinatally infected with HIV. AIDS Patient Care STDS. 2012;26(7):411–22.
36. Van Nuil JI, Mutwa P, Asiimwe-Kateera B, Kestelyn E, Vyankandondera J, Pool R, et al. "Let's talk about sex": a qualitative study of Rwandan adolescents' views on sex and HIV. PLoS One. 2014;9(8):e102933.
37. Kang M, Dunbar M, Laver S, Padian N. Maternal versus paternal orphans and HIV/STI risk among adolescent girls in Zimbabwe. AIDS Care. 2008;20(2):214–7.
38. Bazile J, Rigodon J, Berman L, Boulanger VM, Maistrellis E, Kausiwa P, et al. Intergenerational impacts of maternal mortality: Qualitative findings from rural Malawi. Reprod Health. 2015;12(Suppl 1):S1.
39. Viner RM, Ozer EM, Denny S, Marmot M, Resnick M, Fatusi A, et al. Adolescence and the social determinants of health. Lancet. 2012;379(9826):1641–52.

HIV status disclosure to male partners among rural Nigerian women along the prevention of mother-to-child transmission of HIV cascade

Angela Odiachi[1], Salome Erekaha[2], Llewellyn J. Cornelius[3], Christopher Isah[2], Habib O. Ramadhani[4], Laura Rapoport[5] and Nadia A. Sam-Agudu[2,4*]

Abstract

Background: HIV status disclosure to male partners is important for optimal outcomes in the prevention of mother-to-child transmission of HIV (PMTCT). Depending on timing of HIV diagnosis or pregnancy status, readiness to disclose and disclosure rates may differ among HIV-positive women. We sought to determine rates, patterns, and experiences of disclosure among Nigerian women along the PMTCT cascade.

Methods: HIV-positive women in rural North-Central Nigeria were purposively recruited according to their PMTCT cascade status: pregnant-newly HIV-diagnosed, pregnant-in care, postpartum, and lost-to-follow-up (LTFU). Participants were surveyed to determine rates of disclosure to male partners and others; in-depth interviews evaluated disclosure patterns and experiences. Tests of association were applied to quantitative data. Qualitative data were manually analysed by theme and content using the constant comparative method in a Grounded Theory approach.

Results: We interviewed 100 women; 69% were 21–30 years old, and 86% were married. There were 25, 26, 28 and 21 women in the newly-diagnosed, in-care, postpartum, and LTFU groups, respectively. Approximately 81% of all participants reported disclosing to anyone; however, family members were typically disclosed to first. Ultimately, more women had disclosed to male partners (85%) than to family members (55%). Rates of disclosure to anyone varied between groups: newly-diagnosed and LTFU women had the lowest (56%) and highest (100%) rates, respectively ($p = 0.001$). However, family ($p = 0.402$) and male partner ($p = 0.218$) disclosure rates were similar between cascade groups. Across all cascade groups, fear of divorce and intimate partner violence deterred women from disclosing to male partners. However, participants reported that with assistance from healthcare workers, disclosure and post-disclosure experiences were mostly positive.

(Continued on next page)

* Correspondence: nsamagudu@ihvnigeria.org
[2]International Research Center of Excellence, Institute of Human Virology Nigeria, Abuja, Nigeria
[4]Institute of Human Virology, University of Maryland School of Medicine, Baltimore, USA
Full list of author information is available at the end of the article

(Continued from previous page)

Conclusion: In our study cohort, although disclosure to male partners was overall higher, family members appeared more approachable for initial disclosure. Across cascade groups, male partners were ultimately disclosed to at rates > 75%, with no significant inter-group differences. Fear appears to be a major reason for non-disclosure or delayed disclosure by women to male partners. Augmentation of healthcare workers' skills and involvement can mediate gender power differentials, minimize fear and shorten time to male partner disclosure among women living with HIV, regardless of their PMTCT cascade status.

Keywords: HIV, Disclosure, PMTCT, Serodiscordance, Male partner, Nigeria

Plain English summary

For women living with HIV, disclosure to male partners is important in preventing HIV transmission to infants and staying healthy on treatment. Gender inequality plays a key role in low rates of disclosure by women to male partners. In addition, HIV disclosure rates may differ depending on whether the woman was recently or previously diagnosed, or whether she is pregnant or has delivered. We interviewed 100 women living with HIV in rural North-Central Nigeria to evaluate their disclosure history and experiences. The women were pregnant and newly or previously HIV-diagnosed, breastfeeding, or had dropped out of HIV care.

Most women (81%) reported disclosing to anyone; with more disclosing to male partners than relatives (85% versus 55%). However, family members were typically disclosed to, first. Also, newly-diagnosed and out-of-HIV-care women were least and most likely, respectively, to disclose to anyone. Male partner disclosure rates were similar across groups. Women who disclosed to male partners did so to motivate them to test for HIV and to keep open, honest couples' communication. Women across all groups reported avoiding male partner disclosure due to fear of divorce and violence. However, when healthcare workers were involved, disclosure experiences were mostly positive.

Our results show that family members were more approachable than male partners for initial disclosure, and that healthcare workers can, and have been instrumental in improving male partner disclosure experiences among HIV-positive women. Therefore, healthcare workers should be trained and proactively involved in helping HIV-positive women to disclose to male partners.

Background

In 2016, there were an estimated 3.2 million people living with HIV in Nigeria, at a prevalence rate of 2.9% in the general population [1]. Unprotected heterosexual sexual intercourse remains the main mode of HIV transmission in Nigeria [2]. Latest available data show HIV prevalence at 3.5% in adult females versus 3.3% in males; and 3.6% and 3.2% in rural versus urban areas, respectively [2]. In 2016, only 34% of Nigeria's large HIV-positive population were estimated to know their HIV status, and only 30% of those diagnosed received antiretroviral therapy (ART) [1]. Linkage to treatment is important for HIV prevention, because once an HIV-positive client is initiated and is compliant on a suppressive ART regimen, the risk of onward transmission drops significantly [3]. Thus, knowledge of HIV status through massive scale-up of HIV testing, and subsequent linkage to suppressive treatment is critical to containing the HIV epidemic.

Besides personal knowledge of HIV status, disclosure of such status by people living with HIV to others – family, friends, sexual partners – is important for HIV prevention, including the prevention of mother-to-child transmission of HIV (PMTCT) [4]. Disclosure facilitates treatment uptake, drug adherence and retention in care for people living with HIV, including pregnant women [4–10]. For this population, disclosure is important for dual prevention of HIV transmission to sexual partners and for PMTCT, through promoting male partner HIV testing, the adoption of safer sex practices, and partner support for PMTCT service uptake [11, 12].

The PMTCT cascade is a multistep continuum of care package to be completed by HIV-positive mother-exposed infant pairs, and includes maternal HIV testing and treatment, antenatal and delivery care, early infant diagnosis, postnatal services, and linkage to long-term HIV care and support [13]. Women who have disclosed have higher rates of antenatal care (ANC) uptake, facility delivery, and PMTCT ART use compared to women who have not [7]. Non-disclosure has been reported as a predictor of PMTCT cascade dropout [14], while women who disclosed to their partners were up to five times more likely to access and be retained in PMTCT care [15].

Despite the benefits, disclosure rates in PMTCT are widely disparate, particularly in sub-Saharan Africa. Among pregnant and post-partum African women living with HIV, disclosure rates to any person range between 5% and 97% (pooled estimate 67%), and to male partners, 30 to 93% (pooled estimate 64%) [16]. Gender inequities often rooted in socio-cultural factors play a key role in low rates of HIV status disclosure to male partners among women living with HIV [17]. Reasons for male partner non-disclosure among these women include fear of abandonment with the resultant loss of emotional, material and financial support [17–22]; emotional abuse, including name-calling, accusations of infidelity and exposing the family to HIV [19, 20, 22], and sex deprivation [23, 24]. Stigma as well as perceived or enacted discrimination - from male partners and/or the community at large-have also been reported [19, 25]. In extreme cases, women do not disclose for fear of physical violence and other forms of intimate partner violence [17, 19, 26, 27].

As a result of HIV testing in pregnancy, women are often diagnosed before their male partners-regardless of who was infected first-and assume the added burden and responsibility of disclosure [25, 26]. Such gendered asymmetrical disclosure – where only one partner discloses - affects women disproportionately and negatively, as the partner who tests positive first is considered the unfaithful partner and "cause" of the infection, even though the male sexual partner may already be infected [22, 26]. Among HIV-positive women, the first choice of whom to disclose to is often not their male sexual partner(s); rather, where disclosure occurs, it is usually first to a trusted family member who is expected to provide social support [21]. Disclosure to a male partner may occur later or not at all [28, 29]. Despite pre-disclosure fears, many women who disclose report surprisingly positive reactions and support from family and male partners [6, 12, 15, 17, 21, 22, 30, 31]. Nonetheless, negative consequences have also been reported [6, 12, 15, 17, 18, 21, 26, 27].

The reasons for (non)-disclosure and therefore disclosure rates may differ depending on where a woman may be in her PMTCT or HIV treatment journey. Studies in Nigeria have reported HIV disclosure rates from women to male partners between 23.0% and 75.6% in often urban ART clinics [24, 32–34]; and 90.4% among pregnant women [27]. However there is little differentiated data on rates of disclosure among women at different points along the PMTCT cascade, particularly in programmatically challenging rural areas.

Nigeria is an especially important target for scale-up of impactful strategies in maternal and child health and PMTCT. The country has large gaps, especially in rural settings, including low rates of skilled ANC uptake in rural (46.5%) vs urban (86.0%) areas; and facility delivery for only 21.9% of rural, versus 61.7% of urban women [35]. PMTCT gaps include low maternal ART coverage and poor early infant diagnosis uptake of only 30% and 9%, respectively [36]. Studies discussed above highlight the need for evidence to inform robust socio-behavioral interventions targeting key issues like non-disclosure, to augment biomedical PMTCT strategies in Nigeria and similar settings. This study sought to determine the rates, patterns and experiences of disclosure, primarily to male partners, among women at different stages of the PMTCT cascade in rural Nigeria.

Methods

Study design and setting

This cross-sectional, concurrent mixed-methods study was conducted between July and November 2013, and was nested in the MoMent Nigeria PMTCT implementation research project [37]. The study reported here was designed to understand the rates and context of disclosure (or lack thereof) among women living with HIV. The focus on differences along the PMTCT cascade prompted the study to target core PMTCT consumers (women), and not their male partners. The study was conducted in two high HIV-burden states of Nasarawa and the Federal Capital Territory, with 8.1% and 7.5% general population seroprevalence rates, respectively [2]. Both study states are contiguously located in North-Central Nigeria. The study sites comprised 14 primary healthcare centers and two secondary-level facilities located in rural communities participating in the prospective MoMent study [37]. At the time of the study, all sites were implementing World Health Organization (WHO) Option B regimens per national guidelines, including initiation of maternal ART regardless of CD4 count at booking, and infant breastfeeding concurrent with maternal ART [38].

Study participants and recruitment

Eligible women were HIV-positive, ≥ 18 years old, who were receiving or had previously received PMTCT services at the study sites. Participants were recruited in four groups according to their position along the PMTCT cascade at the time of the study:

- Pregnant, newly HIV-diagnosed (within 7 days), not yet on ART *("newly-diagnosed women")*
- Pregnant, on ART, in PMTCT care (*"ANC women"*)
- Post-partum (up to three months), breastfeeding, on ART, in care (*"postpartum women"*)
- Previously in PMTCT care, lost to follow-up (LTFU), not on ART (*"LTFU women"*). LTFU women were defined as those who had not completed a facility visit in three or more consecutive months.

Women who had not been formally enrolled in PMTCT care and did not have medical records at the recruiting study sites were excluded. We targeted a sample size of 100 participants along the PMTCT cascade, based on recruitment capacity estimations derived from enrollments for women living with HIV at the study sites.

Healthcare workers at study sites identified eligible women during routine clinic visits and contacted LTFU women identified from facility service registers by phone. Thereafter, all interested women were approached by study staff for written informed consent. Self-reported HIV status from participants was cross-checked with medical records at each study facility. To ensure that recruitment calls did not put women at risk of confidentiality breaches, all recruitment calls were made by healthcare workers who only provided details about the call if it was answered by the verified potential study participant; otherwise, a cryptic message or excuse was given by the caller. Those who were not reached by phone, especially those LTFU, were tracked with the assistance of Mentor Mothers (women living with HIV serving as peer counselors at study facilities).

Data collection and analyses

A three-section semi-structured interview guide was used to simultaneously collect quantitative and qualitative data. The first section of the guide collected information on participant socio-demographics (including age, religion, marital status and parity). The second section collected disclosure data (including whether patient had disclosed their status, to whom, and in what order), and data on knowledge of male partner HIV status. The third section collected qualitative information that explored each participant's "lived experience" with disclosure as a woman living with HIV. The key question posed to participants was, "Is there anyone who knows you have HIV?" This was followed by other questions to determine the process, and reasons for disclosure or non-disclosure. The guide was pilot-tested among 10 women and then updated and finalized before implementation.

Two trained study staff fluent in English and the dominant Hausa local language conducted each face-to-face interview in either language, using the semi-structured interview guide. While one study staff interviewed, the other observed and took notes. All interviews were audio-taped, and took place in private rooms at study sites or other designated locations by participant request. Each interview lasted 45 min to one hour. Healthcare workers at study sites neither participated in, nor observed the study sessions. Both English and Hausa audio-taped interviews were transcribed (and where relevant, translated) verbatim in English.

Quantitative data analysis

Participants' socio-demographic and disclosure data (including disclosure status and knowledge of male partner HIV status) were first analysed with descriptive statistics. This was followed by tests for associations between the independent categorical variable "PMTCT cascade group," and dependent categorical variables, including "disclosure to male partners/others" and "knowledge of partner HIV status" using Fisher's Exact test. Statistical Package for Social Sciences version 16.0 for Windows was used for analysis, and statistical significance was set at $p \leq 0.05$.

Qualitative data analysis

All interview transcripts and field notes were analysed manually by theme and content using the constant comparative method in a Grounded Theory approach [39]. In this approach, inductive methodology is used to systematically generate theory from the data collected. Qualitative analysis was performed by a panel of eight trained and/or experienced researchers including SE, CI, LR, NASA, and an experienced Social Scientist (LJC). We selected a series of code words-the initial code word being "disclosure"-to develop themes and sub-themes from the qualitative data. This led to an iterative content analysis of the transcripts to examine the overall conceptual issues that emerged.

During this process, each researcher independently used the code list to hand-code assigned transcripts by reviewing and summarizing each line, phrase and paragraph to identify key themes. This was followed by group review, triangulation, and content analysis by iteration until a final consensus on patterns and categorizations was achieved. The research team that facilitated the in-depth interviews was maintained for completing transcription as well as conducting the qualitative analysis. AO additionally independently analyzed the transcripts and coded data based on identified themes from the interview guide, and compared these to themes identified by the paired researchers.

Results

A total of 100 women were recruited in the four targeted PMTCT cascade groups: 25 newly-diagnosed, 26 in ANC, 28 postpartum, and 21 LTFU women (Table 1). Overall, 69% (69/100) study participants were between 21 and 30 years old, and 88.0% (88/100) had at least primary school education. The majority (86%, 86/100) of participants were married. Recruited participants had similar characteristics across all four cascade groups except for marital status: women in the LTFU group were more likely to be single, compared to the other 3 groups (Table 1). We collected data for both quantitative and qualitative analyses from all 100 women.

Table 1 Respondents' socio-demographic characteristics

Characteristic	Newly- diagnosed *N* = 25 n (%)	ANC *N* = 26 n (%)	Postpartum *N* = 28 n (%)	Lost to follow-up *N* = 21 n (%)	*P* value*	Total *N* = 100 n (%)
Age, years						
< 21	4 (16.0)	0 (0.0)	0 (0.0)	3 (13.6)	0.327	7 (7.0)
21–30	18 (72.0)	16 (61.5)	22 (78.6)	13 (59.1)		69 (69.0)
31–40	3 (12.0)	10 (38.5)	6 (21.4)	5 (27.3)		24 (24.0)
Religious affiliation						
Christian	16 (66.7)	18 (69.2)	25 (92.6)	16 (76.2)	1.000	75 (76.5)
Muslim	8 (33.0)	8 (30.8)	2 (7.4)	5 (23.8)		23 (23.5)
No response	1	0	1	0		2
Marital status						
Single[a]	0 (0.0)	3 (11.5)	3 (10.7)	8 (38.1)	0.001	14 (14.0)
Married	25 (100.0)	23 (88.5)	25 (89.3)	13 (61.9)		86 (86.0)
Number of living children						
None	7 (28.0)	7 (27.0)	1 (3.7)	4 (20.0)	0.058	19 (19.5)
1–2	9 (36.0)	13 (50.0)	19 (70.4)	5 (25.0)		46 (46.9)
3–4	7 (28.0)	5 (19.2)	6 (22.2)	8 (40.0)		26 (26.5)
≥ 5	2 (8.0)	1 (3.8)	1 (3.7)	3 (15.0)		7 (7.1)
No response	0	0	1	1		2

Newly-diagnosed: women pregnant and newly HIV-diagnosed within last 7 days
ANC: women pregnant and in antenatal care
Postpartum: Breastfeeding women within 3 months of delivery
Lost-to follow-up: women who had not attended a clinic visit in 3 or more consecutive months
*Fisher's Exact test
[a]Includes single, widowed and divorced women

Table 2 Disclosure by women living with HIV along the PMTCT cascade

Disclosure status	Newly-diagnosed *N* = 25 n (%)	ANC *N* = 26 n (%)	Postpartum *N* = 28 n (%)	Lost to follow-up *N* = 21 n (%)	Total *N* = 100 n (%)	*P* value[a]
Disclosed to anyone						
Yes	14 (56.0)	21 (84.0)	24 (85.7)	21 (100.0)	80 (80.8)	0.001
No	11 (44.0)	4 (16.0)	4 (14.3)	0 (0.0)	19	
No response	0	1	0	0	(19.2) 1	
Disclosed to family[b]	*N* = 14	*N* = 21	*N* = 24	*N* = 21	*N* = 80	
Yes	5 (35.7)	12 (63.2)	12 (52.2)	13 (61.9)	42 (54.5)	0.402
No	9 (64.3)	7 (36.8)	11 (47.8)	8 (38.1)	35	
No response	0	2	1	0	(45.5) 3	
Disclosed to male partner[b]	*N* = 14	*N* = 21	*N* = 24	*N* = 21	*N* = 80	
Yes	13 (92.9)	17 (81.0)	18 (75.0)	20 (95.2)	68 (85.0)	0.218
No	1 (7.1)	4 (19.0)	6 (25.0)	1 (4.8)	12 (15.0)	
No response	0	0	0	0	0	

Newly-diagnosed: women pregnant and newly HIV-diagnosed within last 7 days
ANC: women pregnant and in antenatal care
Postpartum: Breastfeeding women within 3 months of delivery
Lost-to follow-up: women who had not attended a clinic visit in 3 or more consecutive months
[a]Fisher's exact test
[b]Participants responding "No" to "Disclosed to anyone" have been removed from denominator

Results from quantitative data analysis

Rates of HIV status disclosure among participants

Participants were asked about disclosure of their HIV-positive serostatus to male partners or first-order family members (parents and/or siblings). Approximately 81% of participants reported disclosing to anyone; of these, more had disclosed to their male partner than to family members (85.0% vs 54.5%) (Table 2). At 100%, LTFU women had the highest rates of disclosure to anyone. Newly-diagnosed women had the lowest disclosure rates to anyone or family, while postpartum women had the lowest disclosure rates to male partners. Interestingly, while newly-diagnosed women had the lowest disclosure rates to anyone, they had comparable or higher male partner disclosure rates compared to the other cascade groups. Analysis showed significantly different disclosure rates to anyone across the four groups ($p = 0.001$); however there were no significant differences in disclosure rates to family members ($p = 0.402$) or male partners ($p = 0.218$) (Table 2). Similarly, when compared across pregnant (newly-diagnosed + ANC) and non-pregnant (postpartum + LTFU) women, disclosure rates to anyone were lower among pregnant women (56% for newly-diagnosed women and 84% among ANC women), and were significantly different ($p = 0.0007$) compared to non-pregnant women; but not for disclosure to family ($p = 0.653$) or male partners ($p = 1.000$).

Participants' knowledge of male partners' HIV status

Approximately 67% (54/81) of respondents knew their partner's HIV status, while one-third did not (Table 3). There were significant differences in knowledge of male partner's HIV status across the four groups ($p = 0.004$). The newly-diagnosed group had the lowest proportion of women who knew their partner's status, while the LTFU group had the highest. Among 54 women who knew their partner's status, 30 reported he was HIV-negative, indicating an overall serodiscordance rate of 56%.

Results from qualitative data analysis

Figure 1 displays the core themes that emerged from qualitative data analysis.

Effect of fear on disclosure pattern and experience

One consistent theme that emerged in the qualitative analysis was descriptions of worry and stress experienced by participants, either as they considered disclosing, or as a result of disclosure, particularly with respect to male partners. Digging deeper into the data, we found that fear of marital conflict – in the form of intimate partner violence, or divorce – were important factors during the disclosure process across all four groups:: *"I have not even told my husband, because I don't want to lose my marriage. He is a very difficult person"*- Newly-diagnosed woman. *"Of course he will divorce me since the disease is a license to death"*-Newly-diagnosed woman. *"I feared that telling him would cause a fight"*-LTFU woman. *"I am scared of him beating me and divorcing me at the end"*-Postpartum woman. Some women mentioned being afraid, but failed to explain why, even after probing: *"No, I'm just afraid; I do not know how to tell him"*-Postpartum woman. *"I just feel like not telling him... I know I will tell him, but not now...Yes, he needs to know but it is something you take gradually"*-Postpartum woman.

Nearly 20% of study participants had not disclosed to anyone (Table 2), among whom were women who expressed no intention to disclose their status to male partners and/or others, largely due to uncertainty about the nature of ensuing reactions and/or stigma. *"I haven't told anyone because nobody in my family has experienced anything like this and this is a big shock to me, hearing that I have HIV"*-ANC woman. *"If I tell* [anyone], *I do not know what the outcome will be"*-Newly-diagnosed woman. *"Some people believe that HIV is only from promiscuous people"*-ANC woman.

The fear of marital conflict influenced not only whether women disclosed at all, or whom they disclosed to, but also the timing and pattern of disclosure. While

Table 3 Knowledge of Male Partner's HIV status among Women Living with HIV

Partner's HIV Status	Newly-diagnosed N = 25 n (%)	ANC N = 26 n (%)	Postpartum N = 28 n (%)	Lost to follow-up N = 21 n (%)	Total N = 100 n (%)	P value[a]
Positive	4 (19.1)	8 (38.1)	5 (21.7)	7 (43.8)	24 (29.6)	
Negative	2 (9.5)	7 (33.3)	14 (60.9)	7 (43.8)	30 (37.0)	
Unknown	15 (71.4)	6 (28.6)	4 (17.4)	2 (12.4)	27 (33.4)	0.004
No response	4	5	5	5	19	

Newly-diagnosed: women pregnant and newly HIV-diagnosed within last 7 days
ANC: women pregnant and in antenatal care
Postpartum: Breastfeeding women within 3 months of delivery
Lost-to follow-up: women who had not attended a clinic visit in 3 or more consecutive months
[a]Fisher's Exact test

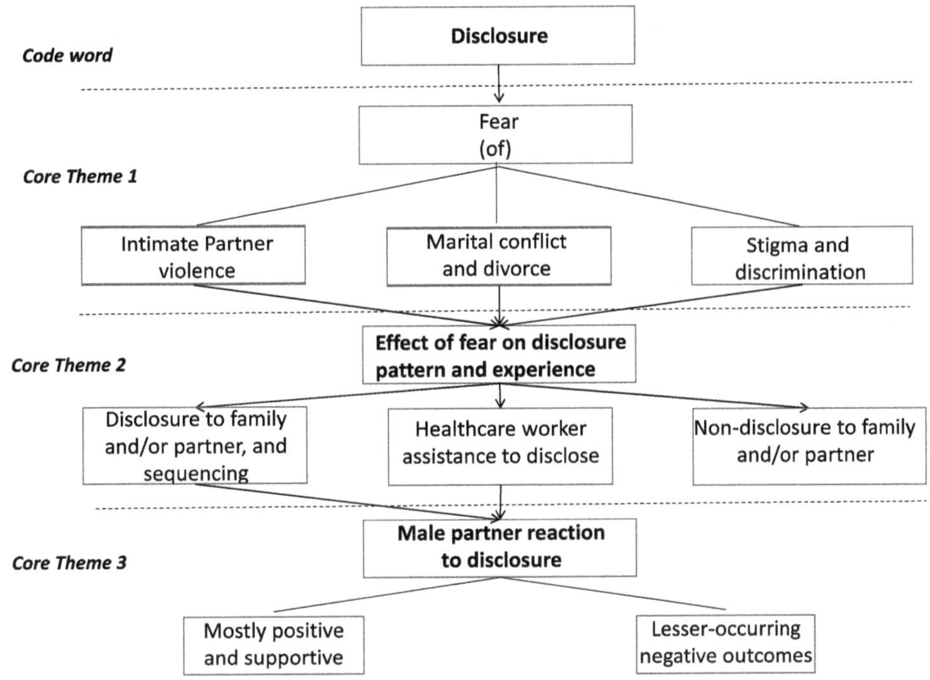

Fig. 1 Core emerging themes from qualitative data analysis

most women who disclosed, disclosed immediately or within days to others, they found it most difficult to disclose to male partners. One respondent stated: "*Only my sister knows. When they told me then I was sad. So I just went straight to her house to tell her...When I told her she was equally sad... I didn't tell him* [husband]"-ANC woman, partner status unknown. "*I called her* [sister] *after I have been told about the diagnosis in the hospital. She later found time to talk with me and encourage me about living with it...*[But] *he* [husband] *is not aware yet*" -Postpartum woman. "*I spoke with her* [friend] *after getting my diagnosis from the hospital. I explained everything to her since I cannot tell my husband. But truly, I am afraid of telling him because it is not something that is easy to disclose*" - Postpartum woman, partner status unknown.

Based on this fear, some women disclosed to only family, and not partners. However, women who first disclosed to male partners were sometimes asked by the latter to refrain from disclosing to anyone else, including family members: "*He begged me not to tell even my family; that we should keep it a secret between the two of us*" -ANC woman, partner HIV-negative. Such partners' requests may be as a result of pride, or fear of stigma "by association," prompting the men to want to protect their families, and their integrity and status in the home and/or community.

Our quantitative analysis showed that nearly half (42%) of newly-diagnosed women had not disclosed to anyone (Table 2), but most stated that they planned to disclose to their male partners: "*I plan to tell my husband very soon.*" "*I will tell him when I reach home.*" Given the immediacy of the HIV-positive diagnosis (seven days or less), there was less data from newly-diagnosed women on disclosure and post-disclosure experiences, especially involving male partners.

Besides fear, some women did not disclose to their male partner due to mistrust, anger and suspicion that he was responsible for their HIV-positive status through infidelity: "[I have not told him] *because I think that he is the one that gave HIV to me, because he doesn't stay at home*"- Postpartum woman. Yet other women withheld their status from partners due to prior refusal to have himself tested. "*I asked him to go and test, but he refused to go*" -Postpartum woman. In these cases, one could postulate that the women were trying to prevent disclosure asymmetry – not wanting to disclose when they did not know their partner's status: "*I didn't tell him immediately, I brought him here for his own test also, so we found out together that we were both positive*" -Postpartum woman. However, reasons for non-disclosure to family were not due to fear, but more to protect family from stress or HIV-related stigma. "*I did not disclose my status to my mother because she is sick and I knew if I told her she would be thinking as if I will die tomorrow*" -ANC woman, partner HIV-negative.

Women who did disclose to male partners did so mainly to maintain honest communication, they did not trust anyone else, and/or wanted to motivate their partner to test for HIV. "*I told him because I cannot live a life of secrecy"* -ANC woman, partner HIV-negative. *"There is no one I can inform about my status except my husband"* -Newly-diagnosed woman. *"I decided to tell him so that he could get tested, so we will know if we are both infected"* -Postpartum woman, partner HIV-negative. *"I told my husband and sister because I encouraged them to go and know their status"* -ANC woman, partner HIV-negative.

The strategic role and influence of healthcare workers in disclosure to male partners

For women who found it especially difficult to disclose to male partners, healthcare workers played a key role in facilitating disclosure and in convincing male partners to test for HIV. "*The day I was told my diagnosis, the nurse asked if she could help me disclose it to my husband, then I said she should go ahead. He was briefed about my HIV diagnosis, and then I spoke to him and asked him to come for the same HIV test too. He didn't refuse it. He was tested too and found out he is HIV-positive"* – Newly-diagnosed woman. *"I didn't tell him, it was the nurses that told him because I told them that if I should disclose it to him, he may not handle the issue well and I may lose my marriage, so they called him and disclosed everything to him"*-Postpartum woman. *"Initially the matron asked me if I would tell him myself and I said yes, but I couldn't do it. She then asked me to tell him to come to clinic. He met with the matron, they discussed my result, he took it in good faith and he was also advised to go for his own test"* -Newly-diagnosed woman.

In some cases, the health care worker was a co-strategist in the disclosure process: "*You know when I came here, the nurses spoke to me and tried to explain that it is important we let our partners know about it. So I told him, when I went for antenatal the previous day, that I saw a woman crying because they told her she had HIV. So he said, 'How would she be crying?' So that now gave me the courage to open up...you don't just say it outright because it is awkward. So I was just looking for a way"* -ANC woman.

Non-disclosure to female partners among HIV-positive male partners

Non-disclosure also seemed to cut both ways, as some participants reported that their male partners were already diagnosed HIV-positive and on treatment but did not disclose to their female partners until prompted by a sentinel event: *"I called him when they told me I was positive. So he came here* [clinic] *and he told us that he is already positive too, and he has been receiving his medication."*-ANC woman. *"He was the first to be diagnosed; he did not tell me. He had tuberculosis, so we went to the hospital where he tested HIV positive. But when we came out of the hospital, instead of him to tell me, he did not. I confronted him and asked him why he did not tell me when he was diagnosed with HIV."* -LTFU woman. In some cases women disclosed to their male partners without asking them to disclose theirs: *"I don't know his status. He didn't disclose it to me, but he knows my status. I wasn't bothered about asking him. I know he did it* [HIV test]*."* -Newly-diagnosed woman. *"I just told him. He told me it is not something we should discuss at that moment. But I don't know his status"*-Newly-diagnosed woman.

Male partner reaction to disclosure

For majority of the women who disclosed to male partners, partner reactions were often more positive and supportive than expected– with the men continuing to provide emotional, material and financial support, despite the initial shock from disclosure. *"I thought he would take it harsh on me. But he has been very caring since I told him that I'm positive and he reminds me when it is time to take my drugs"* -ANC woman, partner HIV-negative. *"From that day* [of disclosure] *he started loving me better. But he asked me not to talk about HIV anymore since we love each other. And he still supports me"* -Postpartum woman, partner HIV-negative. "*When I went home with the news that day, I was so disturbed. So he noticed and tried to find out what was wrong with me. I couldn't really pronounce it... He perceived that something was wrong, and he knew that I went to the hospital for some tests. So he asked if I was confirmed positive, and I said yes. He told me not to feel anxious about it, not to cry and that I should go and take the drugs." ANC woman, partner HIV-negative.*

Very few women who disclosed to male partners reported experiencing the negative consequences feared by many women in the first place, including neglect and separation that could potentially impact on PMTCT outcomes: *"I was sick so he brought me to the clinic. That's how he knew my status. So as we were going home he told me he could not live with me anymore. He then sent me away to my father's house. I was there for four months. He came back six days after I delivered...He refused to give me money for transport to come for my drugs here [clinic]... That's why I was not taking the drugs"* -LTFU woman, partner HIV-negative. "*Since I disclosed to him, he only gives me some money for food and even if I ask him for any other thing, he won't listen. Before now, he wasn't behaving like this"* -LTFU woman, partner's status unknown.

Discussion

Among our study population of women living with HIV in rural North-Central Nigeria, we found overall disclosure rates to anyone to be relatively high, at 81%. Male partner disclosure reported by our study participants was also relatively high at 85%, compared to 23.0%, 86.5% and 90.4% reported in previous studies among women in South-West Nigeria [9, 24, 27]. Across similar African settings, male partner disclosure rates among HIV-positive women ranged between 44% in Kenya to 93% in Zimbabwe [7, 40]. Similar to our findings, a larger proportion of African women living with HIV ultimately disclose to their male partners than to others [7, 15, 21, 41], although our findings suggest, similar to other studies [21], that family members were often the first to be disclosed to.

Fear of divorce, interpersonal/domestic violence, neglect or other forms of psychological abuse deterred women from immediately disclosing to their male partners. However, with time and encouragement, especially from healthcare workers, women in our study population disclosed with surprisingly, largely positive results, as reported elsewhere in Africa [18, 22], even in situations where male partners were reportedly HIV-negative. Among our study cohort, reasons for male partner disclosure included feelings of obligation and to encourage partner HIV testing, as reported from studies in other African countries [15, 28]. For some women, disclosure to anyone occurred on the same day or shortly after diagnosis, as reported in other Nigerian [42] and African studies [18, 29]. Similar to findings in other studies [6, 21, 43], women who did not disclose a positive HIV status to family members were seeking to protect them.

In our study, newly-diagnosed women had significantly lower disclosure rates to anyone or family, compared to women in the other cascade groups who had previously established care ($p = 0.001$). Newly-diagnosed women also had the lowest rate of knowledge of partner serostatus ($p = 0.004$). This is understandable considering that these women were newly-diagnosed and may not have had enough time to process and share their diagnosis with anyone, or seek to know partner's HIV status. This finding is similar to disclosure data for the ART cascade that shows that newly-diagnosed patients had significantly lower disclosure rates than those in established care [5]. Postpartum and breastfeeding women in care, on the other hand, had the lowest disclosure rates to male partners. The reason for this is not clear from our study. However, Brou et al. [12] suggest that breastfeeding status correlates with partner disclosure by HIV-positive women; with women who choose exclusive formula feeding disclosing at a higher rate than those who choose to breastfeed. We were not able to explore disclosure rates in the context of infant feeding practices, as our study objectives did not include in-depth evaluation of infant feeding practices across all four cascade groups.

Pregnant women (newly diagnosed + ANC) had significantly lower disclosure to anyone than non-pregnant women (postpartum + LTFU) ($p = 0.0007$). Again, one likely explanation could be that non-pregnant women may have known their status for a longer duration. However, we were not able to accurately establish when previously-diagnosed women were diagnosed, as many women in our small rural community study setting did not enrol at the facility where they were first HIV-diagnosed: They often presented at multiple other facilities as "testing-naive" patients. Additionally, when asked, they were often unsure of the exact day or month of testing. This phenomenon was noted in the MoMent prospective study as well [44]. We are therefore limited in explaining if, or how time of HIV testing, and infant feeding practice influenced disclosure across the PMTCT cascade. Further research is needed on these aspects. There were no observed differences across the cascade groups with respect to male partner or family disclosure. However, our small sample size may have precluded the discovery of potential differences in our quantitative results.

Addressing the lack of, or delayed disclosure among couples is important for our study population and the larger HIV community in our study setting because of the relatively high reported HIV serodiscordance rate of nearly 56%, and unknown partner HIV status of 33%. Among our cascade groups, newly-diagnosed and ANC women were less likely to know their partner's status, compared to postpartum and LTFU women, and this difference was statistically significant. Previous Nigerian studies reported a similar serodiscordance rate for North-Central Nigeria of 51.9% [23] and lower rate of 38.5% for South-East Nigeria [45]. Proportions of HIV-positive women with unknown male partner status of 62.4% and 85% have been reported from studies in North-Central and South-East Nigeria, respectively [24, 45], which are much higher than for our study. Studies in similar sub-Saharan African settings have reported serodiscordance rates between 22.9% and 39% [15, 46, 47], and unknown male partner status between 32.7% and 80% among women living with HIV [11, 15, 48, 49]. Since we could not establish time of HIV diagnosis for our cascade groups, it is not possible to determine how and if this played a role in the observed differences in serodiscordance, and knowledge of partner status. For serodiscordant couples, early partner testing, notification and treatment can avert seroconversion in the HIV-negative partner [23].

Similar to previous findings [15, 43] our study highlights that healthcare workers play key motivating and supporting roles in disclosure among women living with HIV, especially to male partners, and actively facilitate partner HIV testing. Pre-existing and longstanding gender inequities in our study communities and similar settings have necessitated women needing more support (including to overcome fear) in order to disclose HIV-positive status to male partners. Intimate partner violence, inequitable laws and harmful traditional practices, including limited decision-making for women, reinforce unequal power dynamics between men and women [50]. Healthcare workers can, and have mediated these power dynamics by increasing their involvement in disclosure, especially by women to male partners. By supporting couples counselling and education on testing and treatment, healthcare workers play a crucial authoritative role in minimizing negative partner reactions for women who have accepted testing and tested positive. This is especially important, as studies show that men living with HIV whose wives know their seropositive status are often less likely to be violent or react negatively to news of female partner's seropositivity; thus, stressing the need for mutual HIV testing and disclosure [20, 26]. Couple testing and disclosure will also lessen the burden on the partner, which in the PMTCT context is the woman, who would otherwise test first and/or positive [51, 52].

As much as healthcare workers in our study setting assisted in disclosure, they and mentor mothers could only provide counselling and psychosocial support: they were not trained to provide professional mental health services. As such, professional mental services were not available to our study participants, especially newly-diagnosed women. Mental health services, if available, are often very expensive and located at large and/or tertiary centers located in urban areas at great traveling distance from rural communities. Thus, the study team could not refer participants for these services. Furthermore, such mental health referrals are not included in routine PMTCT care at the study facilities.

While no respondent in our study reported experiencing physical violence from their male partner as a result of disclosure, fear of such intimate partner violence as well as emotional/financial neglect and divorce/separation were expressed by women across cascade groups as reasons for non-disclosure. Therefore, prevention and management of marital conflict and intimate partner violence in the context of HIV disclosure remain important issues to address in PMTCT programming.

Surprisingly, male partner disclosure rates were no different among LTFU women compared to other cascade groups in our study. This is contrary to previous findings where nondisclosure has been reported as a correlate of PMTCT cascade dropout among women living with HIV [14] [53]; however, the disclosure evaluated in these studies were to anyone and not specifically disaggregated for disclosure to male partners or other individuals. Larger, and more robust studies are needed to examine the relationship between male partner-specific disclosure rates among women in and out of care along the PMTCT cascade.

Study limitations

This study was conducted in rural Nigeria with a purposive sample, therefore study findings may not be generalizable to all HIV-positive women in the study communities, nor to urban settings in Nigeria or elsewhere. There was also significant missing data for knowledge of male partner status: 19 of 100 women did not respond to this question. Analysis was therefore based on the remaining 81 who did. Furthermore, as explained earlier, we were unable to collect reliable data for all study participants on specific initial date of HIV diagnosis. Thus, we could not evaluate if timing of diagnosis was a correlate of overall disclosure rates, and rates between cascade groups. Socio-economic status and male partner socio-demographic data could also not be evaluated vis-à-vis disclosure rates, since we did not collect these data. Disclosure and male partner HIV-status was as reported by participants; it was not possible to verify this information and as such may not reflect reality. Lastly, limitations in cascade-based recruitment (especially for the two post-partum groups) in our rural study settings resulted in a relatively small sample size for each cascade group; this limited robust statistical comparisons between and within groups.

Conclusions

With support from healthcare workers and irrespective of cascade status, male partner disclosure was ultimately achieved with largely positive results for the majority of women in our study. Thus, strategies to increase healthcare worker skills and active involvement are likely to yield high rates of successful male partner disclosure in rural communities - a strategy that is especially important where there are high rates of serodiscordance. Concurrent strategies to enable healthcare workers make successful contact with male partners, either at the facility or in the community, will also be needed to facilitate the disclosure process for women at any stage of the PMTCT cascade. Comprehensive healthcare worker-supported interventions that target male partner disclosure in particular and context-specific women's empowerment in general are important to maximize outcomes in communities with high HIV burdens and low PMTCT performance. Lastly, while mental health and gender-based violence programs are limited in Nigeria and similar settings, the need is well-demonstrated [50], and it is important to establish these services in conjunction with PMTCT program scale-up.

Abbreviations

ANC: Antenatal care; ART: Antiretroviral therapy; HIV: Human immunodeficiency virus; LTFU: Lost to follow-up; PMTCT: Prevention of mother-to-child transmission of HIV

Acknowledgements

The authors would like to thank all the women who volunteered to participate in this study and shared their experiences. We also appreciate the efforts of research staff who assisted with data collection and transcription. Lastly, we thank the funders: World Health Organization, Global Affairs Canada, and the Fogarty AIDS International Training and Research Program for providing financial support for this study.

Funding
The MoMent Nigeria study was funded by the World Health Organization through an award for the Integrating and Scaling up PMTCT through Implementation Research (INSPIRE) initiative from Global Affairs Canada. Additional funding was provided by Fogarty AIDS International Training and Research Program grant number 5D43TW001041.

Authors' contributions
AO performed quantitative and qualitative analysis, drafted the manuscript and conducted final review. SE collected data, performed quantitative and qualitative analysis and contributed to manuscript development and final review. LJC designed the study, performed qualitative analysis and contributed to manuscript development and final review. CI performed quantitative and qualitative analysis and contributed to manuscript development and final review. HOR performed quantitative analysis and contributed to manuscript development and final review. LR collected data, performed qualitative analysis and contributed to manuscript development and final review. NASA conceptualized and designed the study, performed qualitative analysis and contributed to manuscript development and final review as well as provided overall supervision for the study. All authors read and approved the final manuscript.

Consent for publication
Not applicable.

Competing interests
The authors declare that they have no competing interests.

Author details
[1]Abuja, Nigeria. [2]International Research Center of Excellence, Institute of Human Virology Nigeria, Abuja, Nigeria. [3]School of Social Work and College of Public Health, University of Georgia Athens, Athens, USA. [4]Institute of Human Virology, University of Maryland School of Medicine, Baltimore, USA. [5]Harvard T. H. Chan School of Public Health, Boston, USA.

References

1. UNAIDS. UNAIDS Data 2017. Geneva: Joint United Nations Programme on HIV/AIDS; 2017.
2. CHAI Nigeria. SMS printer program report. 2012.
3. WHO. Programmatic Update. Antiretroviral treatment as prevention (TASP) of HIV and TB. Geneva: World Health Organisation; 2012.
4. Hodgson I, Plummer ML, Konopka SN, Colvin CJ, Jonas E, Albertini J, et al. A systematic review of individual and contextual factors affecting ART initiation, adherence, and retention for HIV-infected pregnant and postpartum women. PLoS One. 2014;9(11):e111421.
5. Ostermann J, Pence B, Whetten K, Yao J, Itemba D, Maro V, et al. HIV serostatus disclosure in the treatment cascade: evidence from northern Tanzania. AIDS Care. 2015;27(Suppl 1):59–64.
6. Winchester MS, McGrath JW, Kaawa-Mafigiri D, Namutiibwa F, Ssendegye G, Nalwoga A, et al. Early HIV disclosure and nondisclosure among men and women on antiretroviral treatment in Uganda. AIDS Care. 2013;25(10):1253–8.
7. Spangler SA, Onono M, Bukusi EA, Cohen CR, Turan JM. HIV-positive status disclosure and use of essential PMTCT and maternal health services in rural Kenya. J Acquir Immune Defic Syndr. 2014;67(Suppl 4):S235–42.
8. Falang KD, Akubaka P, Jimam NS. Patient factors impacting antiretroviral drug adherence in a Nigerian tertiary hospital. J Pharmacol Pharmacother. 2012;3(2):138–42.
9. Ekama SO, Herbertson EC, Addeh EJ, Gab-Okafor CV, Onwujekwe DI, Tayo F, et al. Pattern and determinants of antiretroviral drug adherence among Nigerian pregnant women. J Pregnancy. 2012;2012:851810.
10. Charurat M, Oyegunle M, Benjamin R, Habib A, Eze E, Ele P, et al. Patient retention and adherence to antiretrovirals in a large antiretroviral therapy program in Nigeria: a longitudinal analysis for risk factors. PLoS One. 2010; 5(5):e10584.
11. Peltzer K, Jones D, Weiss SM, Villar-Loubet O, Shikwane E. Sexual risk, serostatus and intimate partner violence among couples during pregnancy in rural South Africa. AIDS Behav. 2013;17(2):508–16.
12. Brou H, Djohan G, Becquet R, Allou G, Ekouevi DK, Viho I, et al. When do HIV-infected women disclose their HIV status to their male partner and why? A study in a PMTCT programme, Abidjan. PLoS Med. 2007;4(12):e342.
13. Stringer EM, Chi BH, Chintu N, Creek TL, Ekouevi DK, Coetzee D, et al. Monitoring effectiveness of programmes to prevent mother-to-child HIV transmission in lower-income countries. Bull World Health Organ. 2008;86(1):57–62.
14. Woldesenbet S, Jackson D, Lombard C, Dinh TH, Puren A, Sherman G, et al. Missed opportunities along the prevention of mother-to-child transmission services Cascade in South Africa: uptake, determinants, and attributable risk (the SAPMTCTE). PLoS One. 2015;10(7):e0132425.
15. Sendo EG, Cherie A, Erku TA. Disclosure experience to partner and its effect on intention to utilize prevention of mother to child transmission service among HIV positive pregnant women attending antenatal care in Addis Ababa, Ethiopia. BMC Public Health. 2013;13:765.
16. Tam M, Amzel A, Phelps BR. Disclosure of HIV serostatus among pregnant and postpartum women in sub-Saharan Africa: a systematic review. AIDS Care. 2015;27(4):436–50.
17. Medley A, Garcia-Moreno C, McGill S, Maman S. Rates, barriers and outcomes of HIV serostatus disclosure among women in developing countries: implications for prevention of mother-to-child transmission programmes. Bull World Health Organ. 2004;82(4):299–307.
18. Kiula ES, Damian DJ, Msuya SE. Predictors of HIV serostatus disclosure to partners among HIV-positive pregnant women in Morogoro, Tanzania. BMC Public Health. 2013;13:433.
19. Alemayehu M, Aregay A, Kalayu A, Yebyo H. HIV disclosure to sexual partner and associated factors among women attending ART clinic at Mekelle hospital, northern Ethiopia. BMC Public Health. 2014;14:746.
20. Colombini M, James C, Ndwiga C, Mayhew SH. The risks of partner violence following HIV status disclosure, and health service responses: narratives of women attending reproductive health services in Kenya. J Int AIDS Soc. 2016;19(1):20766.
21. Visser MJ, Neufeld S, de Villiers A, Makin JD, Forsyth BW. To tell or not to tell: south African women's disclosure of HIV status during pregnancy. AIDS Care. 2008;20(9):1138–45.
22. Rujumba J, Neema S, Byamugisha R, Tylleskar T, Tumwine JK, Heggenhougen HK. "Telling my husband I have HIV is too heavy to come out of my mouth": pregnant women's disclosure experiences and support needs following antenatal HIV testing in eastern Uganda. J Int AIDS Soc. 2012;15(2):17429.
23. Onovo AA, Nta IE, Onah AA, Okolo CA, Aliyu A, Dakum P, et al. Partner HIV serostatus disclosure and determinants of serodiscordance among prevention of mother to child transmission clients in Nigeria. BMC Public Health. 2015;15:827.
24. Adekanle DA, Olowookere SA, Adewole AD, Adeleke NA, Abioye-Kuteyi EA, Ijadunola MY. Sexual experiences of married HIV positive women in Osogbo, southwest Nigeria: role of inappropriate status disclosure. BMC Womens Health. 2015;15:6.
25. Crankshaw TL, Voce A, King RL, Giddy J, Sheon NM, Butler LM. Double disclosure bind: complexities of communicating an HIV diagnosis in the context of unintended pregnancy in Durban, South Africa. AIDS Behav. 2014;18(Suppl 1):S53–9.
26. Mulrenan C, Colombini M, Howard N, Kikuvi J, Mayhew SH. Exploring risk of experiencing intimate partner violence after HIV infection: a qualitative study among women with HIV attending postnatal services in Swaziland. BMJ Open. 2015;5(5):e006907.
27. Ezechi OC, Gab-Okafor C, Onwujekwe DI, Adu RA, Amadi E, Herbertson E. Intimate partner violence and correlates in pregnant HIV positive Nigerians. Arch Gynecol Obstet. 2009;280(5):745–52.
28. Maman S, van Rooyen H, Groves AK. HIV status disclosure to families for social support in South Africa (NIMH project accept/HPTN 043). AIDS Care. 2014;26(2):226–32.
29. Abdool Karim Q, Dellar RC, Bearnot B, Werner L, Frohlich JA, Kharsany AB, et al. HIV-positive status disclosure in patients in care in rural South Africa: implications for scaling up treatment and prevention interventions. AIDS Behav. 2015;19(2):322–9.

30. Ogoina D, Ikuabe P, Ebuenyi I, Harry T, Inatimi O, Chukwueke O. Types and predictors of partner reactions to HIV status disclosure among HIV-infected adult Nigerians in a tertiary hospital in the Niger Delta. Afr Health Sci. 2015; 15(1):10–8.
31. Atuyambe LM, Ssegujja E, Ssali S, Tumwine C, Nekesa N, Nannungi A, et al. HIV/AIDS status disclosure increases support, behavioural change and, HIV prevention in the long term: a case for an Urban Clinic, Kampala, Uganda. BMC Health Serv Res. 2014;14:276.
32. Titilope AA, Adediran A, Umeh C, Akinbami A, Unigwe O, Akanmu AS. Psychosocial Impact Psychosocial Impact Of disclosure of HIV Serostatus in heterosexual relationship at the Lagos University teaching hospital, Nigeria. Nigerian Med J. 2011;52(1):55–9.
33. Ebuenyi ID, Ogoina D, Ikuabe PO, Harry TC, Inatimi O, Chukwueke OU. Prevalence Pattern and Determinants of disclosure of HIV status in an anti retroviral therapy Clinic in the Niger Delta Region of Nigeria. African J Infect Dis. 2014;8(2):27–30.
34. Adebayo AM, Ilesanmi OS, Omotoso BA, Ayodeji OO, Kareem AO, Alele FO. Disclosure To sexual partner and condom use among HIV positive clients attending ART clinic at a tertiary health facility in south West Nigeria. Pan Afric Med J. 2014;18:245.
35. International NaI. Nigeria Demographic and Health Survey 2013. Abuja, Nigeria, and Rockville, Maryland: National Population Commission (NPC) [Nigeria] and ICF International; 2014.
36. UNAIDS. On the fast track to an AIDS-free generation: the incredible journey of the global plan towards the elimination of new HIV infections among children by 2015 and keeping their mothers alive joint. Geneva: United Nations Programme on HIV/AIDS; 2016.
37. Sam-Agudu NA, Cornelius LJ, Okundaye JN, Adeyemi OA, Isah HO, Wiwa OM, et al. The impact of mentor mother programs on PMTCT service uptake and retention-in-Care at Primary Health Care Facilities in Nigeria: a prospective cohort study (MoMent Nigeria). J Acquir Immune Defic Syndr. 2014;67(Suppl 2):S132–8.
38. Federal Ministry of Health Nigeria. National Guidelines for Prevention of Mother-to-Child Transmission of HIV. Abuja: Federal Ministry of Health Nigeria; 2010.
39. Glaser BG, & Strauss, Anselm L.. The discovery of grounded theory: Strategies for qualitative research: Transaction Publishers; 2009.
40. Shamu S, Zarowsky C, Shefer T, Temmerman M, Abrahams N. Intimate partner violence after disclosure of HIV test results among pregnant women in Harare, Zimbabwe. PLoS One. 2014;9(10):e109447.
41. Patel R, Ratner J, Gore-Felton C, Kadzirange G, Woelk G, Katzenstein D. HIV disclosure patterns, predictors, and psychosocial correlates among HIV positive women in Zimbabwe. AIDS Care. 2012;24(3):358–68.
42. Amoran OE. Predictors of disclosure of sero-status to sexual partners among people living with HIV/AIDS in Ogun state, Nigeria. Niger J Clin Pract. 2012; 15(4):385–90.
43. Madiba S, Letsoalo R. HIV Disclosure to partners and family among women enrolled in prevention of mother to child transmission of HIV program: implications for infant feeding in poor resourced communities in South Africa. Glob J Health Sci. 2013;5(4):1–13.
44. Sam-Agudu NA, Ramadhani HO, Isah C, Anaba U, Erekaha S, Fan-Osuala C, et al. The impact of structured mentor mother programs on 6-month postpartum retention and viral suppression among HIV-positive women in rural Nigeria: a prospective paired cohort study. J Acquir Immune Defic Syndr. 2017;75(Suppl 2):S173–S81.
45. Lawani LO, Onyebuchi AK, Iyoke CA. Dual Method use for protection of pregnancy and disease prevention among HIV-infected women in south East Nigeria. BMC Womens Health. 2014;14(1):39.
46. Feyissa TR, Melka AS. Demand for modern family planning among married women living with HIV in western Ethiopia. PLoS One. 2014;9(11):e113008.
47. Kaida A, Matthews LT, Kanters S, Kabakyenga J, Muzoora C, Mocello AR, et al. Incidence and predictors of pregnancy among a cohort of HIV-positive women initiating antiretroviral therapy in Mbarara, Uganda. PLoS One. 2013;8(5):e63411.
48. Matthews LT, Smit JA, Moore L, Milford C, Greener R, Mosery FN, et al. Periconception HIV risk behavior among men and women reporting HIV-Serodiscordant partners in KwaZulu-Natal, South Africa. AIDS Behav. 2015;19(12):2291–303.
49. Matthews LT, Moore L, Crankshaw TL, Milford C, Mosery FN, Greener R, et al. South Africans with recent pregnancy rarely know partner's HIV serostatus: implications for serodiscordant couples interventions. BMC Public Health. 2014;14:843.
50. AVERT. Gender Inequality and HIV. 2017. https://www.avert.org/professionals/social-issues/gender-inequality. Accessed 27 Jan 2018.
51. Ateka GK. HIV status disclosure and partner discordance: a public health dilemma. Public Health. 2006;120(6):493–6.
52. Roxby AC, Matemo D, Drake AL, Kinuthia J, John-Stewart GC, Ongecha-Owuor F, et al. Pregnant women and disclosure to sexual partners after testing HIV-1-seropositive during antenatal care. AIDS Patient Care STDs. 2013;27(1):33–7.
53. Watson-Jones D, Balira R, Ross DA, Weiss HA, Mabey D. Missed opportunities: poor linkage into ongoing care for HIV-positive pregnant women in Mwanza, Tanzania. PLoS One. 2012;7(7):e40091.

Permissions

All chapters in this book were first published in RH, by BioMed Central; hereby published with permission under the Creative Commons Attribution License or equivalent. Every chapter published in this book has been scrutinized by our experts. Their significance has been extensively debated. The topics covered herein carry significant findings which will fuel the growth of the discipline. They may even be implemented as practical applications or may be referred to as a beginning point for another development.

The contributors of this book come from diverse backgrounds, making this book a truly international effort. This book will bring forth new frontiers with its revolutionizing research information and detailed analysis of the nascent developments around the world.

We would like to thank all the contributing authors for lending their expertise to make the book truly unique. They have played a crucial role in the development of this book. Without their invaluable contributions this book wouldn't have been possible. They have made vital efforts to compile up to date information on the varied aspects of this subject to make this book a valuable addition to the collection of many professionals and students.

This book was conceptualized with the vision of imparting up-to-date information and advanced data in this field. To ensure the same, a matchless editorial board was set up. Every individual on the board went through rigorous rounds of assessment to prove their worth. After which they invested a large part of their time researching and compiling the most relevant data for our readers.

The editorial board has been involved in producing this book since its inception. They have spent rigorous hours researching and exploring the diverse topics which have resulted in the successful publishing of this book. They have passed on their knowledge of decades through this book. To expedite this challenging task, the publisher supported the team at every step. A small team of assistant editors was also appointed to further simplify the editing procedure and attain best results for the readers.

Apart from the editorial board, the designing team has also invested a significant amount of their time in understanding the subject and creating the most relevant covers. They scrutinized every image to scout for the most suitable representation of the subject and create an appropriate cover for the book.

The publishing team has been an ardent support to the editorial, designing and production team. Their endless efforts to recruit the best for this project, has resulted in the accomplishment of this book. They are a veteran in the field of academics and their pool of knowledge is as vast as their experience in printing. Their expertise and guidance has proved useful at every step. Their uncompromising quality standards have made this book an exceptional effort. Their encouragement from time to time has been an inspiration for everyone.

The publisher and the editorial board hope that this book will prove to be a valuable piece of knowledge for researchers, students, practitioners and scholars across the globe.

List of Contributors

Khalid Yassin
Faculty of Medicine, Alnelain University, Khartoum, Sudan

Hadeel A. Idris
Federal Ministry of Health, Khartoum, Sudan

AbdelAziem A. Ali
Faculty of Medicine, Alnelain University, Khartoum, Sudan
Department of Obstetrics and Gynecology, Faculty of Medicine, Kassala University, Kassala, Sudan

Tina Khanna, Murari Chandra, Ajay Singh and Sunil Mehra
MAMTA Health Institute for Mother and Child, B-5, Greater Kailash Enclave-II New Delhi 110048, India

Wakgari Binu
Department of Midwifery, Arba Minch College of Health Sciences, Arba
Minch, Ethiopia

Taklu Marama
Department of Midwifery, College of Health Sciences and Medicine, Wolaita Sodo University, Wolaita Sodo, Ethiopia

Mulusew Gerbaba and Melese Sinaga
Department of Population and Family Health, College of public Health and Medical Sciences, Jimma University, Jimma, Ethiopia

Heba H. Hijazi and Mohammad S. Alyahya
Department of Health Management and Policy, Faculty of Medicine, Jordan University of Science and Technology, Irbid 22110, Jordan

Amer M. Sindiani
Department of Obstetrics and Gynecology, Faculty of Medicine, Jordan University of Science and Technology, Irbid 22110, Jordan

Rola S. Saqan
Department of Pediatrics and Neonatology, Faculty of Medicine, Jordan University of Science and Technology, Irbid 22110, Jordan

Abdulhakeem M. Okour
Department of Public Health and Community Medicine, Faculty of Medicine, Jordan University of Science and Technology, Irbid 22110, Jordan

Julius Ntwenya and Stephen Kibusi
Department of Public Health, College of Health Sciences, The University of Dodoma, Dodoma, Tanzania

Deogratius Bintabara
Department of Public Health, College of Health Sciences, The University of Dodoma, Dodoma, Tanzania
Department of Global Health Entrepreneurship, Division of Public Health, Graduate School of Tokyo Medical and Dental University, 1-5-45 Yushima, Bunkyo-ku, Tokyo 113-8519, Japan

Isaac I. Maro
Department of Global Health Entrepreneurship, Division of Public Health, Graduate School of Tokyo Medical and Dental University, 1-5-45 Yushima, Bunkyo-ku, Tokyo 113-8519, Japan

Daniel W. Gunda
Department of Internal Medicine, Catholic University of Health and Allied Sciences, Mwanza, Tanzania

Bonaventura C. T. Mpondo
Department of Internal Medicine, College of Health Sciences, The University of Dodoma, Dodoma, Tanzania

Kärt Allvee
Estonian Medical Birth Registry, National Institute for Health Development, Hiiu 42, 11619 Tallinn, Estonia

Mati Rahu and Kaja Rahu
Department of Epidemiology and Biostatistics, National Institute for Health Development, Hiiu 42, 11619 Tallinn, Estonia

Kai Haldre
Centre for Reproductive Medicine, West Tallinn Central Hospital Women's Clinic, Sõle 23, 10614 Tallinn, Estonia

Helle Karro
Department of Obstetrics and Gynecology, Institute of Clinical Medicine, University of Tartu, L. Puusepa 8, 51014 Tartu, Estonia
Tartu University Hospital's Women's Clinic, L. Puusepa 8, 51014 Tartu, Estonia

Hong Yu
School of Journalism and Information Communication, Huazhong University of Science and Technology, 1037 Luoyu, Road, Wuhan 430074, People's Republic of China

Precious Madula
School of Journalism and Information Communication, Huazhong University of Science and Technology, 1037 Luoyu, Road, Wuhan 430074, People's Republic of China
Mzuzu University, Private Bag 201, Luwinga, Mzuzu 2, Malawi

Fatch Welcome Kalembo and Atipatsa Chiwanda Kaminga
Mzuzu University, Luwinga, Mzuzu 2, Malawi

Gily Coene
Centre of Expertise on Gender, Diversity and Intersectionality (RHEA), Vrije Universiteit Brussel, Pleinlaan 2, 1050 Elsene, Belgium

Susan Dierickx and Ladan Rahbari
Centre of Expertise on Gender, Diversity and Intersectionality (RHEA), Vrije Universiteit Brussel, Pleinlaan 2, 1050 Elsene, Belgium
Centre for Research on Culture and Gender, Ghent University, Rozier 44, 9000 Ghent, Belgium

Chia Longman
Centre for Research on Culture and Gender, Ghent University, Rozier 44, 9000 Ghent, Belgium

Fatou Jaiteh
Medical Anthropology Unit, Department of Public Health, Institute of Tropical Medicine, Nationalestraat 155, 2000 Antwerp, Belgium
Amsterdam Institute of Social Science Research, Nieuwe Achtergracht 166, 1018 Amsterdam, The Netherlands
Medical Research Council Unit The Gambia at the London School of Hygiene and Tropical Medicine, Fajara, The Gambia

Isabella Epiu
NIH Fogarty Global Health Fellow, University of California Global Health Institute, San Francisco, CA, USA
Health Solutions International, Kampala, Uganda

Josaphat Byamugisha
Makerere University, Kampala, Uganda

Andrew Kwikiriza
Mbarara University, Mbarara, Uganda

Meg Amy Autry
University of California San Francisco, CA, USA

Chancy S. Chimatiro
Department of Health Systems and Policy, School of Public Health and Family Medicine, College of Medicine, University of Malawi, Blantyre, Malawi
Africa Center of Excellence in Public Health and Herbal Medicine(ACEPHEM), University of Malawi, College of Medicine, Blantyre, Malawi

Precious Hajison
PreLuHa consult, Namiwawa Street, Newroard location, Zomba, Malawi

Effie Chipeta
Department of Public Health, School of Public Health and Family Medicine, College of Medicine, University of Malawi, Blantyre, Malawi
Centre for Reproductive Health (CRH), University of Malawi, College of Medicine, Blantyre, Malawi

Adamson S. Muula
Department of Public Health, School of Public Health and Family Medicine, College of Medicine, University of Malawi, Blantyre, Malawi
Centre for Reproductive Health (CRH), University of Malawi, College of Medicine, Blantyre, Malawi
Africa Center of Excellence in Public Health and Herbal Medicine(ACEPHEM), University of Malawi, College of Medicine, Blantyre, Malawi

Tesfaye Yitna Chichiabellu
Department of Nursing, College of Health Science and Medicine, Wolaita Sodo University, Wolaita Sodo, Ethiopia

Baze Mekonnen
Department of Nursing, School of nursing and midwifery, Addis Ababa University, Addis Ababa, Ethiopia

Feleke Hailemichael Astawesegn
School of Public Health, College of Medicine and Health Science, Hawassa University, Hawassa, Ethiopia

Birhanu Wondimeneh Demissie
Department of Nursing, College of Health Science and Medicine, Wolaita Sodo University, Sodo, Ethiopia

Antehun Alemayehu Anjulo
Department of Medical Laboratory, College of Health Science and Medicine, Wolaita Sodo University, Sodo, Ethiopia

Mirjam P. Fransen, Miriam E. Hopman and Laxsini Murugesu
Amsterdam UMC, University of Amsterdam, Department of Public Health, Public Health Research Institute, Meibergdreef 9, Amsterdam, The Netherlands

Ageeth N. Rosman
Rotterdam University of Applied Sciences, School for Healthcare Studies, Department of Master Physician Assistant Midwifery, Rochussenstraat 198, 3015, EK, Rotterdam, The Netherlands

Sian K. Smith
The University of New South Wales, Psychosocial Research Group, Prince of Wales Clinical School, Faculty of Medicine, Lowy Research Centre, Sydney, NSW 2052, Australia

Berhan Tsegaye and Andargachew Kassa
Department of Midwifery, College of Medicine and Health Sciences, Hawassa University, Hawassa, Ethiopia

Jackline Oluoch-Aridi
Regional Research Programs Manager, The Ford Program in Human Development Studies and Solidarity, University of Notre Dame, Regional Office, East Africa, Nairobi, Kenya

Vania Smith-Oka
Department of Anthropology, University of Notre Dame, 248 Corbett Family Hall, Notre Dame, IN 46556, USA

Ellyn Milan
Eck Institute for Global Health, University of Notre Dame, 120 Brownson Hall, Notre Dame, IN 46556, USA

Robert Dowd
The Ford Program in Human Development Studies and Solidarity, Kellogg Institute of International Affairs, University of Notre Dame, 2167 Nanovic-Jenkins Hall, Notre Dame, IN 46556, USA

Yibeltal Alemu and Amanu Aragaw
Department of Reproductive Health, College of Medicine and Health Science, Bahir Dar University, Bahir Dar, Ethiopia

Griffins O. Manguro
Kenyatta National Hospital, Mombasa 80103, Kenya

Linnet N. Masese
Department of Epidemiology, University of Washington, Seattle, WA, 98195, USA

Kishor Mandaliya
Pathcare Laboratories, Mombasa, Kenya

Susan M. Graham and R. Scott McClelland
Departments of Epidemiology, Global Health, and Medicine, University of Washington, Seattle, WA, USA
Institute of Tropical and Infectious Diseases, University of Nairobi, Nairobi, Kenya

Jennifer S. Smith
University of North Carolina at Chapel Hill, Chapel Hill, NC, USA
Lineberger Cancer Center, Chapel Hill, NC, USA

Meaghan O'Connor, Kayla McGowan and R. Rima Jolivet
Maternal Health Task Force, Women and Health Initiative, Harvard T.H. Chan School of Public Health, 651 Huntington Avenue, Boston, MA 02115, USA

Gro Møller Christoffersen
University of Copenhagen, Faculty of Health and Medical Sciences, Blegdamsvej 3, 2200 Copenhagen N, Denmark

Peter James Bruhn
Department of Surgical Gastroenterology, Copenhagen University Hospital North Zealand, Dyrehavevej 29, 3400 Hillerød, Denmark

Rosanna de Neergaard
Department of Emergency Medicine, Zealand University Hospital Slagelse, Ingemannsvej 50, 4200 Slagelse, Denmark

Susanne Engel
Department of Culture, Municipality of Sermersooq, Kuussuaq 2, 3900 Nuuk, Greenland

Vibeke Naeser
Department of Obstetrics and Gynecology, Zealand University Hospital Næstved, Ringstedgade 61, 4700 Næstved, Denmark

R. Rima Jolivet and Mary Nell Wegner
Maternal Health Task Force, Women & Health Initiative, Department of Global Health and Population, Harvard T.H. Chan School of Public Health, 651 Huntington Avenue, Boston, MA 02115, USA

Bella Vasant Uttekar and Kanchan Lakhwani
Centre for Operations Research and Training, 402 Woodland Apartment, Race Course Circle, Vadodara, Gujarat 390 007, India

Meaghan O'Connor
Maternal Health Task Force, Women & Health Initiative, Harvard T.H. Chan School of Public Health, 651 Huntington Avenue, Boston, MA 02115, USA

Jigyasa Sharma
Department of Global Health and Population, Harvard T. H. Chan School of Public Health, 677 Huntington Ave, Boston, MA 02115, USA

Prasanna Raj Supramaniam, Monica Mittal and Lee Nai Lim
Oxford University Hospitals NHS Foundation Trust, John Radcliffe Hospital, Headley Way, Headington, Oxford OX3 9DU, UK

Enda McVeigh
Nuffield Department of Women's and Reproductive Health, University of Oxford, Level 3, Women's Centre, John Radcliffe Hospital, Oxford OX3 9DU, UK

Sumiyo Okawa and Masamine Jimba
Department of Community and Global Health, Graduate School of Medicine, The University of Tokyo, Tokyo, Japan

Sylvia Mwanza-Kabaghe
Department of Educational Psychology, Sociology, and Special Education, School of Education, University of Zambia, Lusaka, Zambia
Paediatric HIV Centre of Excellence, University Teaching Hospital, Lusaka, Zambia

Mwiya Mwiya and Chipepo Kankasa
Paediatric HIV Centre of Excellence, University Teaching Hospital, Lusaka, Zambia

Kimiyo Kikuchi
Institute of Decision Science for a Sustainable Society, Kyushu University, Fukuoka, Japan

Naoko Ishikawa
Bureau of International Health Cooperation, National Center for Global Health and Medicine, Tokyo, Japan

Angela Odiachi
Abuja, Nigeria

Salome Erekaha and Christopher Isah
International Research Center of Excellence, Institute of Human Virology Nigeria, Abuja, Nigeria

Nadia A. Sam-Agudu
International Research Center of Excellence, Institute of Human Virology Nigeria, Abuja, Nigeria
Institute of Human Virology, University of Maryland School of Medicine, Baltimore, USA

Llewellyn J. Cornelius
School of Social Work and College of Public Health, University of Georgia Athens, Athens, USA

Habib O. Ramadhani
Institute of Human Virology, University of Maryland School of Medicine, Baltimore, USA

Laura Rapoport
Harvard T. H. Chan School of Public Health, Boston, USA

Index

www.ingramcontent.com/pod-product-compliance
Lightning Source LLC
LaVergne TN
LVHW080713210926
848485LV00003B/457
* 9 7 8 1 6 3 9 2 7 4 6 8 0 *